Examination Obstetrics and Gynaecology

Examination Obstetrics and Gynaecology

Third edition

Judith Goh
MBBS, FRANZCOG, CU, PhD
Urogynaecologist
Greenslopes Private Hospital, Queensland
Professor, Griffith University, Gold Coast, Queensland

Michael Flynn
MBBS, FRANZCOG, FRCOG
Pindara Private Hospital, Gold Coast, Queensland

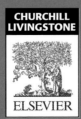

CHURCHILL
LIVINGSTONE

ELSEVIER

Sydney   Edinburgh   London   New York   Philadelphia   St Louis   Toronto

Churchill Livingstone
is an imprint of Elsevier

ELSEVIER

Elsevier Australia. ACN 001 002 357
(a division of Reed International Books Australia Pty Ltd)
Tower 1, 475 Victoria Avenue, Chatswood, NSW 2067

National Library of Australia Cataloguing-in-Publication Data

---

Author: Goh, Judith.

Title: Examination obstetrics and gynaecology / Judith Goh & Michael Flynn.

Edition: 3rd ed.

ISBN: 9780729539371 (pbk.)

Notes: Includes index.

Subjects: Obstetrics. Gynecology. Women--Medical examinations.

Other Authors/Contributors: Flynn, Michael (Michael B.)

Dewey Number: 618

Publisher: Sophie Kaliniecki
Developmental Editor: Neli Bryant
Publishing Services Manager: Helena Klijn
Project Coordinator: Geraldine Minto
Edited by Ruth Matheson
Proofread by Sarah Newton-John
Cover design by Stan Lamond
Internal design adapted by Lamond Art & Design
Typeset by TNQ Books and Journals
Illustrations by Alan Laver
Index by Michael Ferreira
Printed by 1010 Printing International Limited.

Dedications

To my family and friends, for their endless support and encouragement.

JTWG

To Karen, who shared with me the wonder of childbirth. And to Molly, Daniel and Grace, who remind me daily!

MBF

Contents

Preface

When writing the first edition of *Examination Obstetrics and Gynaecology* in 1996 we aimed to present a practical guide for medical students, junior medical staff, specialist trainees and general practitioners. The book not only became a checklist for those undergoing their undergraduate and specialist examinations, but also a handy point-form backup for daily clinical work.

The need has not changed over the second and now third editions for clear, concise explanations and management; however, obstetrics and gynaecology has. The specialty has evolved from an art to a practice with an evidence-based platform. This is a very positive change in our profession and reflecting this we have invited a number of contributors to this edition. Each in their own way has focused on their special area of obstetrics and gynaecology to impart a greater depth to the topic, but retain the note and checklist format. Many chapters have entirely changed to reflect this. Many references now also contain web addresses to long-term ongoing trials, reflecting the fluid nature of our specialty.

A clear focus of the book is passing exams and so sample Objective Structured Clinical Examination (OSCE) cases have been provided from examiners.

Our ultimate goal would be for the reader to not only pass an exam, but also to get the feel for the passion, enjoyment and great satisfaction of a truly wonderful specialty.

Michael Flynn
Judith Goh

Contributors

Based on their respective expertise, the following people have contributed content to chapters and we would like to extend our gratitude to them for dedicating their time, knowledge and input to ensure the success of this project.

Dr Jackie Chua
MBBS, DRCOG (UK), FRANZCOG, DDU, COGU
Queensland Ultrasound for Women, Associate Lecturer, University of Queensland

Professor Caroline De Costa
BA (USyd), MBBS (London University), FRCOG, FRANZCOG, FRCS (Glasgow), MPH (USyd)
Head of Clinical School, James Cook University

Dr Yasmin Jayasinghe
FRANZCOG PhD Scholar, Murdoch Childrens Research Institute
Department of Microbiology, Royal Women's Hospital

Dr Hannah Krause
MBBS, FRANZCOG, CU, MPhil
Gynaecologist, Ramsay Specialist Centre, Greenslopes Private Hospital

Dr Miriam Lee
MBBS, FRANZCOG
Pindara Private Hospital, Benowa, Gold Coast

Dr Amy Mellor
MBBS (UQ), FRANZCOG (medal)
Arrivals Obstetrics Centre, Eve Health and Mater Mothers' Hospital

Dr Justin Nasser
MBBS (Qld), FRANZCOG, DDU
Staff Specialist Obstetrics and Gynaecology, Gold Coast Hospital

Dr Neroli Ngenda
MBBS, MRACOG, FRANZCOG
VMO, Royal Brisbane and Women's Hospital and Sunnybank Private Hospital, Brisbane

Associate Professor Vivienne O'Connor
MEd, MB ChB, MRCOG, FRCOG, FRANZCOG
Associate Dean (Clinical Training), Faculty of Health Sciences and Medicine, Bond University

Dr Gary Swift
MBBS (UQ), FRANZCOG (UQ)
Private Practice at Pindara Private Hospital, Benowa, Gold Coast

Dr Amy Tang
MBBS (Qld), FRANZCOG
Gynaecological Oncology Fellow, Queensland Centre for Gynaecological Cancer, Brisbane

Dr Nikki Whelan
MBBS, FRANZCOG
QMPQC (Qld Maternal and Perinatal Quality Council) member, Clinical Tutor at The Wesley Clinical School, Member of ISSHP (International Society for the Study of Hypertension in Pregnancy) and IADPSG (International Association of Diabetes and Pregnancy Study Groups)

Associate Professor Anusch Yazdani
MBBS (Hons), FRANZCOG CREI
Director of Research and Development, Queensland Fertility Group Research Foundation
Associate Professor of Gynaecology, University of Queensland

Reviewers

Lucy Bowyer
MD, FRANZCOG, FRCOG, CMFM
Obstetrician and Maternal–Fetal Medicine Sub-Specialist, Royal Hospital for Women and the Prince of Wales Private Hospitals, Conjoint Senior Lecturer, University of New South Wales

Ryan Hodges
MBBS (Hons)
Obstetrics and Gynaecology Registrar, PhD student, Monash Institute of Medical Research, Department of Obstetrics and Gynaecology, Monash University, Monash Medical Centre

Yvette Ius
BMed, BAppSci
Second year accredited Obstetrics and Gynaecology Registrar, John Hunter Hospital, Newcastle

Charles Mutandwa
MBChB, FRACGP, FARGP, FACRRM, FACTM, DipCH, Grad Dip Rural General Practice
Senior Lecturer, Flinders University, NT Rural Clinical School, Katherine Senior Rural Medical Practitioner, Katherine Hospital, Northern Territory

Samantha Rothwell
BMed
Obstetrics and Gynaecology Registrar, Hunter Area Health Service

Penelope Sheehan
MBBS, RANZCOG, GDEB
Staff specialist obstetrician, Maternity Unit Head, Royal Women's Hospital, Melbourne
Senior Clinical Research Fellow, Department of Perinatal Medicine Pregnancy Research Centre

Bryony G van Santen
MBBS, MSc
SRMO Obstetrics and Gynaecology, Royal Hospital for Women, Randwick

Abbreviations

17ßHSD III	17-beta-hydroxysteroid dehydrogenase deficiency
3ßHSD II	3-beta-hydroxysteroid dehydrogenase deficiency
5-FU	5-fluorouracil
ACE	angiotensin-converting enzyme
ACL	anticardiolipin antibody
ACTH	adrenocorticotrophic hormone
AFI	amniotic fluid index
AFP	alpha-fetoprotein
AFS	American Fertility Society
AGUS	atypical glandular cells of undetermined significance
AIS	adenocarcinoma in situ
AIS	androgen insensitivity syndrome
ALOs	actinomyces-like organisms
AMH	antimüllerian hormone
APL	antiphospholipid antibodies
APS	antiphospholipid syndrome
APTT	activated partial thromboplastin time
ASC-H	atypical squamous cells, possible high-grade lesion
ASCUS	atypical squamous cells of undetermined significance
BBT	basal body temperature
BGL	blood glucose level
B-hCG	beta-human chorionic gonadotropin
BMI	body mass index
BRCA	breast cancer gene
CAH	congenital adrenal hyperplasia
CC	clomephene citrate
CDC	Centers for Disease Control and Prevention
CIN	cervical intraepithelial neoplasia
CMV	cytomegalovirus
CNS	central nervous system
COCs	combined oral contraceptives
COCP	combined oral contraceptive pill
COX-2	cyclo-oxygenase-2
CRL	crown rump length
CRP	C-reactive protein
CT	computed tomography
CTG	cardiotocograph
CTPA	computed tomography pulmonary angiogram
CVS	chorionic villus sampling
CXR	chest X-ray
DCDA	dichorionic diamniotic
DEXA	dual energy X-ray absorptiometry
DHEAS	dehydroepiandrosterone sulfate
DIE	deep infiltrating endometriosis
DMPA	depot medroxyprogesterone acetate
DSD	disorders of sexual differentiation

DVP	deepest vertical pocket
DVT	deep venous thrombosis
EBV	Epstein-Barr virus
EIA	enzyme immunoassay
EMACO	etoposide, methotrexate, actinomycin D, cyclophosphamide and oncovine
EUA	examination under anaesthesia
fFN	fetal fibronectin
FIGO	Fédération Internationale de Gynécologie et d'Obstétrique
FISH	fluorescence in situ hybridisation
FSH	follicle-stimulating hormone
FTA-ABS	fluorescent treponemal antibody absorption
GFR	glomerular filtration rate
GH	genital hiatus
GnRH	gonadotrophin-releasing hormone
GRIT	Growth Restriction Intervention Trial
HAPO	Hyperglycaemia Adverse Pregnancy Outcome
HbeAg	hepatitis Be antigen
HBV	hepatitis B virus
hCG	human chorionic gonadotrophin
HELLP	syndrome H—haemolysis, EL—elevated liver enzymes and LP—low platelets
HIV	human immunodeficiency virus
hMG	human menopausal gonadotrophin
HNPCC	hereditary non-polyposis colorectal cancer
HPV	human papillomavirus
HRT	hormone replacement therapy
HSIL	high-grade squamous intraepithelial lesion
HyCoSy	hysterosonography
IADPG	International Association of Diabetes in Pregnancy Group
IgA	immunoglobulin A
IGF	insulin-like growth factor
IgG	immunoglobulin G
IgM	immunoglobulin M
IGT	impaired glucose tolerance
INR	international normalised ratio
ITP	idiopathic thrombocytopenic purpura
IUCD	intrauterine contraceptive device
IUD	intrauterine device
IUFD	intrauterine fetal death
IUGR	intrauterine growth restriction
IV	intravenously
IVF	in vitro fertilisation
IVIg	intravenous immunoglobulin
LA	lupus anticoagulant
LCHAD	long-chain 3-hydroxyacyl CoA dehydrogenase
LDH	lactate dehydrogenase
LEEP	loop electrical excision procedure
LH	luteinising hormone
LLETZ	large-loop excision of the transformation zone
LMWH	low-molecular-weight heparin
LNG IUD	levonorgestrel-releasing intrauterine device
LOD	laparoscopic ovarian drilling

LSC	lichen simplex chronicus
LSD	lysergic acid diethylamide
LSIL	low-grade squamous intraepithelial lesion
MCDA	monochorionic diamniotic
MCHC	mean corpuscular haemoglobin concentration
MCV	mean corpuscular volume
MFM	maternal–fetal medical
MMK	Marshall-Marshetti-Krantz
MoM	multiples of the median
MRI	magnetic resonance imaging
MSU	mid-stream urine
NHMRC	National Health and Medical Research Council
NK	natural killer
NPDC	National Perinatal Data Collection
NSAIDs	non-steroidal anti-inflammatory drugs
NST	non-stress test
OCP	oral contraceptive pill
OGTT	oral glucose tolerance test
OHSS	ovarian hyperstimulation syndrome
OR	odds ratio
PAPP-A	pregnancy-associated plasma protein A
PB	perineal body
PCB	polychlorinated biphenyls
PCOS	polycystic ovarian syndrome
PCR	polymerase chain reaction
PE	pulmonary embolism
PEEP	positive end-expiratory pressure
PET	positron emission tomography
PID	pelvic inflammatory disease
POP	progesterone-only pill
(P)PROM	(preterm) prelabour/premature rupture of membranes
PRA	plasma 17-rennin activity
PROST	pronuclear stage tubal transfer
PSANZ–PDC	Perinatal Society of Australia Perinatal Death Classification
PTU	propylthiouracil
Rh	Rhesus
RhD	Rhesus D
RI	resistance index
RMI	Risk of Malignancy Index
RNA	ribonucleic acid
ROA	right occipito anterior
RR	relative risk
SERMs	selective oestrogen receptor modulators
SHBG	sex hormone-binding globulin
SIDS	sudden infant death syndrome
sIUGR	selective intrauterine growth restriction
SLE	systemic lupus erythematosus
SRY gene	sex-determining region on the Y chromosome
SSRIs	selective serotonin reuptake inhibitors
STD	sexually transmitted disease
SVD	spontaneous vaginal delivery
TAH	total abdominal hysterectomy
TAH–BSO	total abdominal hysterectomy–bilateral salpingo-oopherectomy

TENS	transcutaneous electrical nerve stimulation
TOA	tubo-ovarian abscess
TPHA	*Treponema pallidum* haemagglutination assay
TRAP	twin reversed arterial perfusion sequence
TS	Turner's syndrome
TSH	thyroid-stimulating hormone
TSS	toxic shock syndrome
TSST-1	TSS toxin 1
TTTS	twin-to-twin transfusion syndrome
TVL	total vaginal length
TZDs	thiazolidinediones
UDCA	ursodeoxycholic acid
UH	unfractionated heparin
VAIN	vaginal intraepithelial neoplasia
VDRL	Venereal Disease Research Laboratory
VEGF	vascular endothelial growth factor
VIN	vulvar intraepithelial neoplasia
V/Q	ventilation-perfusion
VTE	venous thromboembolism
VZV	varicella zoster virus
WHI	Women's Health Initiative
WHO	World Health Organization
WT1	Wilms' tumour 1

Gynaecology

Chapter 1

History and examination

Michael Flynn

History

The gynaecological history and examination are a modification of standardised history taking designed for the efficient elucidation of the presenting problem, concluding with a provisional or differential diagnosis and a plan for further management. This guide to taking a gynaecological history may need to be modified, depending on the presenting complaint:

- name and age
- presenting complaint
- menstrual history
  - age of menarche/menopause
  - date of last menstrual period
  - length of menstruation and cycle
  - frequency/regularity of cycles
  - menstrual loss, presence of clots or flooding
  - duration of dysmenorrhoea and its relationship to periods
- abnormal bleeding
  - intermenstrual
  - postcoital
  - postmenopausal
- abnormal discharge
  - colour, pruritus, offensive odour
- cervical cytology
  - date of last examination and result
- sexual history
  - dyspareunia (superficial, deep, related to menstruation)
  - contraception
  - previous sexually transmitted diseases
- hormonal therapy
  - oral or injectable or intrauterine contraceptives
  - hormone replacement therapy
- menopausal symptoms
- pain
  - onset, duration, nature, site
  - relationship to menstrual cycles
  - symptoms of prolapse, such as an uncomfortable lump in the vagina
- urinary problems
  - incontinence (stress or urge)
  - nocturia, frequency, dysuria

- other systems review
- past obstetric and gynaecological history
- past medical and surgical history
- social history
- cigarette smoking and alcohol intake
- medications, other drug use, allergies

Examination

Examination always begins with inspection, then palpation, followed by percussion and auscultation.

General
- appearance, colour
- blood pressure, pulse
- breast examination
- presence of lymphadenopathy
- abdominal examination

Genital examination
- inspection of the external genitalia, urethral meatus
- evidence of oestrogen deficiency, prolapse, unusual masses, ulcers
- speculum: inspection of the vagina and cervix; checking for presence of a discharge; taking specimens for cervical cytology and microbiological swabs; using Sims' speculum to assess uterovaginal prolapse
- assessing for urinary incontinence with coughing and prolapse reduced
- bimanual examination to assess: uterine size, shape, ante/retroversion, mobility, tenderness; cervical motion pain; adnexal tenderness, masses; pelvic masses and their relationship to the uterus (e.g. separate from uterus, moving with uterus); uterosacral ligament tenderness, presence of nodules; pouch of Douglas (presence of tumour nodules); rectovaginal septum

Conclusion

- summary of history and clinical findings
- provisional diagnosis, further investigations and management

Chapter 2

Amenorrhoea

Michael Flynn

Puberty

Definition. Puberty is the physiological developmental stage of becoming capable of reproduction (ovulation in the female and spermatogenesis in the male).

Endocrinology of puberty
In the fetus, the hypothalamic–pituitary axis responsible for pubertal development is able to function normally, but chronic inhibitory tone secondary to high levels of sex hormones from the fetoplacental unit inhibits fetal gonadotrophin release. After birth, increasing central nervous inhibition prevents gonadotrophin secretion. Puberty occurs when the gradual rise in gonadotrophin-releasing hormone (GnRH) secretion stimulates the pituitary to release gonadotrophin. With the lowering in central nervous system inhibition, there is an increase in hypothalamic generation of GnRH and increasing ovarian sensitivity to gonadotrophins.

Secondary sexual characteristics
Major physical changes during puberty
- development of secondary sexual characteristics
- changes in body mass and fat distribution
- rapid skeletal growth, with fusion of epiphyses

Secondary female characteristics
These include the enlargement of the ovaries, uterus, vagina, labia and breasts, and the growth of pubic hair.
- **Breast development** (thelarche) is classified into Tanner stages 1–5. Development normally starts between 8 and 13 years of age. It is the first physical sign of puberty and is primarily controlled by ovarian oestrogens.
- **Pubic hair growth** usually begins with the appearance of breast buds. It is under the control of adrenal androgens. There is a high correlation between breast and pubic hair stages.
- **Growth in height** usually occurs, with the peak growth velocity coinciding with Tanner stages 2–3 (at about 12 years of age). In the year of maximum growth, 6–11 cm is added to the height.
- **Axillary hair growth** begins at about 12.5–13 years of age. It takes about 15 months from the first appearance of axillary hair to achieve adult distribution.
- **Menarche** occurs at the average age of 13 years (range 12.2–14.2 years). It occurs within 2 years of the onset of breast development, regardless of the age at which this occurs. Menarche occurs after the peak of the growth spurt in height.
- **Skeletal age** corresponds better to maturity than chronological age.

- **Vaginal length** increases before the development of secondary sexual characteristics. There is also enlargement of the vulva.
- **Uterine growth** is mainly due to enlargement of the myometrium.

Primary amenorrhoea

Definition. Primary amenorrhoea is defined as no spontaneous uterine bleeding by age 16 years when normal growth and secondary sexual characteristics are present, or no sexual development by age 14.

The average age of menarche is 12.7 years. The requirements for having menses are:
- a functional outflow tract and uterus
- normal ovarian hormone production and follicular development
- anterior pituitary stimulation
- hypothalamic/central nervous system regulation

Management of primary amenorrhoea
When to investigate
- no sexual development by age 14 years
- no spontaneous menstruation by age 16 years or within 2 years of onset of breast development
  Before evaluation, exclude:
- pregnancy
- chronic disease

History
- secondary sexual characteristics, sequence of events
- weight gain or loss
- excessive physical activity
- galactorrhoea
- medication and drugs
- past medical history
- family history, genetic anomalies
- anosmia, colour blindness

Examination
- height, weight, blood pressure
- webbed neck, inguinal hernia
- secondary sexual characteristics (feminising, masculinising, infantile)
- genitalia (avoid vaginal examination if the patient is not sexually active; instead, part the labia to observe, for example, an imperforate hymen)

Investigations
Investigations will depend on historical and clinical findings:
- ultrasound scan of the pelvis, magnetic resonance imaging (MRI)
- follicle-stimulating hormone (FSH), luteinising hormone (LH), prolactin, thyroid function tests
- karyotype
- androgens (testosterone, androstenedione, dehydroepiandrosterone sulfate (DHEAS), 17-hydroxyprogesterone)
- endometrial cultures, such as tuberculosis and schistosomiasis where indicated

Classification of primary amenorrhoea
This classification is based on secondary sexual characteristics.

Sexually infantile
- short stature (Turner's syndrome, hypothalamic/pituitary causes, hypothyroidism)
- normal stature (true gonadal dysgenesis, hypogonadotrophic hypogonadism)

Feminising secondary sexual characteristics
- constitutional delay
- testicular feminisation
- müllerian anomalies

Masculinising secondary sexual characteristics
- polycystic ovarian syndrome
- congenital adrenal hyperplasia
- 5-alpha-reductase deficiency
- ovarian tumours
- true hermaphroditism

Causes of primary amenorrhoea
Hypogonadotrophic hypogonadism
Causes of hypogonadotrophic hypogonadism include physiological delay, weight loss, anorexia and excessive exercise, GnRH deficiency with anosmia, and central nervous system defects/trauma.

Investigate with the GnRH test: administer GnRH; if the LH response is appropriate, this indicates hypothalamic failure; in the absence of LH response, pituitary failure is most likely.

The commonest cause of isolated hypogonadotrophic hypogonadism due to deficient GnRH secretion is Kallman's syndrome. This is an autosomal dominant condition, more common in males than females. There is associated anosmia secondary to defective development of the olfactory bulb and tract. Management is by ovulation induction with gonadotrophins or GnRH, and hormone replacement therapy.

Hypergonadotrophic hypogonadism (gonadal dysgenesis)
This is due to genetic or enzymatic abnormality, resulting in failure of gonadal development or abnormal functioning of the ovary.

Causes. Causes include: structural abnormalities of the X chromosome, 45XO; pure gonadal dysgenesis with 46XX, 46XY; 46XX with 17-hydroxylase deficiency (this enzyme is required for oestrogen synthesis); and other causes of premature ovarian failure (*see Ch 12*).

Investigations. Karyotyping is performed; as for premature ovarian failure (*see Ch 12*).

Management. The patient is infertile, and pregnancy can be achieved only with donor eggs and assisted reproductive techniques. For breast development, use oestrogen (ethinyloestradiol 0.01 mg or conjugated equine oestrogen 0.3 mg every second day for 6 months, then daily oestrogen for 6 months, and then the combined oral contraceptive pill).

Androgen insensitivity syndrome (testicular feminisation)
Prevalence. Prevalence is 1 in 20,000 to 1 in 64,000.

Genetics. This is an X-linked inheritance condition, so a family history is important.

Endocrinology. To use testosterone, peripheral tissues need to convert testosterone to dihydrotestosterone via the enzyme 5-alpha-reductase. Testicular feminisation is associated with a variety of defects in androgen receptors (e.g. total absence of androgen receptors, abnormal binding of androgen to receptors and postreceptor binding abnormalities).

Presentation. Primary amenorrhoea; absent uterus and ovaries; sparse pubic/axillary hair; breast development is present; inguinal hernia, possibly with testes present at hernial orifice; vaginal pouch/pit is present; tall stature.

Investigations. The karyotype is male (XY); serum testosterone is above the normal female range and is in the male range.

Management. The patient is phenotypically female; remove gonads after pubertal development (age 18–20 years) because of a risk of malignant change in the gonads. Hormone replacement therapy is required with the use of oestrogen alone. The patient is infertile with no possibility of pregnancy.

Müllerian anomalies
Presentation is one of primary amenorrhoea with secondary sexual characteristics present (*see Ch 15*).

Other causes of primary amenorrhoea
- hyperprolactinaemia
- polycystic ovarian disease
- agonadism
- 46XY with 17-hydroxylase deficiency
- premature ovarian failure

Constitutional delay in puberty
Definition. This is constitutional delay of growth occurring in an otherwise healthy adolescent. Height is below chronological age, but generally appropriate for bone age and stage of pubertal development, both of which are usually delayed. If the normal pattern of growth and puberty is lost, the delay in puberty is likely to be due to an endocrinological abnormality. There is delayed growth in patients with severe systemic disease (e.g. asthma, renal disease, coeliac disease, inflammatory bowel disease and long-term use of corticosteroids).

Principles of management of primary amenorrhoea
Prevent serious/life-threatening disease by:
- removing gonad if Y chromosome is present
- using hormone replacement therapy (initially unopposed oestrogen for 12 months, starting with low-dose oestrogen for breast development and to avoid premature epiphyseal closure)
- treating underlying disease (e.g. anorexia nervosa)

Fertility
- induction of ovulation, donor eggs
- adoption

Physical/emotional development
- secondary sexual characteristics
- sexual function
- stature

Secondary amenorrhoea

Definition. Secondary amenorrhoea is defined as no menses for over 6 months in the absence of pregnancy, lactation, hysterectomy, endometrial ablation/resection or hormonal manipulation. The definition of oligomenorrhoea varies from a cycle length of over 35 days to a woman experiencing fewer than or equal to five periods per year.

Causes of secondary amenorrhoea
Oestrogen deficiency
- gonadal failure
- hypothalamic causes (e.g. stress, exercise, anorexia)
- pituitary lesions
- hyperprolactinaemia

Unopposed oestrogen
- polycystic ovarian syndrome/chronic anovulation
- follicular cysts
- androgen excess

Other causes
- Asherman's syndrome
- congenital adrenal hyperplasia (late-onset)
- other medical conditions (e.g. thyroid disease)

History
- menstrual history (Have all periods occurred while taking hormone therapy?)
- medication: oral contraceptive pill
- weight: anorexia, exercise
- stress: physical, emotional
- hirsutism, acne
- galactorrhoea, visual changes
- hot flushes, dry vagina
- past history of curettage

Examination
- general observations, weight, blood pressure
- sexual characteristics
- hirsutism
- galactorrhoea
- thyroid
- genital/vaginal examination

Investigations
- to exclude pregnancy
- FSH, LH
- thyroid function test, serum prolactin
- if hirsute, perform tests, including serum testosterone, DHEAS, 17-hydroxyprogesterone
- hysteroscopy/hysterosalpingogram

Management and further investigations of secondary amenorrhoea
Premature ovarian failure
(See Ch 12.)
- investigations: chromosomes, autoantibody tests
- management: hormone replacement therapy

Hypothalamic amenorrhoea
Investigations reveal normal serum prolactin levels, normal thyroid function tests, normal or low LH and FSH, and reduced oestrogen levels.

Management depends on the cause of amenorrhoea (e.g. anorexia nervosa requires psychiatric referral).

Polycystic ovarian syndrome
(See Ch 5.)

Asherman's syndrome
• hysteroscopic resection of adhesion
• may use various means to reduce the risk of readherence of endometrial walls (e.g. oestrogen supplementation, intrauterine device)

Medical problems
• Treat and/or refer to other specialist as appropriate.
• Hyperprolactinaemia: treat with pharmacological agents or surgery.

Tumours
• Adrenals: these patients have greatly raised DHEAS and 17-hydroxyprogesterone.
• Ovarian tumours are associated with raised testosterone and androstenedione levels.

Further reading

Edmonds DK 2003 Congenital malformations of the genital tract and their management. Best Practice and Research Clinical Obstetrics and Gynaecology 17:19–40
Lalwani S, Reindollar RH, Davis AJ 2003 Normal onset of puberty: have definitions of onset changed? Obstetrics and Gynecology Clinics of North America 30:279–286
Timmreck LS, Reindollar RH 2003 Contemporary issues in primary amenorrhoea. Obstetrics and Gynecology Clinics of North America 30:287–302

Chapter 3

Menstruation disorders

Anusch Yazdani
Judith Goh

Terminology for describing menstruation disorders has been under review recently with some authors advocating eradication of the older terms such as 'menorrhagia' and 'dysfunctional uterine bleeding'. As there is currently no consensus on this issue, this chapter will continue to use the previous terminology.

Menorrhagia

Definition. Menorrhagia is a menstrual blood loss greater than 80 mL per cycle (the average menstrual loss is 35 mL per cycle).
  Incidence. Menorrhagia occurs in about 10%–20% of women.

Causes of menorrhagia
Dysfunctional uterine bleeding
This is abnormal bleeding (heavy, prolonged or frequent) from the uterus, not due to organic disease/malignancy or pregnancy. It accounts for 50%–60% of cases of menorrhagia. It is subdivided for treatment purposes into:
- anovulatory cycles, which occur at the extremes of menstrual life, in polycystic ovarian syndrome and obesity—due to abnormalities in the hypothalamic–pituitary–ovarian axis
- ovulatory cycles—mainly due to defects in regulation of blood loss/prostaglandin disorders during menstruation

Systemic causes
- hypothyroidism, most likely from anovulation
- coagulation/bleeding disorders such as von Willebrand's disease, platelet function disorders, and use of anticoagulants (about 2% prevalence of bleeding disorders in the general community, but it affects up to 20% of women with proven menorrhagia and rates are higher in adolescents)

Local/gynaecological causes
- endometriosis/adenomyosis
- chronic pelvic inflammatory disease
- uterine tumours: benign submucosal leiomyoma, endometrial polyps, malignant lesions (hyperplasia, carcinoma)
- ovarian tumours

- intrauterine contraceptive devices, which can double menstrual loss in about 50% of patients

History and investigation of menorrhagia
History
- menstrual history, contraception, thyroid disease, bleeding tendency
- exclusion of pregnancy, cervical pathology
- pictorial chart of menstrual loss, number of pads/tampons used

Investigations
- full blood count, iron studies, thyroid function test
- follicle-stimulating hormone (FSH), luteinising hormone (LH), human chorionic gonadotrophin (hCG)
- platelet function studies for platelet/coagulation disorders (which cause up to 20% of adolescent admissions for menorrhagia)
- cervical cytology
- ultrasound scan of pelvis as a first-line diagnostic tool to exclude structural anomalies
- hysteroscopy and endometrial curettage (especially in women >45 years old with failed treatment)
- tests for ovulation (day 21 serum progesterone)

Medical management of menorrhagia
The general treatment for menorrhagia depends on many factors, including the woman's choice, contraindications and future fertility needs.

Prostaglandin inhibitors
- mefenamic acid
- naproxen or other non-steroidal anti-inflammatory drugs (can reduce menstrual loss by 20%–50%, which may be improved if used in conjunction with the oral contraceptive pill; also beneficial in women with dysmenorrhoea)

Antifibrinolytics and haemostatics
- tranexamic acid, aminocaproic acid
- ethamsylate, which reduces capillary fragility and inhibits prostaglandin synthesis

Hormonal therapy
Combined oral contraceptive pill
This reduces menstrual blood flow by inhibiting ovulation and decreasing endometrial thickness.

Progesterone
- Routes of administration are oral, intramuscular, intrauterine and subcutaneous implants.
- It may cause irregular bleeding.
- Cyclical oral progesterone therapy:
  - This reduces menstrual loss, but is not as effective as transexamic acid or Mirena device (Cochrane review).
  - High doses of norethisterone are commonly used to reduce or arrest bleeding in emergency treatment of dysfunctional uterine bleeding.
- Levonorgestrel-releasing intrauterine system has the added advantage of being an effective form of contraception and reducing progesterone systemic side effects. A common side effect is irregular bleeding for the first 6 months.

Surgical management of menorrhagia
Hysteroscopic removal of polyps and fibroids
- Hysteroscopy and curettage is an essential diagnostic tool.
- Endometrial polyps and submucosal fibroids may be removed via the hysteroscope.

Endometrial ablation/resection
- an option for a woman who has completed her childbearing and has dysfunctional bleeding
- endometrial ablation/resection (produces amenorrhoea or an acceptable reduction in blood loss during periods in 90% of patients)
- considered with normal uterus and fibroids less than 3 cm

Hysterectomy
- has the advantage of no risk of menstrual loss following the procedure
- is the option when other treatment options have failed
- possible loss of ovarian function even if ovaries conserved

Uterine artery embolisation
This is an option for a woman who has a large fibroid and wishes uterine conservation.

Dysmenorrhoea

Definition. Dysmenorrhoea means painful menstruation. One-half of all women experience some discomfort during menstruation.

Incidence. In up to 10%–20% of women in their late teens or early 20s, dysmenorrhoea affects their daily activities.

Mechanism. True dysmenorrhoea is related to uterine muscle contraction and cervical dilatation. It usually occurs a few hours before and after the onset of menstruation. The pain is in the hypogastrium, radiating to the inner and front of the thighs. During severe attacks, there is associated sweating, nausea, vomiting and diarrhoea.

Causes
- cervical obstruction due to cervical stenosis
- hormonal imbalance: dysmenorrhoea occurring in ovular cycles; pain resulting from excessive amounts of prostaglandins
- endometriosis, a cause of secondary dysmenorrhoea; ache/pain commences perimenstrually and peaks on day 1–2 of the cycle
- fibroids

Treatment
There is a large quantity of treatments published for the management of dysmenorrhoea, including:
- general health and dietary advice
- medical
  - simple oral analgesia
  - antispasmodics
  - non-steroidal anti-inflammatory drugs (these work best if commenced just before the period)
  - oral contraceptive pill and levonorgestrel-releasing intrauterine system control endometrial growth so less prostaglandins released
  - vitamin B_{12}

- others: transcutaneous electrical nerve stimulation, acupuncture, fish oil, herbal
- surgical
  - laparoscopy used to treat endometriosis
  - hysterectomy, but pain may still persist; used in most severe cases as last resort

Premenstrual syndrome

Definition. It is a syndrome of psychological, behavioural and physical symptoms occurring in the premenstrual phase of the menstrual cycle.

Prevalence. It affects over 90% of women in the reproductive age and in about 5% it significantly affects daily activities.

Symptoms
- Symptoms/signs are cyclical and recur in the premenstrual phase. They are present to some degree in each cycle.
- During the follicular phase, the woman is symptom-free.
- Symptoms affect lifestyle.
- Symptoms/signs increase in severity before or during menstruation.
- Effects include cognitive, emotional, physical and sensory modalities.
- Symptoms are varied and include anxiety and depression, behavioural/performance-related changes, breast tenderness/fullness/pain, abdominal fullness/discomfort, increase in appetite, acne, sweats, headache and backache.

Causes
The precise mechanism is unknown. There are a number of suggestions, including:
- progesterone involvement, suggested by onset just prior to menstruation
- abnormal immunological reaction to hormonal changes in the menstrual cycle
- hormonal imbalance between oestrogen and progesterone (low progesterone in luteal phase)
- central opioid abnormality, abnormal hypothalamic–pituitary–adrenal axis
- abnormal aldosterone function (causing sodium and water retention)
- abnormal prostaglandin production
- nutritional deficiency, environmental factors

Management
Numerous treatment regimes have been tried with a significant placebo effect.

General
- Encourage the woman to keep a daily record of symptoms over two or three cycles.
- Provide information on the syndrome, exercise and nutrition.
- Develop stress management skills.

Pharmacological
- vitamin B_6, calcium carbonate
- antiprostaglandins, such as mefenamic acid
- hormonal (oral contraceptive pill, oestrogen, danazol)
- selective serotonin reuptake inhibitors

Others
- acupuncture, manipulation, bright-light therapy, relaxation, evening primrose oil, exercise
- hysterectomy, oophorectomy

Further reading

El-Hemaidi I, Gharaibeh A, Shehata H 2007 Menorrhagia and bleeding disorders. Current Opinion in Obstetrics and Gynecology 19:513–520

Farage MA, Osborn TW, MacLean AB 2008 Cognitive, sensory and emotional changes associated with the menstrual cycle: a review. Archives of Gynecology and Obstetrics 278:299–307

Farquhar C, Brown J 2009 Oral contraceptive pill for heavy menstrual bleeding. Cochrane Database of Systematic Reviews. Issue 4. Art. No.: CD000154. DOI: 10.1002/14651858

Chapter 4

Endometriosis

Gary Swift

Definition. Endometriosis is defined as the presence of endometrial-like tissue outside the uterus, which induces a chronic inflammatory reaction and is associated with pain, subfertility and impaired quality of life.

Cyclical bleeding into deposits causes inflammation, scarring and adhesions, leading to pain, anatomical distortion and pelvic organ dysfunction. Dysmenorrhoea, dyspareunia, non-cyclical pelvic pain, dysuria, dyschezia and infertility result from the disease, though it may be asymptomatic in a minority. Symptoms in women subsequently found to have endometriosis may commence soon after menarche, with the disease varying widely in severity, symptomatology, and clinical and social impact. The disease ranges from relatively trivial superficial deposits causing few symptoms to severe deep infiltrating endometriosis (DIE) affecting the muscularis of pelvic viscera and/or the rectovaginal septum with associated quality of life implications.

Prevalence. An estimated 10% of reproductive-age women, in all social and ethnic groups, have endometriosis; 30% of women presenting with infertility have endometriosis; 50%–60% of women presenting with pelvic pain have endometriosis.

Risk factors

- higher risk with early menarche, short cycles and heavy menstrual flow (>8 days relative risk (RR) 2.4)
- reduced incidence with smoking (reduced oestrogen) and exercise (increased sex hormone-binding globulin (SHBG) and reduced luteal oestrogen levels)
- relative risk greatly increased with first-degree relative afflicted
- dietary factors: reduced risk with high fruit (odds ratio (OR) 0.6) and vegetable (OR 0.3) intake and fish oil (animal studies); increased risk with high red meat consumption (OR 2.0).
- increased risk with higher levels of vitamin D
- inverse association between endometriosis and body mass index (BMI)
- possible increased risk with alcohol, caffeine, and polychlorinated biphenyls (PCB) and dioxin exposure

Aetiology

The exact aetiology is still not known. The most widely accepted theory is related to viable endometrial cells reaching the peritoneal cavity through retrograde menstruation along the fallopian tubes (Sampson 1927). At least 90% of women with patent fallopian tubes will have evidence of retrograde menstruation; yet, in the majority, the menstrual debris is rapidly and efficiently cleared, by macrophages and natural killer (NK) cells.

Alternative theories of 'coelomic metaplasia' and 'embryonic cell rests' are less favoured.

Increased susceptibility is possibly related to:
- increased exposure to menstrual debris
- abnormal eutopic endometrium
- altered peritoneal environment
- reduced immune surveillance
- increased angiogenic capacity

Genetics

Genes influence susceptibility to endometriosis.
- considered to be a complex heritable trait with many genes contributing to risk, with the contribution of any one individual gene likely to be small
- genomic linkages found on chromosomes 7, 10 and 20 so far
- relative increased risk with sibling affected: 2.34 to 15 times (higher risk in more severe forms of the disease)

Pathology

The lesions of endometriosis vary from superficial to deep and in appearance from clear to white to red to black in proportion to degree of inflammation, vascularity and haemosiderin deposition. Newly formed lesions tend to be clear to red, with older lesions more deeply pigmented, with variable proportions of pale scarring and fibrosis. With increasing fibrosis, lesions become nodular. Lesions in postmenopausal or hormonally suppressed women will tend to be paler.

The inflammation and fibrosis leads to adhesions and anatomical distortion. Shortening and thickening of uterosacral ligaments reduces uterine mobility and causes fixed retroversion. Shortening and thickening of ovarian ligaments displaces ovaries medially. Pouch of Douglas obliteration follows involvement of rectal serosa and sometimes muscularis.

Endometriomas or 'chocolate cysts' are specific lesions that form in the ovaries. They are thought not to be true cysts but invaginations of the ovarian cortex lined by typical endometriotic tissue. The thick altered blood content resembles melted chocolate. These lesions have high recurrence rates if not excised completely. Endometriosis deposits are histologically similar to eutopic endometrium, but not identical. Plaques contain oestrogen, progesterone and androgen receptors, and grow in the presence of oestrogen and atrophy with androgens.

Abnormal levels and function of growth factors, macrophages and proinflammatory cytokines have been observed in the peritoneal fluid and serum of women with endometriosis.

Pathogenesis
- Angiogenic processes are fundamental to the establishment of endometriosis.
- Polymorphisms in the vascular endothelial growth factor (VEGF) gene increase susceptibility to endometriosis in humans.
- There are current searches for endometriosis-specific angiogenic mechanisms.

Clinical presentation

Symptoms include:
- dysmenorrhoea
- deep dyspareunia
- chronic pelvic pain
- ovulation pain
- cyclical or perimenstrual bowel and/or bladder disturbance with or without abnormal bleeding (dysuria, dyschezia)
- infertility
- chronic fatigue
- asymptomatic in minority

Diagnosis

There is no reliable non-surgical diagnostic test for endometriosis. Endometriosis may be suspected clinically with appropriate symptoms and examination findings (nodularity in pouch of Douglas or uterosacral ligaments) or radiologic evidence of endometriomas. Unless endometriotic 'blue dome cysts' are visible in the posterior vaginal fornix, laparoscopy is required for diagnosis, with preferably histological confirmation, and is regarded as the 'gold standard'.

Staging
- combination of clinical, radiological and surgical
- ideal system yet to be developed
- American Fertility Society (AFS) staging is complex and detailed, but is most used in research settings

Treatments

Medical treatment
- primary therapy, postoperative, preventative

Contraceptive
- hormonal medical therapies equally effective in symptom control, but vary in side effects and costs
- no evidence of improved fertility outcomes
- higher recurrence rates after medical treatment compared to surgical

Options
- progesterones: progesterone-only pill (POP), depot medroxyprogesterone acetate (DMPA), oral progestins, progesterone-containing intrauterine contraceptive devices (IUCDs)
- combined oral contraceptive pill
- danazol
- gestrinone
- gonadotrophin-releasing hormone (GnRH) agonists (goserelin, nafarelin, leuprolide)

Surgical treatment

Laparoscopy is the 'gold standard' for diagnosis and therapeutic intervention. If endometriosis is present at laparoscopy, it is recommended that it is surgically removed at the same time as diagnosis, as it is an effective treatment for endometriosis-associated subfertility and pain.

Alternative treatment

- acupuncture, Chinese medicine, naturopathy: potential positive effects on symptom control, but evidence based on randomised controlled trials is lacking

Prognosis

- natural history of early stage disease lacking
- tendency to progressive increase in number and size of deposits until excision, pregnancy, suppressive treatment or menopause

Special areas

Endometriosis in adolescence

Endometriosis can be responsible for admissions with pain in the 10–17-year-old age group. For adolescents with pelvic pain refractory to non-steroidal anti-inflammatory drugs (NSAIDs) and/or combined oral contraceptives (COCs), it is estimated 50% will have underlying endometriosis. First-line medical treatment is appropriate, followed by laparoscopy and surgical management if unsuccessful.

Endometriosis and fertility

Impact on fertility

- spontaneous and assisted conception reduced in proportion to stage of disease and anatomical distortion
- quality of oocytes, ovarian reserve and implantation success reduced
- pain and menstrual disturbance have a negative impact on coital frequency

Medical therapies contraceptive

Surgical management is proven to improve mild and moderate disease stages, with severe forms difficult to evaluate due to variables, but trends to improved fertility, natural and assisted, with optimal surgical management.

Impact on and role of assisted reproductive technology (ART)

Endometriomas are associated with reduced follicle numbers and ovarian responsiveness to gonadotrophin stimulation. Currently, there is debate on excision prior to in vitro fertilisation (IVF). Surgical excision is not proven to improve outcomes with IVF and may reduce ovarian reserve further. Generally, excision is recommended if >=4 cm, there is pain or access to follicles is affected.

Deep infiltrating endometriosis

- defined as deposits invading over 5 mm in depth
- severe form of endometriotic disease forming a subset with infiltrating deposits in bowel and/or bladder muscularis and rectovaginal septum
- management is complex with advanced surgical techniques required
- referral to centre with necessary expertise strongly recommended

Extrapelvic disease

This is rare, but it can affect any organ. Deposits have been documented in the umbilicus, lungs and central nervous system. It should be considered in any symptoms with a cyclical pattern, especially if it is associated with pain and/or bleeding.

Future issues

- Animal models show inhibition of endometriosis by substances that block angiogenesis (vascular endothelial growth factor (VEGF) antibodies, selective cyclo-oxygenase-2 (COX-2) inhibitors) (Hull et al 2003).
- Human Genome Project: genome-wide association studies are expected to provide greater insight into the genetic basis of endometriosis in the future.

Further reading and references

American Society of Reproductive Medicine (ASRM) Guidelines. Available at: www.asrm.org/

D'Hooghe TM, Debrock S 2003 Future directions in endometriosis research. Obstetrics and Gynecology Clinics of North America 30:221–244

Eskenazi B, Warner ML 1997 Epidemiology of endometriosis. Obstetrics and Gynecology Clinics of North America 24:235–238

European Society of Human Reproduction and Embryology (ESHRE) Guidelines. Available at: www.eshre.eu/

Garcia-Velasco JA, Somigliana E 2009 Management of endometriomas in women requiring IVF: to touch or not to touch. Human Reproduction 24:496–501

Hull ML, Charnock-Jones DS, Chan CLK et al 2003 Antiangiogenic agents are effective inhibitors of endometriosis. Journal of Clinical Endocrinology and Metabolism 86:2889–2899

Kennedy S 1998 The genetics of endometriosis. Journal of Reproductive Medicine 43 (Suppl 3): S263–S268

Kennedy S, Bergqvist A, Chapron C et al on behalf of the ESHRE Special Interest Group for Endometriosis and Endometrium Guideline Development Group 2005 ESHRE Guideline for the diagnosis and treatment of endometriosis. Human Reproduction 20:2698–2704

Parazzini F, Chiaffarino F, Surace M et al 2004 Selected food intake and risk of endometriosis. Human Reproduction 19:1755–1759

Rogers MS, D'Amato RJ 2006 The effect of genetic diversity on angiogenesis. Experimental Cell Research 312:516–574

Sampson JA 1927 Peritoneal endometriosis due to the menstrual dissemination of endometrial tissue to the peritoneal cavity. American Journal of Obstetrics and Gynecology 14:422–469

Treloar SA, Wicks J, Nyholt DR et al 2005 Genome-wide linkage study in 1176 affected sister pair families identifies a significant susceptibility locus for endometriosis on chromosome 10q26. American Journal of Human Genetics 77 (3):356–376

Zondervan KT, Treloar SA, Lin J et al 2007 Significant evidence of one or more susceptibility loci for endometriosis with near-Mendelian autosomal inheritance on chromosome 7p13–15. Human Reproduction 22:717–728

Chapter 5

Polycystic ovarian syndrome

Anusch Yazdani

Definition. The definition of polycystic ovarian syndrome (PCOS) was revised in 2003 (Rotterdam Consensus criteria). The diagnosis is based on two out of three of the following criteria:
- oligo or anovulation
- clinical and/or biochemical signs of hyperandrogenism
- polycystic ovaries, defined as at least one of the following:
  - 12 or more follicles measuring 2–9 mm in diameter
  - increased ovarian volume (>10 cm³)

If there is evidence of a dominant follicle (>10 mm) or a corpus luteum, the scan should be repeated during the next cycle. Only one ovary fitting this definition or a single occurrence of one of the above criteria is sufficient to define the PCOS. It does not apply to women taking the oral contraceptive pill. Regularly menstruating women should be scanned in the early follicular phase (days 3–5). Oligomenorrhoeic and amenorrhoeic women should be scanned either at random or between days 3 and 5 after a progestogen-induced bleed *and* the exclusion of other aetiologies (congenital adrenal hyperplasia, androgen-secreting tumours, Cushing's syndrome).

Prevalence. Prevalence is 5%–7% overall, 85% of oligomenorrhoeic females, 90% of women with hirsutism and 30% of infertile women.

Clinical presentation

- menstrual irregularities
  - amenorrhoea or oligomenorrhoea
  - variable menstrual loss
- infertility
- androgen excess, such as hirsutism or acne

Aetiology

- Aetiology is multifactorial.
- About 50% of women with PCOS have affected sisters.
- Multiple candidate genes have been identified, but it is likely that a number of different pathways, both genetic and environmental, contribute to the same phenotype.

Pathophysiology

PCOS is characterised by ovarian, hypothalamic–pituitary, peripheral and adrenal dysfunction. The phenotype develops through chronic anovulation of any aetiology and a clear sequence of events is therefore not identifiable.

Ovaries
- High luteinising hormone (LH) levels drive ovarian androgen production.
- High intraovarian androgen concentrations inhibit follicular maturation and lead to inactive granulosa cells with minimal aromatase activity.
- The large number of ovarian follicles produces a high inhibin B, which inhibits follicle-stimulating hormone (FSH).

Hypothalamus–pituitary
- Hypothalamic dysfunction is associated with increased gonadotropin-releasing hormone agonist (GnRH) frequency and tonic (i.e. non-cyclic) LH release, elevating the LH/FSH ratio. The increase in LH is more pronounced in lean patients.
- The large number of ovarian follicles produces a high inhibin B, which inhibits FSH, but as FSH is not fully suppressed, continuous follicular recruitment and stimulation proceeds, but not to the level of full maturation and ovulation.
- Increased oestrogen production stimulates an increase in prolactin.

Peripheral compartment
- Reduced sex hormone-binding globulin (SHBG) concentrations perpetuate hyperandrogenaemia:
  - hyperinsulinaemia
  - obesity
  - hepatic dysfunction
- Peripheral alteration in insulin-like growth factor (IGF-1), androgen and oestrogen levels perpetuate hypothalamic dysfunction.
- Obesity reduces SHBG and increases peripheral aromatisation of androgens (androstenedione), which produces a chronic hyperoestrogenic state with reversal of the oestrone:oestradiol ratio.

Adrenal compartment
- dysregulation of cytochrome p-450c17 (as in the ovaries), but dehydro-epiandrosterone sulfate (DHEAS) (of adrenal origin) is only increased in 50% of PCOS
- exaggerated adrenarchal response

Consequences of PCOS

Reproductive consequences
- anovulation/oligo-ovulation leading to
  - menstrual disturbances
  - infertility
  - reproductive failure
- abortion
  - controversial
  - may be related to hyperinsulinaemia

Metabolic consequences
- obesity
  - at least 50% of women with PCOS are obese
  - most are also hyperinsulinemic and insulin resistant, independent of obesity
- metabolic syndrome: present in up to 40% of PCOS patients
- hyperinsulinaemia/diabetes
  - hyperinsulinaemia: 80% of obese PCOS; 30% of lean PCOS
  - diabetes
    - increased prevalence of impaired glucose tolerance (IGT) (35%) and type 2 diabetes (10%) in women with PCOS compared with age-matched and weight-matched populations of women without PCOS (Legro 2006)
    - a 5–10 times increased risk of type 2 diabetes
    - 10%–30% of women will develop type 2 diabetes within 3 years
    - conversion from IGT to type 2 diabetes is accelerated in PCOS
    - risk is increased further if positive family history
  - gestational diabetes: increased risk of gestational diabetes, regardless of body mass index (BMI)
- hyperlipidaemia: conflicting data

Neoplasia
- increased endometrial hyperplasia and perhaps carcinoma
  - hyperplasia: women with anovulatory infertility are at increased risk of endometrial hyperplasia
- carcinoma
  - reported three times increased risk of endometrial carcinoma
  - the evidence for an increased risk of endometrial carcinoma in PCOS is incomplete and contradictory
- increased breast cancer: data inconclusive

Cardiovascular disease
- poor data
- limited epidemiological data to support increased coronary heart disease

Other
- increased sleep apnoea
- non-alcoholic steatohepatitis

Differential diagnosis

- constitutional obesity
- idiopathic hirsutism
- Cushing's syndrome
- congenital adrenal hyperplasia
- hypothyroidism
- androgen producing tumours

Assessment

Assessment is based on clinical presentation and investigations to validate the diagnostic criteria, and exclude other endocrinopathies and sequelae.

History
- menstrual history
- reproductive history
- weight gain
- hirsutism, acne
- galactorrhoea, headaches

Examination
- hirsutism
- evidence of virilisation
- evidence of Cushing's syndrome, thyroid disorders
- acanthosis nigricans (a marker of insulin resistance)

Investigations
- FSH, oestradiol (LH/FSH ratio is not clinically useful)
- thyroid function test
- prolactin
- fasting glucose, insulin, lipids
- testosterone levels: if above 6 nmol/L, further investigations are required to check for adrenal or virilising tumours
- DHEAS: levels above 18 nmol/L necessitate exclusion of Cushing's syndrome
- 17-hydroxyprogesterone: if the morning level is <5.5 nmol/L, no further investigations are needed; if the levels are raised, check for congenital adrenal hyperplasia
- endometrial sampling, especially if history or prolonged amenorrhoea or heavy menses
- ultrasound scan of the pelvis
  - more than 80% of women with PCOS have a classic ultrasound appearance
  - morphologic changes have been found in different studies in different settings:
    - in 90% of women with hirsutism
    - in 90% of women with oligomenorrhea
    - in 40% of women with a history of gestational diabetes
    - in 25% of women who considered themselves normal and reported regular menstrual cycles
    - in 15% of women on a combined oral contraceptive pill (COCP)

Management

Management is dictated by the clinical presentation (e.g. menstrual changes, hirsutism and/or infertility).

Supportive
- lifestyle changes: the most important intervention
- weight reduction: 5%–10% of body weight over 6 months is sufficient to reestablish ovarian function in more than 50% of patients
- hirsutism: see management of hirsutism (*Ch 6*)

Not wanting to conceive
COCP
- protects endometrium
- oestrogen increases SHBG, resulting in reduced free testosterone
- progestins inhibit 5-alpha-reductase in the skin, resulting in decreased hirsutism
- progestins suppress LH, resulting in decreased androgen production

Progesterone (cyclical oral or depot medroxyprogesterone acetate (DMPA))
- negative feedback decreases GnRH production, resulting in decreased oestrogen and androgen
- protects endometrium

Insulin-sensitising drugs
- thiazolidinediones (TZDs)
  - insulin sensitisers
  - specifically contraindicated for conception and associated with an increased risk of weight gain; unlikely to become a major component of PCOS management
- metformin
  - no change in BMI, waist:hip ratio
  - no effect on clinical hyperandrogenaemia (e.g. hirsutism)
  - reduced fasting glucose (statistically but not clinically significant)
  - reduced fasting insulin
  - reduced biochemical androgens
  - altered lipids
  - increased nausea and gastronintestinal side effects, but nil serious
- oral contraceptive pill (OCP) and metformin
  - OCP is more effective than metformin in improving menstrual pattern and reducing serum androgen levels
  - limited evidence demonstrating that the addition of metformin to the OCP is more effective than the OCP alone in improving hirsutism score and increasing serum SHBG levels
  - insufficient evidence to demonstrate any benefit to adding metformin to the OCP in terms of reducing body weight, reducing serum androgen levels, and reducing fasting serum levels of metabolic parameters such as insulin, glucose or lipids

Wanting to conceive
See Figure 5.1.

Medical
- clomiphene
- selective oestrogen receptor modulator
- central oestrogen receptor antagonism leads to reflex elevation in FSH and thereby ovulation
- commence on low dose
- 85% ovulation
- 50% conception: possibly due to negative effect of clomiphene on endometrium/mucus
- 7% multiple pregnancy

Metformin
- metformin: increased ovulation rate but not clinical pregnancy rate
- clomiphene and metformin
  - increased live-birth rate: effective also in clomiphene resistance
  - increased ovulation rate
- metformin and gonadotrophin treatment: does not increase pregnancy rate, but reduces total FSH requirement and risk of ovarian hyperstimulation syndrome (OHSS)

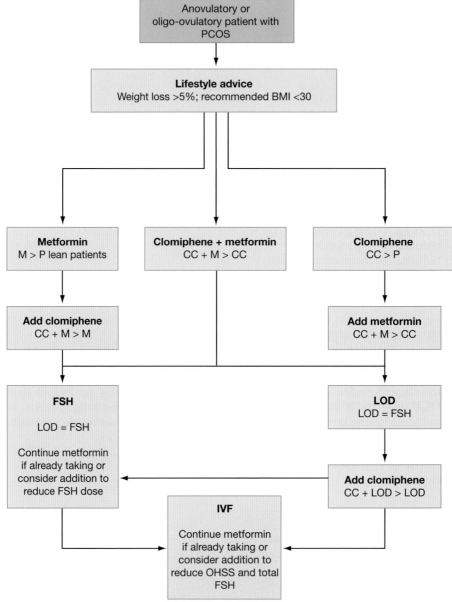

Notes: BMI = body mass index, CC = clomid, FSH = follicle-stimulating hormone,
IVF = in vitro fertilisation, LOD = laparoscopic ovarian drilling, M = metformin,
OHSS = ovarian hyperstimulation syndrome, P = placebo,
PCOS = polycystic ovarian syndrome

Figure 5.1 **Patients with a diagnosis of PCOS wishing to conceive**

Other medical treatment
- ketoconazole: limited benefit
- aromatase inhibitors
  - effective in ovulation induction
  - no difference between letrozole and anastrozole

- mechanism is selective reversible inhibition of aromatase (a product of the CYP19 gene, part of the cytochrome P450 complex), which catalyses the rate-limiting step in the production of oestrogens
  - supposed benefit over clomiphene is reduced negative effects on target tissues such as endometrium and cervix
- increased benefit from addition of dexamethasone to clomiphene: resulted in a significant improvement in the pregnancy rate
- pulsatile GnRH (Cochrane): insufficient evidence from trials to show the effectiveness of pulsatile GnRH in PCOS
- FSH: chronic low-dose stimulation protocol has lower OHSS and multiple pregnancy rate
- in vitro fertilisation (IVF)
  - 7% of PCOS patients need IVF
  - high risk of OHSS (20%)
- surgical
  - wedge resection: high incidence of adnexal adhesions
  - laparoscopic golf balling/pepper potting/ovarian drilling (LOD) (see Table 5.1)
  - high incidence of adnexal adhesions
  - unknown long-term effect on ovarian function
  - effect may be permanent
  - consider in failed ovulation induction

Table 5.1 Comparison of laparoscopic ovarian drilling and FSH stimulation in fertility management in patients with PCOS

	Laparoscopy	FSH
Benefits	Comparable success rates	Comparable success rate
	One treatment affects multiple cycles	Non-operative
	Usually produces mono-ovulation	
	No increased risk of OHSS	
	May lower miscarriage rate	
	No medications required	
	No intensive monitoring required	
	Lower cost	
Problems	Surgical risks	Multiple cycles required
	Adhesion	Intensive monitoring required
	Ovarian atrophy	Increased risk of multiple pregnancy
	Long-term effect on ovarian function uncertain	Increased risk of OHSS
		Increased cost

Further reading and references

Ehrmann DA 2005 Polycystic ovary syndrome. New England Journal of Medicine 352:1223

Legro RS 2006 Type 2 diabetes and polycystic ovary syndrome. Fertility and Sterility 86 (Suppl1):S16–S17

Rotterdam ESHRE/ASRM-sponsored PCOS consensus workshop group 2004 Revised 2003 consensus on diagnostic criteria and long-term health risks related to polycystic ovary syndrome (PCOS). Human Reproduction 19 (1):41–47

Chapter 6

Hirsutism

Judith Goh

Definition. *Hirsutism* is the growth of coarse/terminal hair in amounts that are socially unacceptable to a woman. For the woman, this is typically in a male pattern (sexual hair). The Ferriman-Gallwey (see below) hirsutism score is over 8. Under 5% of women (various ethnic origin) in the reproductive age group have scores over 7. *Hypertrichosis* is generalised excess hair growth that may be hereditary. This is in a non-sexual pattern and is not related to, but may be aggravated by, excess androgens. *Virilism* is a condition usually secondary to hyperandrogenism and is associated with one or more of clitoral hypertrophy, breast atrophy, male baldness and deepening of the voice.

    Prevalence. About 15% of women normally have terminal hair on their faces, and this tends to increase with age. Up to 4% of women seek treatment for hirsutism.

Physiology of hair growth

There are three major groups:
- lanugo: fine, lightly pigmented hair
- vellus hair: short, fine, unpigmented
- terminal hair: longer, thicker and pigmented

    Non-sexual hair is present on the scalp, eyebrow and distal extremities. Its growth is not affected by androgens. **Ambisexual hair** is present in both sexes on the axilla and lower pubic triangle. Small amounts of androgens are required for its growth. **Sexual hair** is present on the upper pubic triangle, face, chest, ear and nose. It is induced and maintained by androgens.

Hair growth and hirsutism

In the skin, plasma testosterone is converted by 5-alpha-reductase to dihydrotestosterone, which is required for the local stimulation of vellus hair follicles to produce terminal hair. Sensitivity of hair follicles is affected by local metabolism of androgens. Once the hair follicle has been stimulated by androgens to produce terminal hair, the changes persist even in the absence of androgen excess.

Causes of hirsutism

Ovarian
- polycystic ovarian disease, the commonest cause of hirsutism (these women have normal 17-hydroxyprogesterone, raised luteinising hormone (LH) and follicle-stimulating hormone (FSH) ratio (LH:FSH ratio) and elevated prolactin levels)

- tumour: arrhenoblastoma, hilus cell, lipoid, luteoma
- ovotestis

Adrenals
- congenital adrenal hyperplasia, with reduction in the enzyme 21-hydroxylase, an autosomal recessive disease (the women present with ambiguous genitalia and raised levels of 17-hydroxyprogesterone and dehydroepiandrosterone (DHEAS))
- androgen-secreting tumours: over 50% are malignant
- Cushing's disease with overproduction of adrenocorticotrophic hormone (ACTH)

Others
- endocrinopathies: thyroid dysfunction, acromegaly and hyperprolactinemia
- drugs such as anabolic steroids, danazol and valproic acid

Idiopathic
- normal androgen levels

Investigation and diagnosis

History
- onset, duration, pattern of growth
- weight gain, acne, change in voice
- menstrual changes
- diabetes, Cushing's syndrome, thyroid disease
- medication, family history

Examination
- general, blood pressure, weight, acne
- Ferriman-Gallwey score for hirsutism
- signs of virilisation
- abdominal and pelvic examination

The diagnosis is a clinical one and the hirsutism score does not necessarily correlate to androgen levels. This is thought be due to the variable response of follicles to androgen.

Investigations
The aim is to exclude serious disease and establish the source of androgens.
- pregnancy test
- ultrasound scan of ovaries for polycystic ovaries or tumour
- early follicular phase tests of serum LH, FSH and prolactin
- glucose tolerance test
- serum levels of free testosterone, DHEAS, androstenedione and 17-hydroxyprogesterone
- assess for Cushing's syndrome, thyroid function or acromegaly if clinically indicated

Management

Exclude or treat causes (see above).

Principles
- androgen suppression
- peripheral androgen suppression
- removal of unwanted hair
- weight control

Counselling
- reassurance that it is a common condition
- weight loss
- fertility not excluded

Hair therapy
- bleaching to mask hairs
- temporary removal of hair
- epilation, such as plucking or waxing
- depilation, such as shaving, is the removal of hair shaft from the skin surface
- chemicals: may be used to dissolve the hair

Permanent hair reduction
- electrolysis by thermal or chemical methods: causes destruction of hair follicle
- photoepilation using lasers or non-laser light sources: destroys hair follicles

Topical treatment
- eflornithine: an irreversible inhibitor of ornithine decarboxylase, an enzyme necessary for hair growth; reduces hair growth rate but does not remove hair

Pharmacological
Oral contraceptives
- Due to teratogenic potential of antiandrogens (see below), contraception should be used.
- Oral contraceptives also reduce hyperandrogenism by reducing LH (which reduces ovarian androgens), and increase sex hormone-binding globulin (which reduces free serum androgen). Some progesterones (e.g. cyproterone acetate) also act as androgen receptor antagonists.

Spironolactone
- an aldosterone antagonist with dose-dependent inhibition of androgen receptor
- inhibition of 5-alpha-reductase activity
- dose: spironolactone 100–200 mg daily
- contraception required: spironolactone may feminise a male fetus

Cyproterone acetate
- a potent androgen receptor antagonist
- inhibits androgen receptor and inhibits 5-alpha-reductase in the skin
- a potent progesterone that inhibits gonadotrophin and androgen levels
- dose: combined ethinyloestradiol 20–50 µg with cyproterone acetate 50–100 mg
- available as oral contraceptive pill with smaller dose of cyproterone acetate
- side effects include fatigue, reduced libido, weight gain

Finasteride
- inhibition of type 2, 5-alpha reductase activity (types 1 and 2 5-alpha-reductase is involved in hirsutism)

- mixed reports of efficacy compared to spironolactone, with finasteride having either equal or reduced efficacy

Flutamide
- an antiandrogen, inhibiting androgen receptors
- small studies show similar efficacy to spironolactone
- major risk is hepatic toxicity with reported liver failure

Insulin-lowering medications
- The place of these medications (e.g. metformin) in women without menstrual or metabolic dysfunction is controversial.
- Trials have shown reduced efficacy in treating hirsutism compared to spironolactone.

Glucocorticoids
- in small doses, reduce adrenal androgens
- dose is dexamethasone 0.25–0.5 mg/day.
- with antiandrogens, the male fetus may be feminised
- side effects include hypertension, weight gain, skin striae, decrease in bone density

Gonadotropin-releasing hormone agonist (GnRH) agonist
- GnRH analogues: usually combined with oral contraceptive pill and androgen blocker
- rationale: reduce LH and FSH and thus reduce ovarian androgens

Further reading

Martin KA, Chang RJ, Ehrmann DA et al 2008 Evaluation and treatment of hirsutism in premenopausal women: an Endocrine Society Clinical Practice Guideline. Journal of Clinical Endocrinology and Metabolism 93:1105–1120

Chapter 7

Contraception

Caroline De Costa
Michael Flynn

A standard measure of contraceptive effectiveness is the Pearl index—the number of pregnancies per 100 woman-years in those at risk of pregnancy. One woman-year equals 12 menstrual cycles.

Natural methods

Natural methods are based on avoiding sexual activity that might lead to conception at the time when the ovum can be fertilised. It is necessary to predict the time of ovulation (generally by observing changes in body temperature) and to allow for the time that the sperm can survive with fertilising potential in the female genital tract. Intercourse is prohibited until 72 hours after the rise in basal body temperature. The Pearl index is 25/100 woman-years; with coitus interruptus, it is 18/100.

Barrier methods

Diaphragm
The diaphragm lies diagonally across the cervix, vaginal vault and anterior vaginal wall (extends from posterior vaginal fornix to behind pubic bone). Types of design are arcing, coil or flat; it is manufactured from natural rubber, latex or silicone.

Function
- acts as retainer of spermicide
- keeps sperm away from alkaline cervical mucus, as sperm die in the acidic pH of the vagina
- prevents physical aspiration of sperm into the cervix and uterus

Effectiveness
- with perfect use, Pearl index 6/100 (normally increased by 3–7 times)
- may be protective against some sexually transmitted diseases, but not human immunodeficiency virus (HIV)
- not suitable for women with anatomical abnormalities of the genital tract and those with large cystoceles, rectoceles or uterine prolapse

Cervical/vault caps
- three types: cervical, vault, vimule (both cervix and vault); manufactured from latex, silicone
- function: to occlude the cervix
- spermicides recommended with use
- Pearl index 7/100

Advantages
- can be used in the presence of genital prolapse
- no rim; therefore, not felt by partner
- fitting not changed by changes in the size of the vagina

Sponge
- function: release spermicide; absorb the ejaculate; block the cervix
- Pearl index 17/100

Condoms
- reduce transmission of sexually transmitted diseases, including HIV
- non-latex condoms (polyurethane) available
- Pearl index, with perfect use, 2/100

Female condoms
- cover the vulva and may protect against infections such as herpes simplex and human papillomavirus

Spermicides
- most commonly used is nonoxynol-9; newer agents: octoxynol, benzalkonium chloride
- act by disrupting sperm cell membrane, causing rupture of spermatozoa
- available in gels, foams, creams, pessaries and capsules
- variable efficacy depending on doses, formulations and compliance
- may protect against sexually transmitted disease, and have in vitro anti-HIV properties

Intrauterine contraceptive devices

Types
- copper, to increase effectiveness and reduce the surface area (e.g. Multiload 375, Slimline TT380)
- progestogen-containing device (e.g. levonorgestrel-releasing intrauterine device (LNG IUD))

Mechanisms of action
- both types: prevent fertilisation of the ovum
- both types: foreign body response in myometrium interferes with implantation of the blastocyst
- both types: interfere with sperm transport
- LNG IUD only: causes endometrial atrophy, thickening of cervical mucus, prevents or delays ovulation in some women; oligomenorrhoea or amenorrhoea a normal side effect

Effectiveness
- Copper devices have a Pearl index in the first year of 2–3/100, later falling to lower than 1/100.

- They can be used as a postcoital contraceptive.
- Progesterone devices have a failure rate of 0.2%.

Counselling
- Take a past medical, surgical and social history.
- Discuss risks.
- The ideal patient for the intrauterine contraceptive device is a multiparous, monogamous woman with regular, normal periods.

Before insertion
- Explain procedure and risks, and acquire consent.
- Conduct a general physical examination.
- Perform a vaginal/pelvic examination.
- Obtain bacteriological, *Chlamydia* swabs, and cervical cytology if indicated.

Insertion
- Preferably insert at menses or up to day 10 of the cycle.
- For postcoital contraception, it may be effective up to 5 days postcoitus.
- For postpartum contraception, insert at 6 weeks after delivery.
- Training in insertion procedure is essential.

Change of the contraceptive device
- Multiload 375 devices require a change every 5 years.
- Progesterone (LNG IUD) is effective for 5 years.

Risks
- increased menstrual blood loss and dysmenorrhoea in copper devices
- incidence of uterine perforation (usually at time of insertion) 1 in 1000
- infection: for pelvic inflammatory disease, relative risk in the first 6 months 1.6; *Actinomycosis israelii* is usually an incidental finding at cervical cytological examination; may be associated with use of an intrauterine contraceptive device (*see Ch 11*)
- no protection against sexually transmitted infections
- increased risk of abortion, premature labour and delivery if a pregnancy occurs while the device is present
- ectopic pregnancy more frequent than in women not using an intrauterine contraceptive device (as device does not prevent ectopic)
- no reduction in fertility after using an intrauterine contraceptive device

Oral contraceptives

Combined oral contraceptive pill (COCP)
Two formulations
- monophasic: contain same oestrogen/progestogen throughout 21 or 24 days of course
- trisphasic: variations in oestrogen/progestogen content to reduce side effects

Mechanisms of action
- inhibit the oestrogen-mediated positive feedback that is required for the mid-cycle luteinising hormone (LH) surge
- inhibit follicle-stimulating hormone (FSH) release, thus preventing follicular maturation
- produce a change in cervical mucus
- reduce endometrial receptivity to the blastocyst

Assessment before commencing COCP
- Assess for and advise/manage risk factors such as hypertension, cigarette smoking and abnormal bleeding, and risk factors for thrombosis.
- Perform cervical cytology and breast examination.
- Contraindications include the presence of an oestrogen-dependent tumour, unexplained vaginal bleeding, pregnancy, breastfeeding, previous thromboembolism or cerebrovascular accident, known thrombophilia, hepatic dysfunction, severe migraine, >15 cigarettes daily in women >35 years, type 2 diabetes with complications, body mass index (BMI) >40.
- The woman must understand method and solutions to problems (see below).

Side effects and risks
- deep venous thrombosis
  - significant increased risk with use of ethinyloestradiol at doses of 100 μg or higher
  - hypercoagulation (may occur, but will reverse within 1 week of cessation of the oestrogen)
- cardiovascular disease: no statistically significant increased risk of hypertension in non-smokers
- malignancy: reduced relative risk of endometrial and ovarian cancer, which may continue for some time after cessation of use
- decrease in functional ovarian cysts; useful in managing polycystic ovarian syndrome (PCOS)
- carbohydrate metabolism: ethinyloestradiol doses lower than 40 μg little or no effect
- decreased menstrual loss and dysmenorrhoea
- improvement in acne

Missed pills
The high-risk time to miss pills, in terms of risk of pregnancy, is at the end of a packet or at the start of a new packet. Manage by continuing oral contraception and use other forms of contraception for 7 days. If these 7 days continue beyond the current 21-day packet, then start the next packet without a normal break (i.e. do not take the inactive pills).

Problems and solutions
- androgenic side effects: use desogestrel, gestodene, drospirenone, cyproterone acetate; increase oestrogen content
- anticonvulsant therapy: use monophasic 50 μg ethinyloestradiol
- breakthrough bleeding, amenorrhoea, dry vagina: increase oestrogen content
- breast tenderness: increase progestogen, reduce oestrogen
- antibiotics: little effect on contraceptive efficacy except for rifampicin; when using antibiotics, continue oral contraception and use other methods during and for 7 days after treatment; hormone-free interval should be omitted if <7 active pills remain in packet (i.e. continue directly with active pills in next packet)
- lactation: combined oral contraceptives may interfere

Progestogen-only pills
These pills contain progestogen only (levonorgestrel or norethisterone). All pills are active, and are taken continuously with no breaks. The mechanism of action is thickening of the cervical mucus, preventing sperm transport, rather than inhibiting ovulation (also possible interference with tubal motility and implantation). The pill should be taken at the same time each day, as efficacy is less than COCP. It is useful in breastfeeding women and those with certain medical contraindications to COCP.

Contraceptive implants

Depot medroxyprogesterone acetate (DMPA)
- dose: 150 mg by intramuscular injection every 12 weeks
- start first injection within 3 days of menstrual period
- Pearl index below 1/100 (i.e. as effective as COCP)

Mechanisms of action
- inhibits ovulation
- atrophies endometrium
- increases viscosity of cervical mucus
- reduces motility of fallopian tubes

Side effects
- irregular vaginal bleeding, especially in first 3 months
- amenorrhoea in 50% of women by 12 months
- restoration of ovulation taking up to 18 months

Subcutaneous progestogen implants
Etonogestrel's mechanisms of action are similar to those of DMPA. It represents a rapidly reversible contraception method. Training in insertion and removal procedures is essential.

Combined vaginal ring
This is a combined hormonal contraceptive ring inserted vaginally by the woman and left in place for 3 weeks and removed for a 7-day interval, as with placebo pills in COCP packs (e.g. NuvaRing). It inhibits ovulation, thickens the cervical mucus preventing sperm migration, and may interfere with implantation. It is a rapidly reversible method of contraception. Efficacy is equivalent to COCP.

Assessment
- as for COCP
- useful for women having difficulty with daily pill taking and women with inflammatory bowel disease
- contraindicated in immediate postpartum period
- the woman must understand method and how to insert ring

Side effects and risks
- may be accidentally expelled (e.g. in presence of prolapse, chronic constipation)
- possible increased vaginal discharge, vaginal infections
- decrease in menstrual loss and dysmenorrhoea
- contraindicated for first 6 months of breastfeeding
- late removal or late reinsertion of ring: cover insertion of new ring with condoms or other methods for 7 days

Pregnancy interception (emergency contraception)

Hormonal methods
- effectiveness dependent on time interval from unprotected intercourse to administration of medication; more effective when taken earlier
- effective preovulation; probably ineffective postovulation
- Yuzpe regimen: oral ethinyloestradiol 100 µg and levonorgestrel 500 µg with an antiemetic; repeat dose in 12 hours; take within 72 hours of coitus; needs follow-up

for failure of method, future contraception, risk of ectopic pregnancy and risk of sexually transmitted infections
- progestogen-only: levonorgestrel 750 µg immediately; repeat dose in 12 hours, or 1.5 mg single dose
- antiprogesterone: mifepristone RU-486 (not yet available in Australia)
- intrauterine contraceptive device (copper): effective up to 5–8 days after coitus

Male contraception

Gonadotropin-releasing hormone (GnRH) analogues
- reduce testosterone levels and libido
- GnRH with testosterone may block spermatogenesis

Steroids
- androgens cause a negative feedback that results in a fall in gonadotrophins
- progesterone and testosterone result in oligospermia

Antiandrogen (cyproterone acetate)
- inhibits spermatogenesis
- reduces potency and libido

Gossypol
- interferes with the acrosome

Sterilisation

Female sterilisation
Abdominal/laparoscopic
- Methods include fimbriectomy, diathermy, Pomeroy technique, Falope rings, Hulka or Filchie clips.
- Failure rate of 2–4/1000 may rise if performed at caesarean section or immediately postpartum.

Hysteroscopic
- Block fallopian tubes by inserting titanium microinserts via tubal ostia.

Male sterilisation
- Vasectomy is not associated with changes in the endocrine function.
- Pearl index is 0.2/100.

Further readings

Sexual Health and Family Planning Australia (SH&FPA) 2008 Contraception: an Australian clinical practice handbook. Canberra: SH&FP

Chapter 8

Miscarriage and abortion

Caroline De Costa
Michael Flynn

Definition. Termination of pregnancy at less than 20 weeks gestation or with the fetus weighing less than 400 g (exact definitions depend on the jurisdiction). 'Miscarriage' is usually taken to mean spontaneous abortion. 'Abortion' or 'termination of pregnancy' (TOP) usually refers to induced abortion (by surgical or medical means).

Incidence. About 15% of all pregnancies spontaneously abort (miscarry) at 6–13 weeks gestation. Up to 80% of spontaneous abortions are diagnosed at 8–12 weeks gestation.

Aetiology of spontaneous abortion

- genetic: chromosomal abnormalities present in up to 50% of first-trimester abortions (e.g. trisomy, monosomy, triploidy)
- fetal malformations (e.g. neural tube defects)
- immunological disorders
- uterine abnormalities
- cervical incompetence
- endocrine disorders (e.g. luteal phase dysfunction, diabetes mellitus)
- infections: listeria, mycoplasma, ureaplasma
- trauma: surgery, amniocentesis, chorionic villus sampling

Presentation and management

Presentation (spontaneous abortion)
- a period of amenorrhoea, followed by vaginal bleeding and cramping lower abdominal pain
- human chorionic gonadotrophin (hCG) positive

Examination
- general examination: colour, blood pressure, pulse
- abdominal examination
- vaginal examination
  - bleeding through the cervical os
  - bulky uterus
- cervical os may be open, with products of conception at the os or in the vagina

Investigations
- full blood count, blood group
- ultrasound scan of the pelvis

Management
- if bleeding not heavy and patient agrees can 'wait and see' (expectant management); complete abortion process may occur naturally
- uterine curettage if incomplete abortion, non-viable pregnancy on ultrasound or patient request
- misoprostol 800 µg vaginally may assist with expulsion of retained products
- anti-D immunoglobulin if patient Rhesus negative

Recurrent abortions

Definition. 'Recurrent abortions' is defined as three or more consecutive spontaneous abortions to the same partner.
   Prevalence. Prevalence is 1%–2%.

Risk of abortion
- After one abortion, the risk of another abortion at the next pregnancy is 20%–25%.
- After two abortions, the risk rises to 25%.
- After three, the risk is 30%.
- After four, the risk is 35%.
- Despite the many listed causes, most women have no obvious aetiology.

Investigations for recurrent abortions
- depends on history and time of miscarriage, with differing aetiologies presenting at different times
- abnormal parental (both maternal and paternal) karyotype and fetal karyotype; accounts for up to 5% recurrent pregnancy loss and is usually early loss
- assessment of uterine cavity via hysteroscopy or ultrasound
- thyroid function tests
- anticardiolipin and lupus anticoagulant testing
- inheritable thrombophilias (protein C resistance, protein S deficiency, factor V Leiden mutation)

Management of recurrent abortions
- immunosuppresive therapy (prednisone) indications unclear and not supported by trials
- anticoagulation therapy (such as aspirin and/or clexane) if indicated in disorders of inherited thrombophilias

Abortions due to uterine abnormalities
- surgery such as hysteroscopic resection of intrauterine adhesions
- cervical suture

Abortions due to endocrine abnormalities
Treat the cause (e.g. maintain good blood sugar control, and appropriate thyroid replacement).

Support and counselling
Women experiencing spontaneous abortion of a wanted pregnancy, especially those with recurrent abortions, may need effective psychological support and counselling.

Induced abortion

Surgical abortion
- carried out up to 12–13 weeks gestation
- suction curettage, increasingly preceded by misoprostol 400–800 µg 2–4 hours preoperatively to soften and dilate cervix
- cover with antibiotics or take swabs preoperatively and treat infection
- anti-D for Rhesus negative women

Medical abortion
- mifepristone plus misoprostol or misoprostol alone used for late abortion (usually for fetal abnormality or serious maternal conditions) in hospital setting
- misoprostol very effective, but process greatly shortened by the addition of mifepristone
- side effects: nausea, vomiting, diarrhoea from misoprostol; vaginal bleeding and pain from uterine contractions part of abortion process (analgesics should be given)
- anti-D for Rhesus negative women

Support and counselling
- All women undergoing induced abortion need appropriate counselling prior to the procedure, and follow-up, including advice about contraception and safe sex as indicated.
- All women experiencing abortion, whether spontaneous or induced, should be told to report promptly following procedure if pain, fever or offensive discharge occurs. Septic abortion can lead to pelvic inflammatory disease and subsequent infertility.

References

Adelberg AM 2002 Thrombophilias and recurrent miscarriage. Obstetrical and Gynecological Survey 57:703–710

Crenin MD, Potter C, Holovanisin M et al 2003 Mifepristone and misoprostol and methotrexate/misoprostol in clinical practice for abortion. American Journal of Obstetrics and Gynecology 188 (3):664–669

Royal College of Obstetricians and Gynaecologists (RCOG) 2004 National Clinical Guidelines. The care of women requesting induced abortion. London: RCOG

Chapter 9

Ectopic pregnancy

Michael Flynn

Definition. An ectopic pregnancy is implantation of a pregnancy outside the uterine cavity.

Incidence. Incidence varies with geographical location, from 1 in 28 to 1 in 300 pregnancies; 65% occur in the age group 25–34 years. In developed countries, incidence remains static at approximately 11 in 1000 pregnancies. Heterotrophic pregnancy (coexisting intrauterine and ectopic pregnancies) occurs in 1 in 30,000 spontaneous conceptions and in at least 1% of technically assisted conceptions.

Site. 97% of ectopic pregnancies occur in the fallopian tubes; the remainder are abdominal, ovarian or cervical.

Tubal ectopic pregnancy

Aetiology and risk factors
- pelvic inflammatory disease: associated with a seven-fold increased incidence of ectopic pregnancy
- tubal surgery
- past history of ectopic pregnancy: a 10%–15% chance of recurrence, rising to 50% if the contralateral tube is abnormal
- contraception associated with a risk of ectopic pregnancy
  - progesterone-only pill
  - postcoital pill
  - intrauterine contraceptive device (users who fall pregnant have a higher risk of ectopic pregnancy than oral contraceptive users)
- assisted reproductive techniques: 5% of pregnancy cycles
- endometriosis
- abnormal embryo

Presentation
- amenorrhoea
- small amount of vaginal bleeding, often after the onset of pain
- lower abdominal pain, shoulder-tip pain
- cervical motion tenderness, adnexal tenderness/mass

Investigations
Quantitative serum human chorionic gonadotrophin (hCG)
From 10 days postfertilisation, the hCG level doubles every 48 hours. If there is an apparently inadequate rise in hCG levels, suspect a failed pregnancy or ectopic pregnancy. Up to 1% of ectopic pregnancies have hCG levels <25 IU/L.

Ultrasound
Intrauterine pregnancy can be identified by 6 weeks gestation via transabdominal ultrasound scan and by 5 weeks gestation when using transvaginal scans. Abdominal ultrasound scans should identify an intrauterine sac with hCG levels >2000 IU/L; with transvaginal scans, the intrauterine sac may be seen with hCG >1000 IU/L. If no intrauterine sac is present with these levels, ectopic pregnancy is suspected.

Other biochemical investigations
Decreased serum progesterone is a sensitive marker in ectopic pregnancies and non-viable intrauterine pregnancies.

Laparoscopy
This is the gold standard in investigation and diagnosis; 3%–4% of very early tubal pregnancies can be missed.

Management
Surgical (laparoscopic or open procedures)
A laparoscopic approach to surgical management in a stable patient is the preferred approach, with shorter hospital stays, no difference in tubal patency rates and lower repeat ectopic rates. There is no role for medical management in the face of haemodynamic compromise.

Salpingectomy and salpingostomy
- In those managed by removal of the ectopic tissue only, follow-up with weekly quantitative hCG test is required. At least 5% of these cases will have evidence of continuing trophoblastic activity (i.e. persistent ectopic pregnancy).
- There is no randomised control trial evidence specifically comparing salpingectomy and salpingostomy. Cohort studies suggest no difference in subsequent intrauterine pregnancy rates between either procedure, but a tendency towards higher subsequent ectopic pregnancies in the salpingostomy group.

Local injection of ectopic pregnancy
- methotrexate, potassium chloride, prostaglandins
- requires follow-up because of risk of persisting ectopic pregnancy

Medical
Systemic methotrexate
Single-dose methotrexate is successful in over 90% of cases. The dose is calculated on body surface area at 50 mg/m^2. Criteria for use include:
- haemodynamic stability
- no fetal cardiac activity
- hCG level <15,000 IU/L
- ectopic mass ≤3.5 cm

About 15% will require a second dose if hCG levels have failed to fall more than 15% in 4–7 days. The outcome is comparable to that of surgery for unruptured ectopic pregnancy. It is useful for early cervical pregnancy, and has been used in continuing hCG activity after incomplete removal of an ectopic trophoblast.

Expectant management
This has been reported in the woman who does not have abdominal pain and who has falling hCG levels of <1000 IU/L. However, there have been cases of ruptured ectopic pregnancy with low and declining levels of hCG.

Anti-D
Rhesus-negative women with confirmed ectopic pregnancy should be given 250 IU of anti-D.

Contraception and future pregnancies
Because of the heightened risk of future ectopic pregnancies, the woman requires advice for subsequent pregnancies, such as an early hCG test and ultrasound scan.

Avoid contraception, which can increase the risk of ectopic pregnancies (e.g. progesterone-only pill, intrauterine contraceptive device).

Abdominal pregnancy

Incidence. Incidence is up to 1 in 10,000 live births. There is a higher incidence with low socioeconomic status and in developing countries.

Maternal mortality. 2%–10% of abdominal pregnancies (i.e. seven to eight times the risk compared with tubal ectopic pregnancies and 90 times the risk of intrauterine pregnancy).

Management
- If the fetus dies and a lithopedion develops, no treatment is required.
- If the fetus dies, wait 3–8 weeks to allow it to atrophy. However, coagulation disorders may develop.
- If the fetus is alive, intervene early because of the risk of maternal morbidity/mortality.
- Management of the placenta is debatable:
  - If an attempt is made to remove it, there is a risk of bleeding.
  - If the placenta is left in situ, there is a risk of infection and abscess formation.
  - Treat with methotrexate.

Reference

Royal College of Obstetricians and Gynaecologists (RCOG) 2004 Guideline 21: The management of tubal pregnancy. London: RCOG

Chapter 10

Infertility

Anusch Yazdani

Definitions. *Infertility* is the failure to achieve a successful pregnancy after 12 months or more of regular unprotected intercourse. *Primary infertility* is no previous pregnancy, regardless of the outcome. *Secondary infertility* is previous pregnancy, regardless of the outcome. *Fecundability* is the probability of achieving a pregnancy per menstrual cycle. *Fecundity* is the probability of achieving a live birth per menstrual cycle.

Incidence. The overall incidence of primary infertility is 10%–15% of couples. Female fertility declines with age and the incidence of infertility increases: 5% under the age of 25; 10% under the age of 30; 15% under the age of 35; 30% under the age of 40; and 60% over the age of 40.

Conception

Conception requires:
- sperm*
  - adequate (quantity, quality)
  - deposition (in vicinity of cervix, prior to/at ovulation, permeable cervical mucus)
- ovulation*
- at least one patent fallopian tube to allow fertilisation*
- transport to endometrial cavity
- implantation

Probability of conception
The probability of conception is time dependent:
- after 3 months: 60%
- after 6 months: 75%
- after 12 months: 85%
- after 24 months: 95%

Therefore, the majority of couples who have not conceived after 1 year are likely to conceive in the subsequent year.

Aetiology

The requirements for conception determine the aetiological factors that contribute to infertility:
- male factors: 40%
  - pretesticular factors: hypothalamic–pituitary abnormalities

---

*denotes common problem.

- testicular factors: primary testicular abnormalities, varicocoele, torsion, trauma, orchiditis, cytotoxic drug treatment, radiotherapy, undescended testes
  - post-testicular factors: genital tract obstruction, may be congenital (congenital absence of vas deferens), inflammatory, Young's syndrome, postvasectomy, vasectomy
- female factors: 50%
  - tubal and pelvic pathology: 40%
    - endometriosis, adhesions, hydrosalpinges, pelvic inflammatory disease, fibroids, congenital abnormalities
  - ovulatory dysfunction: 40%
    - primary ovarian abnormalities, polycystic ovary syndrome, obesity, age
    - hypothalamic–pituitary disorders
  - other: 20%
- unexplained: 10%

History

Female
- history of infertility
  - primary or secondary infertility
    - previous pregnancies: same or different partner, time to conceive, outcome of pregnancy
  - duration of infertility
- sexual history
  - history of contraception
  - sexual function
    - dyspareunia
    - coital frequency, timing during cycle
- menstrual history
  - regularity, frequency of cycles, evidence of ovulation (such as mucus changes)
  - dysmenorrhoea
- evidence of endocrine disorder
  - galactorrhoea, hirsutism, acne
  - weight gain
- past medical history
  - obesity
  - hypertension, renal disease, gastrointestinal disease
  - thyroid disease
  - pelvic inflammatory disease
  - peritonitis, appendicitis, ovarian or pelvic surgery
  - endometriosis
- medications
- social history, including smoking, alcohol or other substance abuse
- family history, including birth defects, mental retardation or reproductive failure

Male
- history of infertility
  - pregnancies to other partners
- sexual function
  - erectile or ejaculatory dysfunction

- past medical history
  - varicocoele, undescended testicle, mumps
  - orchidopexy, inguinal hernia repair
  - urinary tract infection, sexually transmitted disease
  - testicular injury or infections
- medications
- social history, including smoking, alcohol or other substance abuse
- family history, including birth defects, mental retardation or reproductive failure

Examination

Female
- general
  - pulse rate, blood pressure, body mass index (BMI)
  - dysmorphic features, secondary sexual characteristics
- endocrine
  - breast and thyroid, hirsutism, acne, galactorrhoea, striae, acanthosis
- reproductive
  - vaginal examination
    — cervical cytology, microbiological studies, including *Chlamydia*
    — pelvic assessment (e.g. fixed retroversion of the uterus)

Male
- general
  - pulse rate, blood pressure, BMI
  - dysmorphic features, secondary sexual characteristics
- endocrine
  - gynaecomastia, hair distribution
- reproductive
  - phallus
  - spermatic cord: presence of vas, varicocoele
  - testicular size and consistency

Investigations

Initial investigations
Initial investigations focus on the three main factors causing infertility (ovulatory, pelvic and male factors) and assess the suitability for pregnancy (antenatal screening).
- ovulatory factor assessment
  - a regular cycle with symptoms of ovulation is evidence of ovulation
  - basal body temperature (BBT) chart
    — progesterone is thermogenic and raises BBT after ovulation, which is maintained during the luteal phase
    — 20% of ovulatory women have a monophasic BBT
  - serum progesterone
    — tested in the luteal phase on day 21 of an ideal 28-day cycle or 7 days prior to menses
    — raised progesterone in the luteal range is evidence of ovulation in that cycle
- pelvic factor assessment
  - ultrasound scan of pelvis: ovarian morphology, evidence of pelvic disease, such as fibroids
- antenatal screening tests (include cervical screening, rubella serology)

- male factor assessment
  - seminal analysis
    — requires 3 days abstinence before collection
    — volume >2 mL
    — density >20 million sperm/mL
    — motility >50%
    — morphology >15% normal

Extended investigations

Extended investigations are performed when the initial investigations have not identified a cause or when further elucidation is required.

- ovulatory factor assessment
  - follicle-stimulating hormone (FSH), luteinising hormone (LH) and oestradiol in the follicular phase in those menstruating, or randomly when cycles irregular or absent
  - serum prolactin, thyroid function tests
  - endometrial biopsy in secretory phase
  - if hirsutism is present, serum testosterone, androstenedione, dehydro-epiandrosterone sulfate (DHEAS), sex hormone binding globulin and 17-hydroxyprogesterone
- pelvic factor assessment
  - assessment of tubal function
    — provides information regarding uterine cavity and tubes but no extratubal view: hysterosalpingogram, hysterosonography (HyCoSy)
  - laparoscopy, hysteroscopy, dye pertubation
    — detailed survey of the reproductive organs, hydrotubation to assess (and treat) tubal patency, pelvic adhesions, endometriosis
- male factor assessment
  - seminal analysis: if the initial test is abnormal, repeat in 2–3 months (long development cycle of sperm may be affected by, for example, fever)
  - antisperm antibodies: immunobead test, mixed antiglobulin reaction test
  - endocrine tests
    — FSH/LH/total testosterone: to distinguish between obstructive disorders and primary testicular failure
    — inhibin, prolactin, thyroid-stimulating hormone (TSH)
  - chromosomal analysis
    — indications: azoospermia, raised FSH, reduced testicular volume, prolonged unexplained infertility, congenital abnormalities
    — in infertility clinics, 2% of males are chromosomally abnormal, rising to 15% in the azoospermic male
  - testicular biopsy
    — indication: obstructive azoospermia, diagnostic uncertainty

Management

Management of infertility is directed by the assessment of the three main factors (ovulatory, pelvic and male) as above.

Principles

- optimise conception
  - lifestyle modification if required
  - folic acid supplementation in line with National Health and Medical Research Council (NHMRC) requirements

- appropriate coital timing
- correct any primary pathology
  - treatment of endocrine disorders
- manage any non-correctible factors

Ovulatory factor infertility

Management options include:
- ovulation induction: induce ovulation in anovulatory or oligovoulatory females
- superovulation: induce the formation of two or three mature follicles in women who are ovulating
- controlled ovarian hyperstimulation: induce the formation of multiple mature follicles for the purposes of in vitro fertilisation (IVF)

Clomiphene
- description
  - a non-steroidal agent distantly related to diethylstilbestrol
  - the principally antagonistic effect at the level of the hypothalamus activates the oestrogen–gonadotrophin feedback to the pituitary, causing a rise in FSH and LH (but especially FSH), which leads to induction of ovulation
- dose
  - 50–150 mg/day for 5 days on days 5–9 or days 2–6 of the menstrual cycle
  - a lower dose is often required in polycystic ovarian syndrome
  - a rise in luteal serum progesterone on day 21 confirms ovulation
- adverse reactions
  - vasomotor symptoms, breast and abdominal discomfort, visual changes, alopecia, multiple pregnancies (8%)

Follicle-stimulating hormone (FSH)
- description
  - FSH in stimulation regimen may be derived from two sources:
    — synthetic FSH, a manufactured recombinant glycoprotein
    — purified urinary menopausal gonadotrophins, containing both FSH and LH, though the latter has minimal clinical efficacy
- dose
  - 50–450 IU/day self-administered from days 2–5 of the menstrual cycle
  - dosing determines whether one or multiple follicles are developed
  - response is monitored by ultrasound scanning and oestrogen-level measurement
- adverse reactions
  - breast and abdominal discomfort, multiple pregnancies (25%), ovarian hyper-stimulation syndrome

Gonadotropin-releasing hormone (GnRH) agonist/antagonists
- Unless the pituitary is suppressed, the rising oestrogen levels will cause spontaneous LH surge and ovulation prior to follicles reaching the correct size for an egg pick-up.
- GnRH agonists administered in a non-pulsatile fashion (either as injections or nasal sprays) will cause GnRH receptor down-regulation and suppress the mid-cycle LH surge and ovulation; this effect requires 7–10 days.
- GnRH antagonists act as competitive inhibitors and can therefore be administered only at the time suppression is required.

Human chorionic gonadotrophin (hCG)
- Purified urinary or recombinant hCG may be used to induce final oocyte maturation (analogous to the LH surge in a natural cycle).

- It is a cheaper alternative to LH.
- In ovulation induction or superovulation, ovulation is induced for IVF.
- In IVF, a transvaginal egg pick-up is performed prior to ovulation.

Pelvic factor infertility
Tubal factors
- success of repair depends on the site, nature and severity of the tubal damage
  - interstitial tubal obstruction
    — tubal reimplantation has a poor prognosis and is an indication for IVF
  - proximal tubal obstruction
    — has an excellent prognosis, particularly if resulting from sterilisation
    — tubal reanastomosis requires at least one tube of over 4 cm in length with a healthy ampulla and fimbria
    — best results are with isthmo-isthmic anastomosis
    — pregnancy rate >60%; 10% ectopic
  - distal tubal obstruction
    — has a poor prognosis, as it is most often associated with severe tubal damage
    — neosalpingostomy 25% intrauterine pregnancy and 30% ectopic pregnancy rate
- success rates of tubal surgery must be compared to assisted reproductive techniques
- hydrosalpinges should be corrected or removed prior to any assisted reproduction

Adhesions
Removal of adhesions around the ovary and fimbriae, if the tube is otherwise normal, have a 50% chance of a live birth and a 10% risk of ectopic pregnancy.

Endometriosis
(*See Ch 4.*)

Fibroids
(*See Ch 20.*)

Male factor infertility
Pretesticular factors
- gonadotrophin deficiency: gonadotrophin therapy
- note that testosterone supplementation results in a feedback suppression of gonadotrophins and cessation of spermatogenesis

Testicular factors
- most testicular factors are not correctible
  - if spermatogenesis persists, sperm may be used for insemination, IVF or intracytoplasmic sperm injection (ICSI)
  - in the absence of spermatogenesis, donor sperm will be required
- varicocoele (with abnormal seminal analysis) may be repaired
- sperm auto-antibodies: corticosteroids are rarely useful; IVF–ICSI is now considered the primary treatment of choice

Post-testicular factors
- surgical correction of obstruction may be considered depending upon the level of obstruction
- alternatively, testicular or epididymal sperm retrieval for IVF–ICSI has a high success rate

Coital disorders
- correction of primary pathology
- pharmacotherapy for erectile dysfunction
- psychosexual counselling

Assisted reproduction

Definitions. IVF: in-vitro fertilisation; ICSI: intracytoplasmic sperm injection.
    Success rates. IVF—fresh embryo transfer: 35–40%; frozen embryo transfer: 25–30%.

Steps in assisted reproduction
The aim of assisted reproduction is to induce the development of multiple mature ovarian follicles. There are five steps.

Step 1: Controlled ovarian hyperstimulation
- administration of FSH, commencing on day 3–5 of the cycle
- combined with pituitary down-regulation to prevent a premature LH surge and ovulation
- ovarian response is carefully monitored by oestradiol assays and/or transvaginal ultrasound scans over a period of 9–12 days
- ovarian follicles grow at a predictable rate of approximately 2 mm/day
- once follicles have reached maturity (>18 mm in diameter), an injection of hCG is given to initiate the final process of egg maturation

Step 2: Egg collection
- performed under a local or general anaesthetic using a vaginal ultrasound probe at 36–38 hours following the hCG
- the needle is guided through the top of the vagina into the ovary and each follicle is aspirated
- the follicular fluid is assessed by a scientist for the presence of an egg

Step 3: Fertilisation and embryo culture
- the semen sample (collected by masturbation) or surgically retrieved sperm is prepared in the laboratory
- the oocyte is prepared
  - IVF: the prepared oocytes are cultured with prepared sperm
  - ICSI: the prepared oocytes are directly injected with a single sperm
- fertilisation is completed the following day and the embryo develops in culture
- 2–3 days after egg collection, the embryos have reached the 2–8 cell stage

Step 4: Embryo transfer
- performed in the day theatres without anaesthetic or sedation
- a maximum of two embryos may be transferred, but couples should consider the transfer of a single embryo to prevent a twin pregnancy
- luteal support in the form of hCG injections or progesterone pessaries may be required after the embryo transfer to support the uterine lining

Step 5: Embryo freezing and subsequent cycles
- spare embryos may be frozen and stored for future use
- in subsequent cycles, an embryo is thawed and transferred in synchrony with a natural cycle and drug therapy is usually not required

Ovarian hyperstimulation syndrome

Ovarian hyperstimulation syndrome (OHSS) is an exaggerated response to ovulation/ovulation triggers characterised by increased vascular permeability, intravascular depletion and third space fluid sequestration. It is usually an iatrogenic, self-limiting disorder associated with ovulation induction/ovarian stimulation. It may be:

- early onset: related to hCG trigger
  - flare of GnRH therapy
- late onset: related to ensuing pregnancy, especially multiple
  Incidence. Severe OHSS occurs in 0.5% episodes of assisted reproduction.
  Pathophysiology. OHSS occurs in response to endogenous or exogenous LH or hCG, resulting in increased vascular permeability, arterial dilation, fluid shift from vascular to third space, intravascular depletion and circulatory dysfunction.

Risk factors
Patient factors
- young age
- low body weight
- history of OHSS
- polycystic ovaries

Cycle factors
- agonist down-regulated cycles are more likely to result in OHSS
- GnRH antagonists reduce incidence of severe OHSS
- high doses of exogenous gonadotrophins
- high absolute or rapidly rising oestradiol (E2)
- large number of developing follicles or oocytes retrieved (>20)
- high-dose hCG ovulation trigger

Management
Outpatient
Mild forms may be managed as an outpatient.
- simple analgesia
- simple antiemetics
- maintain oral intake
- encourage mobilisation

Inpatient
Moderate to severe forms require admission.
INDICATIONS
- pain
- intractable nausea/vomiting/diarrhoea
- haemodynamic compromise
- respiratory compromise

INVESTIGATIONS
- haematocrit >45 L/L
- white cell count >15 x10^9/L
- hyponatraemia
- hyperkalaemia
- abnormal liver function test
- renal impairment (creatinine >0.12 μmol/L; creatinine clearance <50 mL/minute)

ASSESSMENT
- regular assessment of vital signs (every 2–8 hours)
- daily weight

- daily abdominal circumference
- fluid balance sheet
- pulse oximetry
- ward test of urine

INVESTIGATIONS
- full blood examination
- electrolytes and liver function tests
- coagulation profile
- pelvic ultrasound scan
- chest X-ray if respiratory compromise
- echocardiogram if respiratory or cardiovascular compromise

MANAGEMENT
- bed rest
- analgesia
- antiemetic
- thromboprophylaxis
- fluid management
- oral
- intravenous fluids
- type
- normal saline preferred initial resuscitation
- paracentesis

Intensive care unit admission
Indications are:
- haemodynamic compromise requiring invasive monitoring
- renal compromise requiring invasive monitoring (central venous pressure monitoring), dopamine agonist therapy or dialysis
- respiratory compromise requiring ventilation/positive end-expiratory pressure (PEEP)/oxygen

Further reading

Cahill DJ, Wardle PG 2002 Management of infertility. British Medical Journal 325:28–32
Grudzinskas JG (ed) 2003 The management of subfertility. Best Practice and Research Clinical Obstetrics and Gynaecology 17(2):169–367

Chapter 11

Pelvic infections

Yasmin Jayasinghe

Definition. Pelvic inflammatory disease (PID) is an upper genital tract infection. This includes infection of the uterus, fallopian tubes and other pelvic viscera.

Pathogenesis

Organisms ascend from the lower genital tract.

Physiological barriers to infection
- cervix
  - mechanical: diameter of endocervix, downward flow of mucus
  - biochemical: production of antibacterial lysozymes
  - immunological: local immunoglobulin A (IgA)
- endometrium
  - cyclical shedding
- uterotubal junction: a mechanical barrier

Causes of infection

- organisms introduced to the upper genital tract via procedures such as insertion of an intrauterine contraceptive device, and dilatation and curettage
- motile organisms: spermatozoa acting as carriers of organisms
- coital uterine contractions enhancing the spread of organisms
- spread from other organs (e.g. appendix)
- association with other disease: tuberculosis, schistosomiasis

Risk factors

- increased risk in adolescents and young women due to sexual behaviours and immaturity of the cervical epithelium with wide transformation zone
- early sexual debut, multiple partners, lack of condoms or contraception
- increased risk with sexual activity during menses

Microbiology

It is a polymicrobial infection.

Tubal cultures
Table 11.1 lists the microbiological aetiology of PID.

Neisseria gonorrhoea
- gram-negative diplococcus which invades the columnar epithelium; infection usually occurs in the first half of the menstrual cycle
- incubation period: usually 2–7 days
- period of communicability: months in untreated individuals

Diagnosis
Definitive diagnosis is by culture.
- Collect microbiological swabs from the endocervix (or posterior fornix if pregnant), urethra, rectum and throat.
- Send slide for gram stain, and then place second swab into Amies +/– charcoal transport medium.
- Conduct polymerase chain reaction (PCR) test on endocervical specimens (95% sensitivity, 100% specificity). In women, PCR testing of first pass urine (10–20 mL at least 1 hour after passing urine) is less sensitive (around 50%), and, if positive, should be followed up by collection of further endocervical specimens for PCR and culture, prior to antibiotic therapy. Treatment can be commenced before these repeat results are obtained.

Treatment
- ceftriaxone 500 mg intramuscular injection immediately, mixed with 2 mL 1% lignocaine or ciprofloxacin 500 mg orally; single dose in areas where there is no resistance
- coinfection with *Chlamydia* may occur, so always cover for both
- a notifiable disease

Chlamydia trachomatis
- It is an obligate intracellular organism.
- Its lifecycle has two stages: (a) an infectious and metabolically inactive elementary body which penetrates the cell wall by endocytosis, where it is transformed into (b) the reticulate body, which reproduces by binary fission to form new elementary bodies in the vacuole, which eventually ruptures to release the organism.
- It is the most common notifiable sexually transmitted disease (STD). Incidence is 2.5%–14% in STD clinic patients, 5% in family planning clients and up to 15% in commercial sex workers.
- The incubation period is poorly defined: 7–14 days or longer.
- The period of communicability is unknown: perhaps months to years.

Table 11.1 Microbiological aetiology of PID	
Aetiology	Incidence
Chlamydia trachomatis	40%–60%
Neisseria gonorrhoea	15%–18%
Mycoplasma species	10%–15%
Anaerobic facultative bacteria: *Escherichia coli*, group B streptococcus (GBS), *Bacteroides* species, *Peptostreptococcus* species, *Staphylococcus aureus*	30%

Diagnosis
- endocervical swab into PCR transport tube (or send as dry swab) or first void urine PCR
- both have comparable sensitivity: 87%–99% sensitivity, >95% specificity

Treatment
- first-line azithromycin 1 g orally, single dose, or
- doxycycline 100 mg orally twice daily for 7 days, or
- erythromycin 500 mg orally four times a day for 7 days
- a notifiable disease

Mycoplasma genitalium
- *Mycoplasma genitalium* is strongly associated with PID and is best detected by PCR, to distinguish from other *Mycoplasma* species.
- *Mycoplasma hominis* and *Ureaplasma urealyticum* are associated with bacterial vaginosis, possibly PID, but also may be non-pathogenic commensals.
- Treatment of choice is azithromycin.

Anaerobes: *Bacteroides* and *Peptostreptococcus* species
Treat with metronidazole 400 mg three times a day for 7 days.

Diagnosis of PID

Presentation. It may be acute, subacute or subclinical. Most women with endocervical chlamydial or gonorrhoeal infection are asymptomatic.

Symptomatic PID
- Symptoms are acute pelvic pain, febrile illness, vaginal discharge, postcoital or intermenstrual bleeding; less frequent symptoms include urethral syndrome (dysuria and pyuria), bartholinitis, perihepatitis and proctitis.
- Signs are fever, abdominal tenderness, adnexal tenderness or mass, uterine or cervical motion tenderness, cervical inflammation and vaginal discharge.
- The Centers for Disease Control and Prevention (CDC) 2006 guidelines recommend that empiric treatment be undertaken in sexually active women with lower abdominal pain if they meet at least one of the following criteria: cervical motion, uterine or adnexal tenderness.
- Laparoscopy is the gold standard for diagnosis, and is useful in unwell subjects where diagnosis is unclear, or there is no improvement with antibiotics, and for surgical intervention.
- Findings include erythema and oedema of tubes, purulent discharge, pyosalpinx, tubo-ovarian abscess and pelvic adhesions.

Investigations
- serum human chorionic gonadotrophin (hCG) level
- full blood count, erythrocyte sedimentation rate, C-reactive protein (CRP), blood cultures
- urine for bacteriological studies
- vaginal wet prep:
  - >3 polymorphs on smear has sensitivity of 87%–91%
  - 0 polymorphs has a negative predictive value of 95%
- bacteriological assessment of specimens from the vagina, endocervix, urethra, rectum, throat and pelvis (at laparoscopy), screening for other sexually transmitted

infections, including human immunodeficiency virus (HIV), hepatitis B and syphilis
- transvaginal ultrasound scan: adnexal mass, tubal oedema (thick wall, incomplete septum, cogwheel, beading): sensitivity 32%–85%, specificity 97%–100%

Management of PID

Principles
- broad spectrum antibiotics for 14 days: cure rates of over 90%
- investigation and empiric treatment of sexual partners
- notifiable diseases must be reported to Department of Health
- counsel regarding safe sexual practices
- advise avoidance of sexual intercourse for duration of treatment
- test of cure is not cost-effective where the above advice has been followed; however, may provide reassurance

Outpatient treatment for mild–moderate PID
Outpatient treatment for mild–moderate PID is safe and efficacious.
- azithromycin 1 g orally, immediately
- plus metronidazole 400 mg orally twice daily for 14 days
- plus doxycycline 100 mg orally twice daily for 14 days
- plus ceftriaxone 500 mg intramuscular injection with 2 mL 1% lignocaine if suspect gonorrhoea

Inpatient treatment for severe PID
- cefotaxime 1 g intravenously (IV) 8 hourly, or cefoxitin 2 g IV 6 hourly, or ceftriaxone 1 g IV daily
- plus metronidazole 500 mg IV 8 hourly
- plus doxycycline 100 mg orally twice daily, or roxithromycin 150 mg orally twice daily or 300 mg orally daily as a single dose, until the patient is afebrile and improved; then continue doxycycline or roxithromycin for 2–4 weeks

Outpatient treatment of mild–moderate procedure-related PID
- doxycycline 100 mg orally twice daily for 2–4 weeks, or
- amoxycillin 500 mg orally three times a day, plus metronidazole 400 mg orally three times a day for 2–4 weeks

Inpatient treatment of severe septicaemic procedure-related PID
- amoxycillin 2 g IV 4 hourly, plus gentamicin 1.5 mg/kg IV 8 hourly, plus metronidazole 500 mg IV 8 hourly until afebrile; then doxycycline 100 mg orally twice daily for 2 weeks

Consequences of PID

Short-term
- pyosalpinx
- tubo-ovarian abscess (TOA): accounts for 30% of hospitalisations with PID; treat initially with parenteral antibiotics; surgery if poor response; rupture of TOA is medical emergency
- pelvic peritonitis
- perihepatitis, colitis

- acute infection with *Chlamydia* and gonorrhoea increases susceptibility to HIV infection

Long-term
- recurrent PID: risk increased by two to three times
- infertility: risk of tubal obstruction
  - after one episode of PID: 10%–15%
  - after two episodes: 20%–35%
  - after three episodes: 40%–75%
- chronic pelvic pain (in 20% of cases)
- ectopic pregnancy: risk increased by seven to ten times
- Fitz-Hugh-Curtis syndrome (perihepatitis) (1%–30% of cases)

Actinomyces israelii

- This is a gram-positive, non-acid, mycelium-bearing, anaerobic fungus. It is a normal commensal of mouth and gastrointestinal and genital tract.
- Actinomyces-like organisms (ALOs) may be identified on cervical smears, but this is not diagnostic of pelvic disease.
- They are found in women with and without an intrauterine device (IUD).
- If a woman is symptomatic, or has a pelvic mass, the IUD should be removed, and treatment with antibiotics penicillin, tetracycline or erythromycin, plus or minus surgical intervention, is required.
- There is no evidence to support the routine removal of an IUD in an asymptomatic woman.

Toxic shock syndrome (TSS)

- historically associated with use of superabsorbant tampons in presence of exotoxin producing *Staphylococcus aureus* colonisation
- non-menstrual TSS related to infected wounds, foreign bodies
- menstrual TSS declining, annual incidence 1–2 in 100,000, with a 3% case fatality rate
- incidence of non-menstrual TSS remains relatively constant, with a 6% case fatality rate

Aetiology
- caused most commonly by *S. aureus*, which produces TSS toxin 1 (TSST-1); accounts for 90% of menstrual cases and 60% of non-menstrual cases of TSS or *S. aureus* producing enterotoxin B
- can also be caused by *Streptococcus pyogenes* (group A streptococcus), non-group A beta-haemolytic streptococcus, and *Streptococcus viridans* (more fulminant disease with higher mortality)

Presentation
- fever, hypotension
- erythroderma of palms, soles, hands, desquamation, multiorgan dysfunction including coagulopathy, renal failure, adult respiratory distress syndrome, and abnormalities in electrolytes and liver biochemistry

Investigations
- full septic and biochemical screen
- isolation of TSST-1 pathognomonic for *S. aureus* TSS

Management
- resuscitate, ventilate if required
- intravenous antibiotics
- remove tampon if present
- open and debride infected wounds

Further reading and references

Centers for Disease Control and Prevention 2006 Sexually transmitted diseases treatment guidelines 2006. MMWR Recommendations and Reports 55 (No. RR–11):1–77

Cook RL, Hutchison SL, Østergaard L et al 2005 Systematic review: noninvasive testing for *Chlamydia trachomatis* and *Neisseria gonorrhoeae*. Annals of Internal Medicine 142 (11):914–925

FFPRHC Guidance 2004 The copper intrauterine device as long-term contraception. Journal of Family Planning and Reproductive Health Care 30 (1):29–42

Gainer J, Yost M 2003 Critical care infectious disease. Obstetrics and Gynecology Clinics of North America 30:695–709

Ness RB, Soper DE, Holley RL et al 2003 Effectiveness of inpatient and outpatient treatment strategies for women with pelvic inflammatory disease: results from the Pelvic Inflammatory Disease Evaluation and Clinical Health (PEACH) Randomized Trial. American Journal of Obstetrics and Gynecology 186 (5):924–937

Sexual Health Society of Victoria 2008 National management guidelines for sexually transmissible infections. Royal Australian College of General Practitioners, 18 December. Available: www.racp.edu.au

Victorian Department of Health 2009 Blue book. Available: www.health.vic.gov.au/ideas/bluebook/

Westrom L, Joesoef R, Reynolds G et al 1992 Pelvic inflammatory disease and infertility. A cohort study of 1844 women with laparoscopically verified disease and 657 control women with normal laparoscopic results. Journal of Sexually Transmitted Diseases 19 (4):185–192

Chapter 12

Menopause and premature ovarian failure

Michael Flynn

Definitions. *Natural menopause* is the permanent ceasing of menstruation resulting from the loss of ovarian follicular activity. Menopause is by definition only after 12 months of amenorrhoea with no other pathological cause. Menopause is the final period diagnosed only in retrospect. *Perimenopause* is the time immediately premenopause, as characterised by endocrinological and clinical features, and continuing until the year postmenopause. *Premature menopause* occurs at an age <2 standard deviations from the community mean. In practice, this is menopause prior to the age of 40. The average age of menopause is 50–51 years.

Aetiology

Menopause is due to the exhaustion of primordial follicles, causing a fall in oestrogen and progesterone levels.

Endocrinology in the climacteric and menopause

Three phases of endocrine changes
- hypothalamic–pituitary hyperactivity occurring years before and continuing after menopause
- ovulatory failure
- ovarian follicular failure

Initial changes in ovarian function are due to a failure in ovulation and a deficient luteal phase. Following this is a reduction in serum oestradiol and a rise in follicle-stimulating hormone (FSH) due to the negative hormonal feedback. Rises in luteinising hormone (LH) occur later, but these are not as marked as the rise in FSH. Follicular development and menstrual cycles then become irregular. At menopause, insufficient ovarian follicular development results in insufficient oestrogen to cause endometrial growth. In the postmenopausal state, oestradiol decreases with a normal or slightly raised level of oestrone.

Gonadotrophins after the menopause
- Maximal rises in FSH and LH occur in the first 2–3 years.
- After 20 years, FSH and LH may return to reproductive life levels.

Oestrogens
- Postmenopausal oestrogen sources are derived from the peripheral conversion of androstenedione (produced by the adrenals and ovaries) to oestrone.
- Aromatisation of androstenedione occurs at peripheral sites.

Androgens
- Ovaries continue to secrete androgens: androstenedione and testosterone.

Progesterone
- Levels are lower than premenopausal levels.

Others
- Prolactin levels decrease.
- Inhibin has a specific negative feedback control on FSH and levels are reduced.

Clinical features of menopause

Generally, clinical features are the best guide to menopause: 10%–20% have no symptoms; 60% have mild to moderate symptoms; and 10%–20% have severe symptoms. While vasomotor symptoms predominate, they are not necessary and symptoms are variable. Symptoms are relieved by oestrogen.

Vasomotor symptoms
- A hot flush lasts between 1 and 4 minutes and is associated with a rise in temperature, peripheral vasodilatation and a slight rise in pulse rate.
- There is a possible association with rising and falling oestrogen levels.
- Hot flushes are synchronous with, but are not caused by, LH pulses.
- Up to 50%–80% of women suffer from vasomotor effects at the menopause and climacteric, and 20%–25% of these women continue to have symptoms after 5 years.
- Symptoms include intense heat, flushing and sweating.

Genital and urinary tract symptoms
- Urogenital atrophy results in reduced glycogen and lactobacilli, causing a rise in vaginal pH, dryness and increased risk of infection.
- Vaginal dryness and dyspareunia due to atrophy respond to oestrogen.
- Oestrogen also reduces irritative urinary symptoms and urinary tract infections.
- There is decreased libido.

Psychological changes
- Anxiety, depression, insomnia and irritability may be reduced with oestrogen.

Skin, bone and joint changes
- Formication (or sensation of crawling under the skin) may be present.
- In the long term, there may be osteoporosis and associated complications.
- There may be joint and muscle aches.

Concentration and memory
- Perimenopausal changes in short-term memory are reported.

Premature ovarian failure

Incidence. Incidence is 1%. It is associated with primary amenorrhoea in 10%–30% of cases.

Embryology
Development of oocytes
- Primordial follicles/ovary develop from the gonadal ridge and germ cells migrate there from the primitive endoderm of the yolk sac during the fifth week of embryonic life.
- The 8-week-old embryo has 60,000 germ cells; the 20-week fetus has 6–7 million follicles. At menarche there are 300,000–400,000 follicles.
- Two X chromosomes are needed for definitive ovaries to develop.

Oocyte
- The oocyte commences meiosis, but arrests in the diplotene phase of prophase.
- The primary oocytes, which are surrounded by granulosa cells, are the primordial follicles.
- The first meiotic division is completed at the time of ovulation with the extrusion of the first polar body.

Causes of premature ovarian failure
Genetic
Chromosomal
- Turner's syndrome 45XO; 45XO/XX
- pure gonadal dysgenesis 46XX, 46XY
- trisomy: 13 and 18, 47XXX
- deletions/inversions
- familial

Metabolic
- 17-hydroxylase deficiency, galactosaemia, myotonic dystrophy

Autoimmune
- thyroid disease: Hashimoto's disease, Graves' disease, hypothyroidism, thyroiditis, silent thyrotoxicosis
- Addison's disease
- others: myasthenia gravis, hypoparathyroidism, autoimmune haemolytic anaemia/thrombocytopenia, pernicious anaemia

Infectious
- mumps (the commonest)
- tuberculosis

Environmental
- smoking (there is a dose-related effect of smoking on age of menopause)
- increasing parity
- poor health and nutrition

Iatrogenic
- irradiation, chemotherapy (methotrexate, actinomycin)
- posthysterectomy (ovarian failure may be advanced by 6 years)

Idiopathic
Pathophysiology
- Ovarian biopsy shows a reduced number of preantral follicles. The lack of gonadotrophin receptors may be the underlying cause of premature ovarian failure, because follicles require gonadotrophins and gonadotrophic receptors to develop beyond the preantral stage.

- Resistant ovary syndrome may be an early stage of premature ovarian failure. It implies decreased sensitivity of gonadotrophin receptors or a defect in the adenyl cyclase system.

Diagnosis of premature ovarian failure

Diagnosis is based on a triad of amenorrhoea, raised gonadotrophins and signs/symptoms of oestrogen deficiency.

- age <40 years
- primary or secondary amenorrhoea
- FSH levels of >15 IU/L indicating perimenopausal levels
- hot flush and genital atrophy present in 50% of cases

Examination and investigations

Examination

- stigmata of Turner's syndrome
- secondary sexual characteristics
- body mass index, blood pressure, thyroid
- signs of hypo-oestrogenism

Investigations

- to exclude pregnancy as a cause of amenorrhoea
- gonadotrophin levels
- FSH of >40 IU/L diagnostic
- repeat if results borderline (e.g. three assays at 2–4-week intervals)
- karyotype (required for all patients with primary amenorrhoea and early-onset premature ovarian failure)
- adrenals/thyroid function
- adrenals: dehydroepiandrosterone sulfate (DHEAS), 17-hydroxyprogesterone
- thyroid: thyroid-stimulating hormone, antithyroid antibodies
- autoimmune tests

Consequences and their management

Treat the underlying disease, such as an autoimmune disorder. Consequences:

- short-term: vasomotor symptoms, vaginal dryness, stress incontinence, psychological effects
- long-term: infertility, osteoporosis, cardiovascular effects

Managing infertility

- Pregnancy is possible with follicular forms of ovarian failure and resistant ovary.
- Low-dose hormone replacement therapy may stimulate the development of ovarian FSH receptors.
- Other options are in vitro fertilisation using donor eggs or adoption.
- Psychological support is very important.

Further reading

Van Kastern YM, Schoemaker J 1999 Premature ovarian failure: a systemic review of therapeutic interventions to restore ovarian function and achieve pregnancy. Human Reproduction Update 5:483–492

Chapter 13

Management of the menopause

Michael Flynn

Assessment

History
- past medical/surgical history
- family history
- oestrogen deficiency symptoms
- cigarette smoking (which changes the metabolism of oestrogen and reduces responsiveness to it)

Examination
- general, weight, blood pressure
- breast examination, pelvic examination

Investigations
- cervical cytology
- mammography and, if required, breast ultrasound
- bone density assessments
- vaginal ultrasound
- full blood examination, coagulation studies, lipid profile fasting glucose
- thyroid-stimulating hormone (TSH)

Management

The management of the menopausal woman is aimed at a full treatment regimen to optimise quality of life. The concept of risk and benefit should be fully explained. This includes management of:
- osteoporosis: prevention and treatment
- cardiovascular risk factors
- incontinence advice and treatment
- nutrition and exercise
- psychosexual dysfunction
- symptom relief of oestrogen deficiency symptoms

Oestrogen is the best short-term treatment for most symptomatic women with vasomotor symptoms. Contraindications to oestrogen therapy include history of breast cancer, coronary artery disease, thromboembolic event and stroke, or those at high risk of these complications. In women who have not had a hysterectomy, combined oestrogen and progesterone therapy is indicated.

The aim is to commence at lowest dose therapy for cessation of vasomotor symptoms. Topical vaginal oestrogen is effective in genitourinary symptoms. Testosterone therapy may be of help in some women with significant loss of libido or fatigue.

Trials

The Women's Health Initiative (WHI)
This has been a long-term research program to address the most common causes of death, disability and quality of life in postmenopausal women. There have been many publications using these data.

Nurses Health Study
This study commenced in 1976 and expanded in 1989 with information from nurse participants in the United Kingdom. The primary focus is cancer prevention.

Million Women Study
Coordinated in Oxford, UK, women were recruited between 1996 and 2001 to investigate women's health specifically in those over age 50. It particularly looks at hormone replacement therapy (HRT) and its effects on the breast and other aspects of health.

Within a clinical field where advice is changing as data emerge, the International Menopause Society provides consensus advice on the trials.

Cardiovascular disease and HRT
- HRT does not increase the risk in healthy women aged 50–59 and may even decrease the risk.
- It is unclear if there is an increase in stroke risk in healthy women aged 50–59, as no difference in WHI; however, increased risk was reported in the Nurses Health Study.
- The risk of venous thromboembolism is increased with HRT (less so with transdermal therapy); however, prevalence is low.

Breast disease and HRT
- After 5 years of combined oestrogen and progesterone, the increase in breast cancer is 8 cases per 10,000 women per year.
- Oestrogen-only replacement does not increase breast cancer rates up to 7 years.

Bone and HRT
- HRT is the first-line management in osteoporosis prevention and treatment in women aged 50–59.

Cognition and HRT
- Cognition benefits of HRT may depend upon age of initiation.

Current recommendations
- The main indication for HRT is to control menopausal symptoms.
- Avoid therapy of >4–5 years duration.
- HRT reduces fracture risks and is therefore appropriate for women with osteoporosis.
- HRT is not appropriate for primary or secondary cardioprotection.
- Review each patient's management annually with risk–benefit assessment.

Osteoporosis and treatments

Definition. Osteoporosis is said to be present when there are reduced amounts of normally mineralised bone matrix relative to bone volume. This has an associated increased risk of fracture.

Prevalence. By age 75 years, 1 in 5 Australian women have had an osteoporosis-related fracture.

Affected bone

The skeleton is composed of 80% cortical bone (mainly in peripheral bones) and 20% trabecular bone (mainly in axial skeleton). Trabecular bone turns over more rapidly than cortical bone and is thus more sensitive to changes in resorption and formation.

Risk factors

- family history of osteoporosis or early menopause
- low calcium and protein intake
- lack of exercise
- smoking, alcohol, caffeine
- drug therapies: corticosteroids, gonadotrophin-releasing hormone (GnRH) analogues, antacid, diuretics
- thinness
- medical/surgical conditions
- oophorectomy, hysterectomy
- raised prolactin levels and thyroid function
- insulin-dependent diabetes, hyperparathyroidism

Bone mass

Peak bone mass is reached at between 30 and 40 years of age. Then bone mass falls by 1% per year until menopause. From menopause onwards, about 3% of bone mass is lost per year. The rate of loss decreases to perimenopausal rates 4–10 years after the menopause. Bone mass at any age is a function of:
- peak bone mass achieved
- age at which loss of bone mass commences
- rate at which bone loss proceeds

Specific high-risk patients for osteoporosis
- women who have had an oophorectomy prior to natural menopause
- women who have had a hysterectomy with ovarian conservation: a quarter of these women develop endocrine evidence of ovarian failure within 2 years of hysterectomy (the reasons for this remain unclear, but it is perhaps due to changes in blood flow to the ovary following surgery)
- women with prolonged amenorrhoea, due to raised prolactin levels or hypothalamic causes such as anorexia
- women using GnRH analogues (e.g. in the treatment of endometriosis or fibroids)
- women with coexisting medical conditions or medications (e.g. Cushing's syndrome, use of corticosteroids, thyrotoxicosis, insulin-dependent diabetes)

Prevention and management of osteoporosis
General advice
- diet: including total food calcium of 1500 mf/day and vitamin D requirement of 800 IU/day
- exercise: 30 minutes 3 times a week has shown benefit in hip fracture rates
- stop smoking and reduce alcohol intake

Drug management
Women at high risk of osteoporosis, especially those with a recent fracture, should be evaluated for drug therapy.

Oestrogen
- effective therapy for prophylaxis of hypo-oestrogenic osteoporosis
- reduction in rate of bone mass loss to 0.75% per year
- possible modes of action
  - indirect effect on bone resorption by increasing levels of calcitonin
  - direct bone cell effects via oestrogen receptors on osteoblast-like cells

Bisphosphonates
These slow the rate of bone loss and enchance growth of new bone. Their mechanism of action is inhibition of osteoclast (now often first-line management).

Selective oestrogen receptor modulators (SERMs)
RALOXIFEN
- reduces bone loss, fracture risk and increases bone mineral density
- increases risk of thromboembolism

CALCITONIN
- less efficacious than bisphosphonates or oestrogen
- acts directly on osteoclasts, which have calcitonin receptors (i.e. it directly inhibits osteoclasts)
- useful for treatment of severe bone pain associated with more severe osteoporosis
- suitable as an adjuvant treatment

CALCITRIOL
- is 1,25-dihydroxy-vitamin D_3
- acts by enhancing absorption of calcium
- stimulates osteoclastic and osteoblastic activity by decreasing parathyroid hormone-driven bone resorption and direct stimulation of osteoblast
- should be given lower calcium diet

Monitoring of therapy
- Follow up with bone mineral density scans every 2 years.

Further reading and resources

International Menopause Society 2008 HRT in the early menopause: scientific evidence and common perceptions. Summary of the First Global Summit on Menopause Related Issues:29–30 March
Million Women Study: www.millionwomenstudy.org
Nurses Health Study: www.channing.harvard.edu/nhs
van Kastern YM, Schoemaker J 1999 Premature ovarian failure: a systemic review of therapeutic interventions to restore ovarian function and achieve pregnancy. Human Reproduction Update 5:483–492
Women's Health Initiative (WHI): www.nhibi.nih.gov/whi/index.html
World Health Organization (WHO) 1994 Scientific Group on Research on the menopause in the 1990s. WHO Technical Report Series 866. Geneva: WHO

Chapter 14

Disorders of sexual differentiation

Yasmin Jayasinghe

Definition. Disorders of sexual differentiation (DSD) occur where the development of chromosomal, gonadal or anatomic sex are atypical. The terms 'intersex' or 'hermaphrodite' are no longer accepted. The term now encompasses all atypical development (e.g. müllerian) agenesis.

  Incidence. Incidence is 1 in 5000 live births; therefore, it is rare. However, the situation requires rapid and sensitive assessment, knowledge of which is important.

Normal sexual differentiation

Undifferentiated gonads begin to develop during the fifth week after conception. During the sixth week, migration of primordial germ cells into the gonad is completed. So far, around 20 genes have been found to be involved in testicular and ovarian determination.

Male phenotypic development
Presence of the sex-determining region on the Y chromosome (SRY gene) causes differentiation of the gonad into a testis. (Several other genes are also involved in testicular development, mutations of which will result in 46XY sex reversal or ambiguous genitalia—for example, SRY, SOX9 and Wilms' tumour 1 (WT1).) Testis produces fetal testosterone and antimüllerian hormone (AMH), which act in exocrine fashion causing ipsilateral regression of müllerian ducts and development of wolffian structures. 5-alpha-reductase converts testosterone to dihydrotestosterone in order to virilise the cloaca.

Female phenotypic development
Two X chromosomes are required for normal ovarian development. The absence of SRY and the presence of DAX1 gene on the X chromosome inhibits testicular development. AMH is absent and müllerian development occurs.

Abnormal sexual development

- Sex chromosome abnormalities can interfere with gonadal differentiation (e.g. mutations in WT1 SRY, SOX 9, DAX 1).
- Lack of testosterone is due to failure of testicular differentiation or biosynthetic (Leydig cell) defects.

- Reduction or absence of 5-alpha-reductase causes impaired cloacal response to testosterone, but there is normal response by the wolffian structures.
- An androgen receptor defect (androgen insensitivity) causes lack of cloacal response to androgens, regression of müllerian structures due to AMH, and no development of male internal genitalia (vas deferens, seminal vesicles, epididymis).
- Deficiencies in AMH (produced by Sertoli cells) cause growth of müllerian structures.
- A 46XX male occurs when the SRY gene is present on the X chromosome due to atypical crossover during meiosis.

Classification of DSD

Classification is according to chromosomes, gonadal histology and phenotype.

Sex chromosome DSD
- 45XO Turner's syndrome
- 47XXY Klinefelter's syndrome

Undervirilisation of 46XY individuals
- faults of androgen production (3-beta-hydroxysteroid dehydrogenase deficiency (3ßHSD II), 17-beta-hydroxysteroid dehydrogenase deficiency (17ßHSD III))
- end-organ receptor defect (androgen insensitivity syndrome (AIS))
- defects in testosterone metabolism (5-alpha-reductase deficiency)
- XY gonadal dysgenesis, SOX9 or WT1 mutations
- drugs: spironolactone

Virilisation of 46XX individuals
- congenital adrenal hyperplasia (CAH)
- exposure in utero to androgen-producing tumour (fetal or maternal)
- maternal drugs: danazol, methyltestosterone, androgenic progesterone

Ovotesticular DSD
- Gonads are ovotestis.
- Diagnosis is by gonadal biopsy.
- Commonest chromosomes are 46XX; also associated with 46XX/XY, 45XO/46XY and 46XY.

Unclassified anatomical abnormalities
- Mayer-Rokitansky-Küster-Hauser syndrome (müllerian agenesis)
- cloacal exstrophy

Presentations of DSD

- ambiguous genitalia
- apparent female genitalia: clitoromegaly, posterior labial fusion, inguinal/labial mass
- apparent male genitalia: non-palpable testes, micropenis, hypospadius
- genital karyotype discordance
- delayed puberty, primary amenorrhoea
- inguinal hernia in female
- virilisation
- pelvic tumour

Newborn investigation of ambiguous genitalia

Key points
- There needs to be an immediate referral to experts in a collaborative multidisciplinary DSD team.
- Postpone gender assignment in infants born with ambiguous genitalia prior to expert consultation. An answer is usually available within 2–3 days. Refer to the child as 'the baby' until then. The first interactions families have with healthcare providers are remembered, and have long-lasting consequences.
- Gender identity, gender role and sexual orientation are distinct entities. It is hoped that assigned gender in childhood will be congruent with gender identity; however, gender dissatisfaction may manifest later in life. Gender dissatisfaction is not predictable by karyotype, androgen exposure, degree of genital virilisation or assigned sex.
- Ongoing psychological support, family-centred care and education, and full disclosure to the family and young patient that evolves over a developmental time line, are standards of care.

Investigations
- monitor weight and fluid balance, and check electrolytes and plasma 17-rennin activity (PRA)
- hydroxyprogesterone, testosterone, gonadotrophins, AMH
- karyotype with SRY detection
- abdominopelvic and renal ultrasound
- urogenital sinogram to evaluate urethra and vagina

Gender assignment
Influencing factors include diagnosis, genital appearance, therapeutic options, fertility potential, cultural practices and pressures, and parental views.

Turner's syndrome (TS)

Incidence. Incidence is 1 in 2000 to 1 in 5000 live born.

Clinical presentation
- 45XO or mosaicism 45,X/46,XX or 45,X/46,XY
- clinically short stature and pubertal failure along with other stigmata
- diagnosis: clinical, karyotype (note that follicle-stimulating hormone (FSH) levels may be markedly elevated up to 2 years of age, then nadir to near normal levels at age 4–10 years before rising again)
- spontaneous puberty with menses may occur in 9% of XO (and up to 30%–50% of mosaics)
- 2% may conceive spontaneously; pregnancy may be achieved through oocyte donation, but there is a high risk of pregnancy complications: 30% miscarriage; 7% stillbirth; 34% of live births will have a malformation (e.g. Down syndrome, TS)
- aortic dissection with maternal mortality of 2%
- medical complications must be monitored: osteoporosis, hypertension, diabetes, obesity, thyroid disorders, Crohn's disease, sensorineural hearing loss, cardiovascular anomaly including aortic root dilatation and risk of dissection

Management
- gonadectomy if Y component (present in 6% on karyotype) to avoid malignancy
- growth hormone
- optimal to start oestrogen therapy at bone age of 12 years in those on growth hormone, and 11 if not (although coordination with paediatric endocrinologist is

advised); start with very low doses, and aim to complete feminisation over 2–3 years (may add progesterone when withdrawal bleeding occurs)

Congenital adrenal hyperplasia (CAH)

Incidence. Incidence is 1 in 14,500.

Clinical presentation
Clinical presentation varies, although it is often diagnosed after birth, and includes:
- ambiguous genitalia
- salt-losing crisis
- hypertension
- virilisation and amenorrhoea in late-onset CAH
- >90% identify as females

Pathophysiology
- autosomal recessive disorder
- enzymatic defect in the synthesis of cortisol with loss of adrenal–pituitary feedback control
- result: an increase in adrenocorticotropic hormone (ACTH), adrenal hyperplasia, increase adrenal androgen production

21-hydroxylase deficiency
- accounts for ≥95% of cases of CAH
- due to mutations in CYP21 gene
- classic CAH (both alleles affected) presents in newborn period with ambiguous genitalia and three-quarters are salt losing
- diagnosis: based on raised 17-hydroxyprogesterone, +/– decreased Na, increased K, decreased aldosterone, increased PRA
- treatment: corticosteroids and, if salt-losing, fluorohydrocortisone
- monitor with 17-hydroxyprogesterone and PRA
- increase glucocorticoids during stress, illness, surgery
- surgery: 6 weeks to 6 months: clitoroplasty, labioplasty, vaginoplasty
- in pregnancy, administration of maternal dexamethasone, starting in the first trimester; may prevent virilisation in up to one-third of female babies
  - degree of suppression of the fetal pituitary–adrenal axis can be gauged by maternal oestriol and 17-hydroxyprogesterone levels
  - prenatal testing for mutations in CYP21 is available

11-beta-hydroxylase deficiency
- due to mutations in CYP11B1
- 11-deoxycortisol and 11-deoxycorticosterone levels high, resulting in *salt-retention*
- presentation: with ambiguous genitalia, cryptorchidism, hypertension and hypernatraemia

3-beta-hydroxysteroid dehydrogenase
- mutations in HSD3B2 gene
- very rare, severe adrenal insufficiency, may be salt-losers, mild virilisation of female or undervirilisation of male (testosterone deficiency)

20,22-desmolase deficiency
- addisonian crisis

Androgen insensitivity syndrome (AIS)

Incidence. Incidence is 1 in 20,000 to 1 in 64,000 XY births.

Clinical presentation
- XY karyotype, mutation in androgen receptor gene

Complete AIS
- phenotypic female, testes may be present in inguinal hernias at birth
- testes function normally, resulting in production of AMH; therefore, absent müllerian structures and blind-ending vagina
- normal androgen production; however, target tissues are unresponsive and male phenotype does not develop
- absent axillary and pubic hair
- female gender identity: manage with gonadectomy, vaginal dilators or vaginoplasty when mature enough; hormone replacement therapy

Partial AIS
- spectrum of ambiguous genitalia, pubic and axillary hair present
- gender identity may be male or female

Müllerian agenesis

- XX karyotype, absent uterus, blind ending vagina, axillary and pubic hair present
- often diagnosed in puberty due to primary amenorrhoea
- rudimentary müllerian structures may cause pelvic pain
- managed with vaginal dilators when ready

Surgery

Role of surgery
- goals: restore anatomy for menstruation, sexual function; promote sexuality and reproductive function; prevent urologic complications
- feminising genitoplasty—may involve:
  - clitoroplasty with preservation of neurovascular bundle
  - labioplasty
  - neovaginal construction or simple Y–V flap vaginoplasty
  - gonadectomy in XY containing karyotypes due to risk of dysgerminoma, gonadoblastoma
    - high risk of malignancy (15%–50%): intrabdominal dysgenetic gonads, partial AIS with non-scrotal gonads
    - low risk 2%–3%: complete AIS, ovotesticular DSD
- may defer removal of gonads until after puberty in complete AIS (peripheral conversion of androgens to oestrogen allows spontaneous induction of puberty); however, risk increases over time

Timing of surgery
- At large Australian multidisciplinary centres of excellence, with defined protocols, most surgery in females born with ambiguous genitalia is performed up to and including 6 months of age, collaboratively between the surgeon and gynaecologist, with excellent long-term outcomes compared to other countries (6% require

revision in adolescence, and around 25%–30% may need to use dilators, compared to around 50% revision rates worldwide).
- Parents must be informed that there are those who advocate no sex assignment, allowing the child to choose for themselves when old enough; however, data are limited.
- When diagnosis of vaginal agenesis is made in later childhood or early puberty, vaginoplasty is best deferred, as most women can create a neovagina with the use of dilators alone (80% success rate). If surgery is required, success in the older population depends on successful use of a vaginal mould or dilators postoperatively (inappropriate to perform in young children).

Further reading

Allen L 2009 Disorders of sexual development. Obstetrics and Gynecology Clinics of North America 36:25–45
Creighton SM 2004 Long-term outcome of feminization surgery: the London experience. British Journal of Urology International 93 (Suppl3):S44–S46
Hughes IA 2002 Intersex. British Journal of Urology International 90:769–776
Karnis MF, Reindollar RH 2003 Turner syndrome in adolescence. Obstetrics and Gynecology Clinics of North America 30:303–320
Lean WL, Deshpande A, Hutson J, Grover SR 2005 Cosmetic and anatomic outcomes after feminizing surgery for ambiguous genitalia. Journal of Pediatric Surgery 40:1856–1860
Lee P, Houk CP, Ahmed F et al 2006 Consensus statement on management of intersex disorders. Pediatrics 118:e488–e500
Migeon CJ, Wisniewski AB 2002 Human sex differentiation and its abnormalities. Best Practice and Research Clinical Obstetrics and Gynaecology 17:1–18
Warne G, Grover S, Hutson A et al 2005 A long-term outcome study of intersex conditions. Journal of Pediatric Endocrinology and Metabolism 18:555–567

Chapter 15

Paediatric and adolescent gynaecological disorders

Yasmin Jayasinghe

Gynaecological problems encountered in children and adolescents are unique to these age groups and involve sensitivity and skills differing from those utilised for adults.

Paediatric disorders

- normal genital anatomy in the prepubertal child
- maternal oestrogenisation wanes by 6 months
- hypooestrogenisation causes labia to be atrophic, and hymen to appear erythematous
- hymen may be crescentic, annular (circumferential), microperforate or cribriform
- cervix is often flush with the vaginal vault or protrudes slightly
- uterus may be so small that it may be difficult to identify on ultrasound in inexperienced hands

Examination of a prepubertal child

- examine only with parental consent, and once the child and parent are comfortable with you
- start with a general examination
- appropriate explanation to child and parent is important: it will not involve internal examinations, it should not hurt, there is no use of force, listen to the child if she wants you to stop
- with appropriate rapport and explanation, these examinations are usually tolerated very well; if very resistant, consider deferring examination or performing an examination under anaesthesia (EUA) depending on urgency
- frog-leg position on mother's lap if more comfortable

- genital inspection then lateral and outward traction on labia majora will enable hymen to open; ask child to cough while inspecting lower vagina

Vulvovaginal abnormalities

Vulvovaginitis
- symptoms: pruritis, dysuria, soreness of the vulval area, vaginal discharge, occasionally vaginal bleeding
- usually non-specific inflammation with no identifiable pathogen (80% of cases)
- specific pathogens: group A beta-haemolytic streptococci and *Haemophilus influenzae*, from the upper respiratory tract, are the most common

Causes
- underlying factors: hypo-oestrogenism causing overgrowth of normal flora, close proximity of vagina to anus, alkaline vaginal pH
- moisture: synthetic fibre underwear, obesity
- irritants (bubble baths, irritant soaps)

Differential diagnosis
- threadworms, vulval dermatoses, foreign body, sexual abuse, ectopic ureter, Crohn's disease

Investigation
- only take introital swab if moderate to severe offensive discharge, or bloody discharge

Management
- perineal hygiene (vinegar baths: ½ cup white vinegar in shallow bath as required)
- cotton underwear and change soon after sport
- barrier cream
- antibiotics if severe symptoms, including bloody discharge; if symptoms do not promptly settle, EUA
- treat empirically for *Enterobius vermicularis* (pinworms) if persistent significant pruritis
- reassurance, as symptoms settle with age

Vaginal bleeding
- pathological and warrants further investigation
- consider the following:

Vaginitis
- commonest cause
- if suspected, may treat with antibiotics alone initially, but if recurrent bleeding do EUA to exclude another cause

Foreign body
- commonly toilet paper
- EUA and removal of the object

Sarcoma botryoides (embryonal rhabdomyosarcoma)
- presents with lower abdominal mass and vaginal bleeding
- may sometimes see grape-like lesions at introitus

Genital trauma
- Straddle injuries may cause haematomas and genital lacerations (usually involving labia or fourchette) and associated with bruising of labia or thigh. A consistent history is important.
- Labial fat pads generally protect the hymen and vagina. Hymenal, vaginal or perianal lacerations, without labial or thigh bruising, is suspicious for non-accidental penetrating injury. Note that most children who have been sexually abused have normal clinical findings (<5% have abnormal findings). Any concerns regarding sexual abuse should be immediately referred to a skilled professional in the field so that appropriate investigation, documentation and follow-up can be organised.

Management
- ensure voiding is possible, sitz baths
- EUA if ongoing bleeding expanding haematoma, concerns about anatomical integrity

Urethral prolapse
- precipitants: hypo-oestrogenisation, chronic straining
- treat with oestrogen cream nocte and sitz baths; regression seen over days to weeks
- if persists and symptomatic, may require surgical excision

Other anatomical causes
- vascular lesions
- Crohn's disease

Precocious puberty
- bone age, follicle-stimulating hormone (FSH), luteinising hormone (LH), oestradiol, pelvic ultrasound to look for ovarian activity

Labial adhesions
- labia adherent in mid-line, mid-line raphe seen
- present in 0.6%–3% of prepubertal girls
- usually present 6 months to 6 years, not seen in the newborn
- often asymptomatic, but may cause urinary dribbling due to narrow vaginal opening, vulvitis, and rarely urinary tract infections

Due to hypooestrogenisation
- differential diagnosis: imperforate hymen or disorder of sexual differentiation, where no mid-line raphe will be seen

Management
- reassurance, vinegar baths and barrier cream for symptoms
- manual separation not indicated in hypo-oestrogenised child: 40% recurrence rate
- oestrogen creams may cause breast budding and are also associated with recurrence after cessation of use
- adhesions usually resolve with age and increasing oestrogen levels

Lichen sclerosus
- commonest age of presentation in premenarcheal girls is 5–7 years
- symptoms: pruritus, papules, fissures, erosions, bleeding
- 75% improvement in symptoms after menarche

- 0.05% betamethasone dipropionate for 6–12 weeks until resolution, then maintenance with low potency steroid for 3 months
- recurrences common

Genital ulcers
- may raise suspicion for sexual abuse, but often associated with non-specific viral illness
- differential diagnosis of solitary ulcers syphilis, chancroid (*Hemophilus ducreyi*), Crohn's disease, pyoderma gangrenosum, ulcerative vulvitis (bacterial pathogen or trauma) and malignancy
- multiple ulcers (more common): herpes, chicken pox or shingles (varicella zoster virus (VZV)), mononucleosis (Epstein-Barr virus (EBV))
- secondary syphilis, candidiasis, scabies, Behçet's syndrome, aphthous ulcers due to non-specific viral illness (very common), and fixed drug reactions
- investigation: viral, bacterial fungal swabs, serology (syphilis, EBV, VZV); consider autoantibody screen, biopsy

Genital warts
- Genital warts may raise suspicion for sexual abuse, particularly in children over 3 years; however, they may be transmitted in other ways (e.g. vertical and latent infection may possibly reactivate later in life).
- Warts are found in up to 0.2%–3% of children who have been sexually abused.
- The presence of warts alone without supporting clinical or social information is not diagnostic of abuse.
- Human papillomavirus (HPV) typing is not recommended. The viral subtype alone cannot determine the mode of transmission, as the virus doesn't display 100% site specificity in children.
- DNA fingerprinting to test for clonality is not useful. HPV6 and HPV11 are stable viruses, and do not vary markedly between hosts. Viral variants between the child and an alleged perpetrator are likely to be identical, as they represent circulating type for that area, and would not indicate the mode of transmission or the source.
- Get advice if concerned.

Precocious puberty

Definition. The onset of pubertal development prior to 8 years of age in females may represent precocious puberty (some healthy children begin development before this age). Normal pubertal development often occurs in sequence: growth acceleration, thelarche, adrenarche, menarche. The time between onset of breast development to menarche is around 2 years. The mean age of menarche in Australian girls is 13 years (range 12.2–14.2 years).

Aetiology
Central precocious puberty (gonadotrophin-dependent)
- constitutional precocious puberty
  - no organic abnormality; accounts for 90% of cases
  - caused by premature release of gonadotrophins from the anterior pituitary with no organic lesions
  - signs of puberty appear in correct order
  - bone age and height advanced for chronological age
- intracranial lesions
  - meningitis, encephalitis, tumours, hydrocephalus, tuberous sclerosis
  - caused by premature pituitary release of gonadotrophins

Peripheral precocious puberty (gonadotrophin-independent)
- feminising ovarian tumours
  - include granulosa cell, malignant teratoma
  - signs of puberty do not appear in the normal order: breast enlargement occurs with little body hair because adrenal function is not mature
- McCune-Albright syndrome
  - gonadotrophin-independent autonomous ovarian function
  - polyostotic fibrous dysplasia of bones, and café-au-lait skin lesions are characteristic
  - also associated with hyperthyroidism, hypophosphatemia
  - dominant ovarian cyst develops, which secretes oestradiol
- adrenal cortical tumours
  - include congenital adrenal hyperplasia and cause precocious virilism
- ingestion of drugs containing oestrogen

Management of precocious puberty
History
- current age
- sequence of secondary sexual characteristics
- drugs
- family history, past history

Examination
- general features: feminising, masculinising
- blood pressure, café-au-lait skin lesions
- thyroid, abdominal, neurological examination

Investigations
- growth chart
- bone age, computed tomography/magnetic resonance imaging (CT/MRI) scan of the head, ultrasound scan of the pelvis and adrenals
- oestradiol, FSH, LH, thyroid function
- gonadotrophin-releasing hormone (GnRH) test
- if virilising, test serum dehydroepiandrosterone sulfate (DHEAS), 17-hydroxy-progesterone, testosterone, free androgen index

Treatment of precocious puberty
Centrally mediated precocious puberty
- GnRH analogues: a full 3 months are needed to suppress the hypothalamic–pituitary–gonadal axis. Depot preparations are preferable.
- Medroxyprogesterone acetate and cyproterone acetate are no longer commonly used.

Gonadotrophin-independent
- McCune-Albright syndrome is the commonest cause, and treatment with GnRH analogues is ineffective. Suppress gonadal steroidogenesis directly with aromatase inhibitors (which block conversion of testosterone to oestradiol). Other options are ketoconazole and tamoxifen.

Adolescent gynaecology

Adolescent health principles
- accessible, non-judgmental, confidential, adolescent-friendly care
- only some exceptions to the duty of confidentiality, including the risk of self-harm or harm to others, or abuse

Consent to treatment

A young woman under 18 years can give consent to treatment if judged a 'mature minor', if she is assessed to be mature and competent and where she fully comprehends the nature of the specific condition for which treatment is sought, the purpose, methods, risks, potential benefits of treatment and alternatives to treatment. Assessment of maturity and competence include general maturity of speech, level of schooling, ability to understand the nature and rationale of treatment, and to be able to explain it in words.

Adolescent menorrhagia

- The commonest cause is anovulatory dysfunctional uterine bleeding.

Bleeding disorders

- about 10% of 'healthy' adolescents presenting to a tertiary clinic in Australia with menorrhagia (up to 20% if known bleeding disorders included)
- family history is important risk factor
- menorrhagia may be the only symptom of a bleeding disorder in a young person

Causes

- Von Willebrand disease 5%, platelet function disorders 6%, factor deficiencies rare but severe

Bleeding screen

- Von Willebrand's factor, platelet function analysis, coagulation profile and full blood count

Management

- avoid non-steroidal anti-inflammatory drugs (NSAIDS), all of the usual hormonal measures, menstrual suppression
- cyklokapron, intranasal desmopressin acetate if necessary, although oral contraceptive pill (OCP) and cyklokapron are a good first line

Adolescent metrostaxis (acute heavy loss)

- The commonest cause is still dysfunctional uterine bleeding, but consider pregnancy complication, genital tract trauma, coagulopathy, arterio-venous malformation and malignancy (all rare).
- In the acute phase, vital signs may remain stable despite significant blood loss, and then drop very quickly. Aggressive medical management is required.
- Resuscitate with intravenous fluids, transfuse and get haematological opinion.
- If hypo-oestrogenic (perimenarchal, slim, poor breast development), consider oestrogen first, then may try OCP four times a day over a few days, and then wean slowly to one daily.
- If clinically normo-oestrogenic, then try provera 10 mg every 2 hours until bleeding stops, and then wean slowly over a few weeks.
- Maintenance hormonal treatment with OCP daily thereafter may be beneficial while under investigation for bleeding disorder over ensuing months.
- Surgical investigation is rarely required.

Adolescent dysmenorrhoea

- Prostaglandin-mediated primary dysmenorrhoea is the commonest cause.
- Endometriosis is being diagnosed more commonly with increasing laparoscopy rates (47%–67% prevalence in adolescents with refractory symptoms). The disease tends to be in the cul de sac, and atypical in appearance, and usually early stage.

It is unclear if surgical intervention changes the natural history of disease in adolescents or improves reproductive potential. Current standard of care at Department of Gynaecology Royal Children's Hospital, Melbourne, is to manage with medical therapy and resort to diagnostic laparoscopy in refractory cases.
- Uterine anomaly: always consider in severe refractory primary dysmenorrhoea and pain in an adolescent.

Uterine anomaly
Imperforate hymen
- amenorrhea, cyclic pain, urinary retention, bluish introital bulge with abdominal pressure, treat with cruciate incision
- consider microperforate hymen in someone with scant vaginal loss and similar symptoms

Transverse vaginal septum
- incidence: 1 in 70,000
- amenorrhea, bulge at introitus absent with abdominal pressure, yet haematocolpos seen on ultrasound
- correct diagnosis is crucial, as requires Z-plasty, and possibly use of vaginal dilators preoperatively and vaginal mould postoperatively (can only be done when the young woman is psychologically ready)
- menstrual suppression with the OCP prior to this to manage pain is successful

Obstructed longitudinal vaginal septum, uterine didelphys, renal agenesis
- incidence: 1 in 35,000
- menstruating from normal side, unilateral haematocolpos
- menstrual suppression for pain management until septum resected vaginally
- mould not required

Rudimentary uterine horn
- most are diagnosed in the third decade
- non-communicating horns even with little endometrium may carry a pregnancy and rupture in the second trimester causing fetal loss and significant maternal morbidity
- recommended that rudimentary non-communicating horns be removed prior to childbearing

Vaginal agenesis
- incidence: 1 in 5000
- associated with renal spinal cardiac anomalies and hearing problems
- 80% success with use of dilators to create neovagina (when the young woman is ready)
- modified Sheares vaginoplasty may be used in other cases with use of mould and dilators postoperatively (timing driven by the young woman)
- important not to misdiagnosis late presentation of complete androgen insensitivity syndrome, by performing karyotype, and asking/checking for presence or absence of axillary or pubic hair, inguinal hernias

Adolescent polycystic ovarian syndrome (PCOS)
Incidence is 3% in the adolescent population. While current definitions of PCOS do not vary between adult and adolescent, some feel that the Rotterdam criteria will overdiagnose PCOS in adolescence. Adolescents typically have relative androgenaemia,

insulin resistance, cystic ovaries and anovulatory cycles. Special considerations regarding PCOS in adolescents are:

- Primary amenorrhoea may be a presenting feature of severe PCOS.
- Clues to the presence of PCOS in adolescent women are persistence of menstrual irregularity 2 years postmenarche, premature pubarche and adrenarche, insulin resistance as determined by acanthosis nigracans and a fasting insulin:glucose ratio <7 (as opposed to 4.5 in an adult).
- A follicular phase morning 17-alpha-hydroxyprogesterone is useful to exclude non-classic congenital adrenal hyperplasia.
- Small studies with the use of metformin have shown a favourable effect on ovulation, resumption of menses and reduction of central adiposity, but treatment is generally reserved for those who have failed other lifestyle measures.

Further reading

Black M, McKay M, Braude PR (eds) 2002 Obstetric and gynecologic dermatology, 2nd edn. London: Mosby

Goldstein DP, De Cholnoky C, Emans SJ 1980 Adolescent endometriosis. Journal of Adolescent Health Care 1 (1):37–41

Jayasinghe Y, Garland S 2006 Genital warts in children: what do they mean? Archives of Disease in Childhood 91 (8):696–700

Jayasinghe Y, Moore P, Donath S et al 2005 Bleeding disorders in teenagers presenting with menorrhagia. Australian and New Zealand Journal of Obstetrics and Gynaecology 45 (5):439–443

Jayasinghe Y, Rane A, Stalewski H, Grover S 2005 The presentation and early diagnosis of the rudimentary uterine horn. Obstetrics and Gynaecology 105:1456–1467

Lalwani S, Reindollar R, Davis A 2003 Normal onset of puberty: have definitions of onset changed? Obstetrics and Gynecology Clinics of North America 30:279–286

Laufer MR, Goitein L, Bush M et al 1997 Prevalence of endometriosis in adolescent girls with chronic pelvic pain not responding to conventional therapy. Journal of Pediatric and Adolescent Gynecology 10 (4):199–202

Medical Practitioners Board of Victoria 2004 Consent for treatment and confidentiality in young people, September

Partsch CJ, Heger S, Sippell WG 2002 Management and outcome of central precocious puberty. Clinical Endocrinology 56:129–148

Pfeifer S, Kives S 2009 Polycystic ovary syndrome in the adolescent. Obstetrics and Gynecology Clinics of North America 36:129–152

Templeman C 2009 Adolescent endometriosis. Obstetrics and Gynecology Clinics of North America 36:177–185

Traggiai C, Stanhope R 2003 Disorders of pubertal development. Best Practice and Research Clinical Obstetrics and Gynaecology 17:41–56

Van Eyk N, Allen L, Giesbrecht E et al 2009 Pediatric vulvovaginal disorders: a diagnostic approach and review of the literature. Journal of Obstetrics and Gynaecology Canada 31 (9):850–862

Young D, Hopper J, Macinnis R et al 2001 Changes in body composition as determinants of longitudinal changes in bone mineral measures in 8 to 26-year-old female twins. Osteoporosis International 12:506–515

Chapter 16

Chronic pelvic pain

Michael Flynn

Pelvic pain is the commonest indication for laparoscopy. This is pain present for at least 6 months severe enough to interfere with normal daily activities.

Physiology and innervation

Pain
- Somatic innervation from the vulva, perineum and lower vagina is via the pudendal nerve (S2–S4).
- Visceral innervation from the uterus, tubes, ovaries and visceral peritoneum is via the autonomic nervous system (T10–L1).
- The assessment of pelvic pain requires a detailed pain history and system review.

Origin
- gynaecological
- gastrointestinal
- urological
- musculoskeletal
- neurological

Viscera
- Viscera are not sensitive to thermal and tactile sensation.
- Pain is poorly localised.
- Pain is referred from the overlying peritoneum via dermatomes of the same nerve root.

Stimuli that produce pain
- distension/contraction of an organ
- stretching of organ capsule
- irritation of the parietal peritoneum
- ischaemic tissues
- inflammation, neoplasia or fibrosis stimulating nerves

Examination

- General examination: look for signs of malignancy, lymphadenopathy, oedema.
- Abdominal palpation: feel for masses, ascites, organomegaly.
- Vaginal speculum examination:
  - check for discharge
  - cervical pathology
  - bimanual examination: check uterine size and position, adnexal pathology, cervical motion pain, pouch of Douglas

- uterosacral ligament nodularity, thickening or tenderness
- rectal examination for masses
- lumbosacral and hip joints
- Assess anatomical locations of tenderness and correlate these with areas of pain.

Gynaecological causes of pelvic pain

- cyclical: dysmenorrhoea, ovulation pain, endometriosis, adenomyosis (some aetiologies of pelvic pain can be exacerbated during menses (irritable bowel syndrome and interstitial cystitis))
- chronic pelvic inflammatory disease
- polycystic ovarian syndrome
- residual ovary, ovarian remnant syndrome
- neoplasia
- pelvic venous congestion
- levator muscle spasm
- pelvic adhesions

Non-gynaecological causes of pelvic pain

- gastrointestinal tract
  - diverticulitis, malignancy, obstruction
  - inflammatory bowel disease, irritable bowel syndrome
- urinary tract
  - calculus, infection, retention, malignancy
  - interstitial cystitis (painful bladder)
- musculoskeletal
  - osteoarthritis
  - prolapsed disc
  - fibromyalgia
  - myofascial pain
  - peripartum musculoskeletal pain

Clinical presentation

Cyclical
Dysmenorrhoea is severe in 5% of women and is often associated with endometriosis, adenomyosis.

Ovulation
- Acute onset of lower abdominal pain is followed by a dull ache for several hours.
- The pain corresponds to the luteinising hormone (LH) peak (1 day before ovulation).
- The pain is due to prostaglandin F_2 causing contractility of ovarian perifollicular smooth muscle.

Pelvic inflammatory disease
- Only about 60% can be correctly diagnosed on history alone.
- The gold standard for diagnosis is by laparoscopy.
- Long-term sequelae include chronic infection, pelvic pain, dyspareunia, menstrual changes, infertility and ectopic pregnancy.

Endometriosis
- associated with dysmenorrhoea, dyspareunia and chronic pain

Neoplasia
- benign: degenerating fibroid, ovarian cyst complications
- malignant: weight loss, nausea, abdominal/pelvic pain, ascites, lymphadenopathy, irregular mass in pelvis

Pelvic venous congestion
- has been implicated as a cause of pelvic pain
- may be due to oestrogen causing dilatation of the thin-walled, unsupported pelvic veins

Residual ovary syndrome
- occurs in about 3%–4% of ovaries not removed during hysterectomy
- 75% of patients present with chronic pelvic pain and dyspareunia

Polycystic ovarian syndrome
- pelvic pain/discomfort may be a presenting complaint

Uterovaginal prolapse
- dull ache, dragging lump in vagina

Gastrointestinal
- change in bowel habit, rectal bleeding

Urinary
- infection, calculus causing dysuria, loin pain

Musculoskeletal
- low back ache of musculoskeletal origin, radiating commonly to lower limbs and not abdomen or pelvis

Investigation for pelvic pain

Laparoscopy
- the most informative investigation for chronic pelvic pain

Radiology
- ultrasound scan of the pelvis
- X-ray of lumbosacral spine and hip joints
- other imaging (e.g. upper gastrointestinal series, barium enema, renal tract) if indicated

Others
- mid-stream urine
- *Chlamydia*
- pelvic congestion is difficult to diagnose

Treatment

Identify specific cause if evident and treat appropriately. The management of women with normal laparoscopy and other investigations is especially difficult.

Treatment of chronic pelvic pain
- pharmacological
  - non-steroidal anti-inflammatories
  - oral contraceptive pill
  - gonadotrophin-releasing hormone (GnRH) agonist
- physiotherapy
- psychological: pain clinics and management
- pain assessment forms may benefit in long-term management

Further reading

Gambone JC, Mittman BS, Munro MG et al 2002 Consensus statement for the management of chronic pelvic pain and endometriosis: proceedings of an expert-panel consensus process. Fertility and Sterility 78:961–972

Gelbaya TA, El-Halwagy HE 2001 Chronic pelvic pain in women. Obstetric and Gynecological Survey 56:757–764

Howard FM 2003 Chronic pelvic pain. Obstetrics and Gynecology 101:594–611

Chapter 17

Lower urinary tract symptoms

Judith Goh

Urinary incontinence is the complaint of involuntary urinary leakage. Lower urinary tract symptoms include complaints regarding urinary storage, voiding or postmicturition symptoms. When a woman presents with urinary symptoms, a detailed history on lower urinary tract symptoms is required.

History

- daytime frequency (normally up to 8 times a day): increased frequency is associated with increased fluid intake, detrusor overactivity, poor bladder compliance or increase in bladder sensation
- nocturia: waking up to pass urine
- urinary urgency: sudden desire to pass urine, which is difficult to defer
- urinary stress incontinence: involuntary leakage on effort or exertion
- urinary urge incontinence: involuntary leakage accompanied by urgency
  - may present with frequent losses or large leakage
  - commonly associated with 'triggers' causing urgency and incontinence (e.g. turning on taps, coming home with 'key-in-the-door')
- continuous leakage
- voiding problems
  - slow stream
  - straining to void: effort required to initiate, maintain or improve urinary flow
  - intermittent flow
  - hesitancy: difficulty in initiating micturition
- postmicturition
  - sensation of incomplete emptying
  - postvoid dribble: leaking after voiding (e.g. when standing from the toilet)
- other urinary history
  - dysuria, haematuria, previous urinary tract infections
  - suprapubic pain
  - coital incontinence
- other history
  - constipation
  - caffeine intake
  - symptoms of prolapse: needing to reduce the prolapse to void
  - previous gynaecological/urological procedures

Examination

A physical examination is performed to exclude transient causes and to evaluate other disease and functional ability.
- general, weight
- vulva (excoriation or urine dermatitis)
- gynaecological, vaginal prolapse, vaginal atrophy, urine in vagina
- local neurological
- urethra
  - urethral diverticulum, scarring around urethra and anterior vaginal wall
  - mobility of urethra
  - cough test and/or reduce prolapse and ask the woman to cough to assess for urinary stress incontinence

Investigation

This would depend on the history and examination.
- bladder diary
  - very useful tool
  - over a 2–3 day period, the woman is asked to record the times of micturition and her voided volumes, together with symptoms (e.g. urgency, incontinence)
  - fluid intake is also recorded
- urinalysis and culture, cytology
- postvoid residual volume
- blood sugar, renal function
- dye test: if a urinary tract fistula is suspected

Further evaluation
Further evaluation includes urodynamics assessment, cystoscopy and imaging. Criteria for further evaluation include uncertain diagnosis, failure of response to initial therapy, consideration of surgical intervention and suspicion of other pathology.

Urodynamic assessment
The tests are designed to determine the functional status of the urinary bladder and urethra. The main components of urodynamics assessment are uroflowmetry, cystometry and urethral closure pressure/Valsalva leak point pressure.
- Uroflowmetry is a timed measure of voided urine volume.
  - a simple and non-invasive tool
  - cannot distinguish between obstruction and detrusor weakness as cause of voiding dysfunction without simultaneous measurement of detrusor function
- Cystometry is a test of detrusor function consisting of an observation and/or recording of the pressure/volume relationship during bladder filling.
- Maximal urethral closure pressure is the highest pressure, relative to bladder pressure, generated along the functional length of the urethra.
- Valsalva leak point pressure is the intravesical pressure at which urinary leakage occurs due to an increase in intra-abdominal pressure and in the absence of detrusor contraction.

Common causes of urinary incontinence

- urodynamic stress incontinence
- urge incontinence
  - idiopathic detrusor overactivity (detrusor instability)
  - neurogenic detrusor overactivity (detrusor hyperreflexia)

- mixed incontinence (combined stress and urge)
- overflow incontinence: atonic detrusor, impaired bladder compliance
- extraurethral incontinence: genito-urinary fistula, urethral diverticulum, congenital abnormality
- functional disorders: cognitive impairment, physical disorder, psychological
- reversible causes (temporary causes)
  - conditions affecting lower urinary tract: infection, atrophy, constipation
  - drugs, diuretics, caffeine, alcohol
  - increased urine production: hyperglycaemia, excessive fluids
  - impaired mobility

Treatment of urinary incontinence

Aims are to:
- determine cause of incontinence
- detect and treat related urinary tract pathology
- evaluate the woman and available resources

The extent and interpretation of evaluation must be tailored to the individual. A multidisciplinary team approach optimises outcomes. Not all detected conditions can be cured and simple interventions may be effective even in the absence of a diagnosis. Many women with urinary incontinence develop undesirable bladder habits, which often exacerbate the problem and/or provoke other urinary symptoms (e.g. 'going just in case', voiding too often, reducing oral fluids). There is evidence to suggest that in women with mixed incontinence, detrusor overactivity should be treated prior to continence surgery, as this optimises overall outcomes.

In Australia, resources are available to women, including government-funded or subsidised schemes such as home assessments and continence products. The Continence Foundation of Australia provides a 24-hour helpline for men and women with urinary and faecal incontinence.

Overactive bladder
- overactive bladder is a symptom complex: urgency with or without urge incontinence, usually associated with frequency and nocturia
- detrusor overactivity
  - a urodynamic diagnosis: involuntary detrusor pressure rise during filling/cystometrogram, which may be spontaneous or provoked
  - causes include neurogenic, outflow obstruction, ageing and idiopathic (most common)
- overactive bladder survey in Europe and USA: about 17% of women with symptoms suggestive of overactive bladder; increasing prevalence with increasing age

Overactive bladder and idiopathic detrusor overactivity
The mainstay of treatment is non-surgical.
- initial management (multidisciplinary approach)
  - exclude other causes (e.g. infection, voiding dysfunction, neurological)
  - bladder diary
  - bladder training, pelvic floor rehabilitation
  - treat constipation, weight loss, reduce/avoid caffeine
- pharmacological
  - major portion of neurohumoral stimulus for physiological bladder contraction is acetylcholine-induced stimulation of postganglionic parasympathetic cholinergic receptor sites on bladder smooth muscle

- anticholinergic drugs: contraindicated in closed-angle glaucoma (availability limited in Australia)
  — oxybutynin: oral or patch
  — solifenacin, darifenacin, tolterodine
  - tricyclic antidepressants (have anticholinergic effects): imipramine, amitriptyline
  - oestrogen: topical
- others
  - peripheral nerve stimulation
- surgical
  - intravesical botox injection
  - sacral nerve stimulator implant
  - augmentation cystoplasty, diversion

Urodynamic stress incontinence
Conservative management
- multidisciplinary approach
- treat overactive bladder symptoms
- pelvic floor rehabilitation
- vaginal/urethral devices for urinary incontinence

Surgery
There are over 100 described surgical procedures for the management of urodynamic stress incontinence. Common complications of these procedures include voiding difficulty, injury to lower urinary tract, infection, denovo overactive bladder symptoms and failure to treat the stress incontinence. Better results have been documented for the slings and colposuspension, with an approximately 85% success rate. Commonly performed procedures today are: slings (mid-urethral, pubo-vaginal); retropubic urethropexy (Burch colposuspension, Marshall-Marshetti-Krantz (MMK)); and urethral bulking agent.

Slings
- Traditional slings are placed at the urethro-vesical junction.
- In the mid-1990s the mid-urethral sling was described, which allowed minimally invasive surgery, reduced hospital stays and a quicker return to daily activities, without a reduction in success rates.
- Slings are made of fascia (autologous, human donor or xenographs) or synthetic mesh (e.g. polypropylene). When synthetic mesh is to be used, current evidence recommends a macroporous, monofilamentous mesh. This reduces the risk of mesh extrusion/erosion and infection.
- Mid-urethral slings may be placed in the retropubic space (first generation) or through the obturator foramen (second generation). The third-generation slings are 'exit-less'.

Retropubic urethropexy
- The Burch colposuspension 'hitches' the paravaginal tissue to the iliopectineal ligament, whereas the MMK sutures are placed into the periosteum of the posterior part of the pubic symphysis.
- Colposuspension may be performed laparoscopically or via a laparotomy.

Urethral bulking agent
- This involves periurethral or transurethral injection of a bulking agent, under endoscopic control, imaging or using an introducer.
- Materials used as a bulking agent include bovine collagen, silicone microparticles, Teflon and autologous material (e.g. fat).

- As a primary procedure, the success rates are lower (about 50%).
- Advantages include minimal anaesthesia/analgesia, ability to redo or 'top-up'.

Further reading and resources

Abrams P, Cardozo L, Fall M et al 2002 Standardisation of terminology of lower urinary tract function. Neurourology Urodynamics 21:167–178
Continence Foundation of Australia Helpline: 1800 330 066

Chapter 18

Pelvic organ prolapse

Hannah Krause

Definition. Pelvic organ prolapse is the protrusion of pelvic organs into the vaginal canal. Prolapse of pelvic organs occurs when their attachments, neural connections and supports fail.

    Incidence. Pelvic organ prolapse is common and affects about 1 in 3 women who have had one or more children.

Causes and risk factors

- age, parity, vaginal delivery, connective tissue dysfunction, chronic cough, constipation, size of genital hiatus, congenital factors, obesity

History

- presenting complaint: asymptomatic or symptomatic of prolapse
- symptoms of prolapse include:
  - lump
  - sensation of discomfort or dragging
  - voiding difficulty
  - incomplete bowel emptying (splinting, manual evacuation)
  - dyspareunia
  - vaginal 'wind'
- other pelvic floor history
- urinary symptoms
- sexual function: dyspareunia
- bowel function
- menstrual history: menopausal
- past medical history: may be unsuitable for surgery
- past surgical history: previous prolapse or continence surgery

Examination

- general examination, including body mass index (BMI)
- abdominal: exclude mass lesion
- vaginal
  - genital hiatus: widened
  - cough with and without prolapse reduced: assess for urinary leakage
  - use Sims' speculum: left lateral or lithotomy, Valsalva

• POP-Q assessment (see below)
• vaginal examination for pelvic organ assessment

POP-Q (pelvic organ prolapse quantification) classification

The POP-Q system evaluates descent relative to a fixed reference point, the hymen. Six points are measured in centimetres above or below the hymen, and three further measurements evaluate the genital hiatus, perineal body and total vaginal length (see Fig 18.1). The six points are as follows:

1. Point Aa is located in the mid-line of the anterior vaginal wall, 3 cm above the external urethral meatus.
2. Point Ba is a point that represents the most dependent (distal) position of any part of the upper anterior vaginal wall down to point Aa.
3. Point Ap is located in the mid-line of the posterior vaginal wall, 3 cm above the hymen.
4. Point Bp is a point that represents the most dependent (distal) position of any part of the upper posterior vaginal wall down to point Ap.
5. Point C is the distal edge of the cervix or the vaginal cuff following a hysterectomy.
6. Point D is the location of the posterior fornix in women with a cervix present.

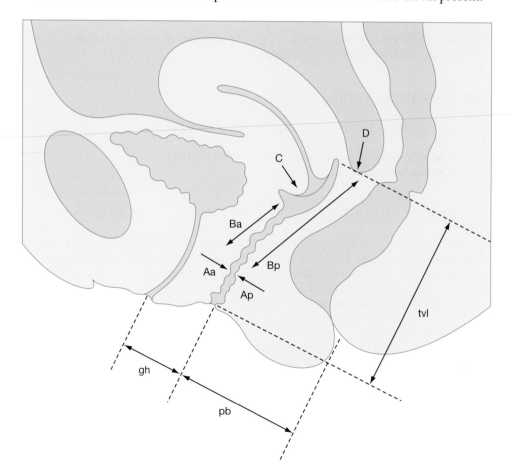

Figure 18.1 **Reference points for the International Continence Society classification (1996) for vaginal prolapse**

The three further measurements are:
1. Genital hiatus (GH) is measured from the middle of the external urethral meatus to the posterior mid-line hymen.
2. Perineal body (PB) is measured from the posterior margin of the genital hiatus to the mid-anal opening.
3. Total vaginal length (TVL) is the length of the vagina when points C or D are reduced to their normal positions.

Stages
- Stage 0: no prolapse is demonstrated.
- Stage 1: most distal portion of prolapse is >1 cm above the level of the hymen.
- Stage 2: most distal portion of prolapse is ≤1cm proximal to or distal to the plane of the hymen.
- Stage 3: most distal portion is >1 cm below the plane of the hymen, but protrudes to no further than 2 cm less than the TVL.
- Stage 4: complete eversion of total length of lower genital tract.

Investigations

- Urodynamics studies are useful to assess for preexisting voiding dysfunction and occult urodynamic stress incontinence.

Conservative management

- pelvic floor exercises: may reduce symptoms of prolapse
- pessary
  - mechanical support for prolapse inserted into vagina
  - numerous types: ring, shelf, cube

Surgical management

Identify which compartments require repair, and repair all defects. Options are vaginal or abdominal approach; conserve uterus or hysterectomy; and native tissue repair or augment with biomaterials. Biomaterials are biological or synthetic. Biological materials are autografts, allografts or xenografts. Synthetic materials are mesh. The mesh should be a macroporous monofilamentous mesh.

Vaginal approach
- anterior compartment defects: anterior native tissue repair, anterior repair with biomaterial augmentation, vaginal paravaginal repair
- posterior compartment defects: posterior native tissue repair, posterior repair with biomaterial augmentation
- vault or uterine descent: sacrospinous colpopexy or hysteropexy with sutures or mesh, high uterosacral placation
- perineorrhaphy

Abdominal approach
- open or laparoscopic
- sacral colpopexy with mesh
- paravaginal repair

Risks and complications
- intraoperative complications: anaesthetic complications, bleeding and transfusion, damage to bladder, ureters or bowel
- immediate postoperative complications: infection, deep venous thrombosis, voiding difficulties, fistula formation
- long-term issues: recurrence of prolapse, dyspareunia
- mesh complications: vaginal mesh exposure, mesh erosion into bladder or bowel, mesh contraction and scarring

Long-term considerations
Depending on the type of pelvic organ prolapse repair performed, there can be significant prolapse recurrence rates of more than 30%. While traditional native tissue repairs do have significant recurrence rates, they do avoid the risks of mesh augmentation such as mesh exposure and erosion. Repair techniques using biomaterial augmentation aim to reduce recurrence rates and are continuing to be developed in order to try to reduce such risks.

When counselling patients regarding prolapse treatment, conservative and surgical options should be fully discussed. An important aspect of counselling is the realistic expectations of outcomes, in particular of surgery.

Further reading

Bump RC, Mattieson A, Bo K et al 1996 The standardization of terminology of female pelvic organ prolapse and pelvic floor dysfunction. American Journal of Obstetrics and Gynecology 175 (1):10–17

Chapter 19

Cervical neoplasia

Amy Tang

Role of human papillomavirus

Over 60 different genotypes of human papillomavirus (HPV) have been identified. In some populations, it is present in over 70% of women and may be a vaginal commensal. Other co-factors, such as smoking, may be required to promote the development to cervical intraepithelial neoplasia (CIN).

Link with cervical cancer
- HPV has been identified in benign conditions and cancer.
- Infection with HPV is present in over 90% of preinvasive or invasive cervical neoplasia.
- High-risk HPV subtypes include types 16, 18, 31, 33 and 35.

Management
- Up to 10% of women will have HPV on cervical cytology at some stage.
- If HPV only on cytology, 35%–40% will have CIN on further investigations.
- There is no risk of cancer in patients with HPV without CIN.
- If only HPV is present and this is not treated, 20%–25% progress to CIN in 2 years, which persists in 30%–40% of these patients.
- If treated, the rate of progression is similar to untreated.
- There is no evidence that examining or treating male partners changes the outcome for women.
- There is no evidence that wearing condoms reduces the progression of HPV to CIN.

Cervical cytology

When to perform cervical cytology
The best time is at mid-cycle. In the absence of abnormal bleeding and previous abnormal cervical cytology or treatment, smears should be taken every 2 years. When sexually active, perform the first smear test within 2 years of the first sexual intercourse or from 18–20 years of age, whichever is later. Cease at age 70 years if there have been two normal smears within the past 5 years. In women who have had a hysterectomy and who previously had normal cytology, no further smears are required.

Screening for CIN
Cervical cytology
- is 99.7% specific (i.e. has a false-positive rate of 0.3%)
- is 80% sensitive (with a false-negative rate of 20%)

Computer-assisted screening
- Liquid-based cytology (ThinPrep) with automated image analysis technology can reduce the number of unsatisfactory smears and improve the sensitivity to detect cervical dysplasia.

Possible reasons for false-negatives
- sampling error
- incorrect fixative (95% ethyl alcohol fixative is required)
- timing of smear (best at mid-cycle)
- amount of sample (too little/too much)
- screening error
- interpretive error

Endocervical cells present
- means that the squamocolumnar junction is reached (i.e. the upper limit of the transformation zone)
- <1% of smears containing no endocervical cells (and no abnormal cells seen) is an abnormal result

Effectiveness against cervical cancer
- If a smear is performed every year and appropriate management is undertaken, cervical cancer is reduced by 93.5%.
- If performed every 2 years, cancer may be reduced by 92.5%.
- If performed every 3 years, cancer may be reduced by 90.8%.

HPV testing
- Preliminary data suggest that HPV testing is a feasible technique for primary screening for cervical cancer. However, it has not been shown to be a cost-effective screening tool in the Australian context.
- It may be useful in the triage of equivocal cytology results or low-grade lesions.
- In Australia, it is used as a 'test of cure' for high-grade cervical dysplasias. Pap smear and HPV typing is carried out at 12 months after treatment and annually thereafter, until both tests are negative on two consecutive occasions. Patients can then have smears every 2 years.

Terminology for cervical cytology/Pap smear reporting
The Bethesda System 2001 for squamous abnormalities
- atypical squamous cells of undetermined significance (ASCUS)
- low-grade squamous intraepithelial lesion (LSIL): includes HPV and CIN1
- atypical squamous cells, possible high-grade lesion (ASC-H)
- high-grade squamous intraepithelial lesion (HSIL): includes CIN2 and CIN3
- squamous cell carcinoma

The Australian Modified Bethesda System 2004
- possible low-grade squamous intraepithelial lesion
- low-grade squamous intraepithelial lesion (HPV and CIN1)
- possible high-grade squamous intraepithelial lesion
- high-grade squamous intraepithelial lesion (CIN2 and CIN3)
- squamous cell carcinoma

Management of abnormal Pap smear
- If LSIL, repeat Pap smear in 12 months; then 24 months if normal result. Otherwise refer for colposcopy
- If possible HSIL or HSIL, refer for colposcopy and biopsy.

Cervical intraepithelial neoplasia (CIN)

Definition. Normally, as cells differentiate and mature they move towards the surface. Abnormalities result in mitotic figures, nuclear pleomorphism, and changes in the nuclear-to-cytoplasmic ratio.

- CIN1: two-thirds or more of the upper epithelium showing good differentiation
- CIN2: maturation/differentiation in the upper half of the epithelium with mitotic figures in the basal half
- CIN3: less than one-third of the upper epithelium showing differentiation

Progression of CIN
- Incidence varies in different studies.
- CIN1 progressing to higher CIN lesions: about 16%–25% in 2–4 years.
- CIN3 to invasive cancer: about 18%–35% in 1–23 years.

Management
Colposcopy
- Aims: identify abnormal area and exclude invasive disease.
- The transformation zone needs to be seen. This is the area between the original and existing squamocolumnar junction. The columnar epithelium undergoes metaplasia as the transformation zone extends. The squamocolumnar junction may recede up the endocervical canal (e.g. in postmenopausal women). The pathological process often occurs in the transformation zone.
- With 3%–5% acetic acid, abnormal epithelium turns acetowhite.
- Schiller's test: columnar or abnormal squamous epithelium has little or no glycogen and does not stain with iodine.
- Colposcopic changes seen with CIN lesions are punctation (vessels are perpendicular to surface), mosaic (capillaries parallel to surface), and atypical vessels irregular in size, shape and course.

Conservative treatment
Current Australian guidelines recommend that histologically proven low-grade squamous abnormalities can be safely managed by repeat Pap smears at 12 and 24 months. If persistent possible or definite LSIL, annual smears should be continued until at least two are negative.

Ablative treatment
- A colposcopic-directed cervical punch biopsy is needed to confirm the diagnosis of CIN and to exclude invasive cancer before ablative treatment.
- Depth of ablation is up to 10 mm, as almost all lesions are <7 mm in depth.
- Postablation, it takes 4–6 months to replace the transformation zone.
- It should not be carried out if presence of glandular lesion or if entire transformation zone is not visualised.

Excision
- Large-loop excision of the transformation zone (LLETZ) or loop electrical excision procedure (LEEP) has a 96% cure rate.
- Its advantage over ablative treatment is the availability of a histological specimen.

Cone biopsy
Indications. At colposcopy, the lesion is not fully visualised, especially the upper limit; suspected adenocarcinoma in situ; colposcopic examination shows no evidence

of dysplasia despite repeated cytology with high-grade dysplasia; or early invasive disease is suspected.

Hysterectomy
- It may be indicated if other gynaecological problems are present.
- Yearly vault smears are required, as there is a risk of vaginal intraepithelial neoplasia.

Cryosurgery
- Freeze for 2–3 minutes to obtain a 4 mm depth.
- About 60% are successful with one treatment.
- It is advisable that women with CIN3 are not treated with cryotherapy.

Pregnancy
- Perform colposcopy by an experienced colposcopist to exclude invasive cancer.
- If CIN, leave treatment until postpartum.
- If invasion is suspected colposcopically, biopsy should be performed.
- Cone biopsy of the cervix is associated with a 5% fetal loss.

Follow-up
- After treatment for HSIL, perform colposcopy and Pap smear at 4–6 months.
- Repeat Pap smear and perform HPV typing at 12 months after treatment and annually thereafter until negative tests on two consecutive occasions.

Cervical intraepithelial glandular neoplasia

Adenocarcinoma in situ (AIS) coexists with CIN in 70% of patients. Up to 15% of CIN is associated with glandular abnormalities. AIS is present in 40%–45% of cervical adenocarcinoma.

Atypical glandular cells of undetermined significance (AGUS) refers to morphological changes in glandular cells beyond those suggestive of a benign reactive process, but insufficient for the diagnosis of AIS. Other terminology under the Australian Modified Bethesda System 2004 includes possible high-grade glandular lesion, endocervical adenocarcinoma in situ and adenocarcinoma.

Management of adenocarcinoma in situ
Colposcopy and biopsy
- Abnormal epithelium is often within the cervical glands with few or no surface changes.
- Most lesions are near the squamocolumnar junction.

Treatment
- Cone biopsy: requires a cone of up to 2.5 cm in length. Risk of skip lesion is about 30%.
- Hysterectomy should be considered if fertility is not desired due to continued risk of residual and recurrent disease.

Cervical cancer

Of cervical malignancies, 85% are squamous cell carcinoma and 15% are adeno-carcinoma. The development of cervical cancer is in either the squamous epithelium or endocervix. Most squamous cancers originate in the transformation zone.

Spread of malignancy
- Direct extension: ureteric obstruction can occur if malignancy extends to the pelvic side wall.
- There may be lymphatic spread to the pelvic nodes.
- Haematogenous spread is less common.

Risk factors
- age: mean age at time of diagnosis is 52 years, with two peak frequencies at ages 35–39 years and 60–64 years
- early age of sexual activity
- multiple sexual partners
- smoking
- partner with previous partner with cervical cancer

Diagnosis and examination
Presenting complaint
- most common: abnormal vaginal bleeding such as menorrhagia, postcoital, irregular and postmenopausal bleeding
- vaginal discharge

Examination
- general, lymphadenopathy
- vaginal/pelvic findings depending on the stage of the disease
- speculum: check vaginal extension of tumour; cervix may be large, ulcerated, irregular, bleeding
- vaginal/pelvic examination: cervix expanded, firm, assess for parametrial spread
- rectal examination

Investigations and staging of cervical cancer
- full blood count, electrolytes, liver biochemistry, renal function
- radiology: chest X-ray, abdominopelvic computed tomography (CT) scan, magnetic resonance image (MRI) of pelvis
- positron emission tomography (PET) scan can delineate extent of disease more accurately
- staging examination under anaesthesia: vaginal/pelvic and rectal examination; cervical biopsy; cystoscopy; curettage and sigmoidoscopy if indicated

FIGO staging for cervical cancer
This is a clinical staging system. See Table 19.1 for correlation of stage and 5-year survival.
- Stage 1: the carcinoma is strictly confined to the cervix; extension to corpus is disregarded.
  - 1A: invasive cancer identified only microscopically
  - 1A1: measured invasion of stroma not >3 mm in depth and 7 mm in diameter
  - 1A2: measured invasion of stroma >3 mm in depth and not >5 mm in depth and 7 mm in diameter
  - 1B: clinical lesions confined to the cervix or preclinical lesions larger than stage 1a
  - 1B1: clinical lesions not >4 cm in size
  - 1B2: clinical lesions >4 cm in size
- Stage 2: the carcinoma extends beyond the cervix, but has not extended onto the pelvic walls. The carcinoma involves the vagina, but not the lower third.
  - 2A: no obvious parametrial involvement
  - 2B: obvious parametrial spread

Stage	+ pelvic nodes	+ para-aortic nodes	5-year survival
1			85%
1A1	<1%	0	
1A2	5%	<1%	
1B	15%	2%	
2A	25%	10%	70%
2B	30%	20%	60%
3	45%	30%	35%
4	55%	40%	<15%

Table 19.1 Correlation of stage and 5-year survival

- Stage 3: the carcinoma has extended onto the pelvic side wall. On rectal examination there is no cancer-free space between the tumour and the pelvic wall. The tumour involves the lower third of the vagina. All cases with hydronephrosis or non-functioning kidney.
  - 3A: no extension to the pelvic wall but involvement of the lower third of the vagina
  - 3B: extension onto the pelvic wall and/or hydronephrosis or non-functioning kidney
- Stage 4: the carcinoma has extended beyond the true pelvis or has clinically involved the mucosa of the bladder or rectum.
  - 4A: spread to adjacent organs
  - 4B: spread to distant organs

Management of cervical cancer
Surgical treatment
- incision: mid-line vertical or Maylard incision
- laparotomy: assessing ascites, liver, kidneys, ureters, nodes, spleen, subdiaphragmatic spaces, paracolic gutters, appendix
- radical surgery: removal of the uterus, cervix, parametrium, upper third of the vagina and pelvic nodes

Complications
- haemorrhage
- prolonged theatre time, which increases risk of infection and thromboembolism (1%–2%)
- atonic bladder, which occurs in up to 3% of cases due to pelvic denervation
- ureteric fistula, which occurs in 1%–2%; vesicovaginal fistula in <1%
- urinary tract infection in 10%
- febrile morbidity, which affects 10%–20%, caused by pulmonary atelectasis, urinary tract infection, wound infection, haematoma, pelvic cellulitis
- pelvic lymphocyst, which affects 1%–2% (incidence may decrease with intraoperative drainage)
- nerve injury (obturator nerve injury causing weakness in adduction of thigh; femoral nerve compression)
- small bowel obstruction, which affects 1%

Radiation therapy
- The limiting factor in getting the maximum dose to the tumour is normal tissue tolerance. Cellular DNA is damaged by a direct action of radiation or indirectly via water free radicals.
- Tumour cells undergo mitotic death and rate of tumour shrinkage is proportional to cell cycle time.
- The typical radical dose is 60 gray; a palliative dose is 30 gray. The total dose is delivered in multiple fractions to allow repair of normal tissues between fractions (e.g. 50 gray may be given in 30 fractions over 6 weeks for pelvic radiotherapy). The chance of eradication of the tumour depends on the dose and number of malignant cells.

Morbidity of pelvic radiotherapy
- About 5% severe morbidity is considered acceptable.
- Acute effects are proctitis, ileitis, diarrhoea, tenesmus, skin reaction (especially skinfolds) and bladder irritability.
- Late effects are chronic proctitis, ileitis with perforation or stricture, fistula or necrosis, lymphoedema, vaginal atrophy and contraction, radiation menopause, femoral head necrosis, induction of malignancy.
- Radiation morbidity may be reduced by field planning, barium contrast and gentle fractionation to allow normal tissue the chance to repair.

Treatment of early-stage cervical cancer
Stage 1A
- Microinvasion <1 mm may be treated with cone biopsy or simple hysterectomy.
- Less than 3 mm invasion may be treated with simple hysterectomy.
- Stage 1a lesions >3 mm invasion require radical hysterectomy and lymphadenectomy, with adjuvant radiotherapy and concurrent chemotherapy if nodes are positive.

Stage 1B
- Identical survival rates obtained if managed primarily by radical hysterectomy/ lymphadenectomy or radiotherapy when surgical margins and lymph nodes are clear.
- Radical hysterectomy and pelvic lymphadenectomy are often used to treat stage 1B1 disease.
- Use radiotherapy and concurrent chemotherapy if the woman is unfit for surgery or as adjuvant therapy if the nodes are positive.
- Radical trachelectomy can be an option for a woman who wants to preserve fertility if the tumour is <2 cm.

Stage 2A
- Surgery can be offered to patients with early stage 2A cervical cancer. Otherwise, primary radiation therapy is the standard treatment for more advanced disease.

Advantages of surgery
- In young women, the ovaries may be left if they appear normal, as the risk of ovarian metastasis is <1% in squamous cell carcinoma of the cervix, stage 1.
- The risk of distant metastasis is influenced by primary therapy (i.e. lower risk with surgery than with radiation).

Management of advanced-stage cervical cancer
- Radiation treatment with concurrent chemotherapy is used for stages 2B or greater. Radiation doses are normally quoted from point A (i.e. 2 cm lateral to the centre of the uterus and 2 cm above the lateral fornix).

- Stage 2B and large (>5 cm) stage 1B cancers may be treated with radiation and chemotherapy followed by hysterectomy. Stage 4A may be treated with pelvic exenteration.

Follow-up management of cervical cancer
- Review the patient 4–6 weeks after surgery, then every 3 months for 2 years, then every 6 months to year 5, then yearly to year 10. Assessment requires general examination (breasts, nodes), vault smear, vaginal and rectal examination, and other investigations as appropriate, such as chest X-ray, colposcopy/biopsy.
- Recurrence usually occurs in the first 12 months, and most patients with recurrent disease die within 2 years.

Post-treatment surveillance
- vaginal cytology: poor sensitivity (15%) but up to 100% specificity
- physical examination: about 60% sensitivity and up to 95% specificity
- suspicious symptoms: 70% sensitivity and up to 95% specificity

Adenocarcinoma of the cervix
- This accounts for 15%–25% of cervical cancer. FIGO prognosis for this condition is poorer than for squamous lesions, due to greater tumour volume.
- Clinical behaviour of the disease is similar to that of squamous cell carcinoma.
- In young women with early-stage disease, the ovaries may be conserved, as <2% metastasises to the ovaries.

Special circumstances
Cervical cancer in pregnancy
- It occurs in about 1 in 1500 pregnancies.
- Vaginal delivery is not advised, as this may disseminate disease through large cervical venous sinuses and dilated lymphatics, cause disease to be transmitted down the vagina or produce haemorrhage.

Small cell cancer
- metastasises early and requires local surgery in conjunction with combination chemotherapy

Further reading

Basil JB, Horowitz IR 2001 Cervical carcinoma. Obstetrics and Gynecology Clinics of North America 28:727–740

Berek JS, Hacker NF (eds) 2005 Practical gynecologic oncology, 4th edn. Philadelphia: Lippincott Williams & Wilkins

Flowers LC, McCall MA 2001 Diagnosis and management of cervical intraepithelial neoplasia. Obstetrics and Gynecology Clinics of North America 28:667–684

Grisby PW, Herzog TJ 2001 Current management of patients with invasive cervical carcinoma. Clinical Obstetrics and Gynecology 44:531–537

Levine L, Lucci JA, Dinh TV 2003 Atypical glandular cells: new Bethesda terminology and management guidelines. Obstetrical and Gynecological Survey 58:399–406

National Health and Medical Research Council (NHMRC) 2005 Screening to prevent cervical cancer: guidelines for the management of asymptomatic women with screen detected abnormalities. Canberra: NHMRC

Chapter 20

Uterine neoplasia

Amy Tang

Benign tumours of the uterus

Uterine polyps
Polyps in the uterine corpus (the commonest site) may be part of a hyperplastic endometrium and present with changes in the menstrual cycle. Presenting symptoms include vaginal discharge and intermenstrual bleeding.

Uterine fibroids (leiomyomas)
These are present in 20%–30% of women and the aetiology is uncertain. Risk factors include nulliparity, family history, African race and hormonal influences, especially oestrogen.

Pathology
- macroscopic: firm, round, whorled masses
- sites: intramural, subserous, submucous, also in cervix and broad ligament
- microscopic: smooth muscle proliferation, fibrous tissue

Degenerative changes
These occur because of poor vascularity, and include:
- hyaline degeneration
- cystic degeneration
- calcification
- necrosis
- red degeneration/necrobiosis
- sarcomatous degeneration, rarely (<0.5%)

Clinical features
- often asymptomatic or variable in presentation; usually shrink after menopause
- presentation: menorrhagia, intermenstrual bleeding, infertility, abdominal swelling, pressure effects on the bladder or on large pelvic veins, which can result in oedema of legs or deep venous thrombosis
- in pregnancy, may grow in size, undergo red degeneration and may obstruct labour

Management
- conservative with small or asymptomatic fibroids
- medical treatment
  - progesterone
  - gonadotrophin-releasing hormone (GnRH) analogues: cause rapid shrinkage of fibroids in the first 3 months, but they regrow to pretreatment size within

3 months of stopping therapy; reduction in volume is proportional to degree of oestrogen suppression; side effects include menopausal symptoms, pelvic pain from acute necrosis of fibroids, reduced bone density (6% trabecular bone loss in lumbar vertebrae after 6 months, but reversed 6 months after stopping therapy)
- surgery: hysterectomy; hysteroscopic resection, myomectomy with or without pretreatment GnRH analogues

Fibroids in pregnancy

Fibroids become soft because of oedema and grow in size in pregnancy. If pedunculated, the fibroid may undergo torsion. There is an increased risk of red degeneration. This causes pain and a slight rise in temperature. Management of red degeneration of fibroids in pregnancy is conservative (rest, analgesia). Pain will abate in about 10 days.

Effect of fibroids on pregnancy
- uterus is larger than dates; the growth of fibroid occurs mostly in the first trimester
- risk of abortion/miscarriage
- when present at lower parts of the uterus and cervix, fibroids can obstruct the presenting part and cause abnormal lie of the fetus
- risk of postpartum haemorrhage
- caesarean section may be difficult if the fibroid is in the lower uterine segment
- rupture of uterus after myomectomy is rare

Endometrial hyperplasia

Definition. Hyperplasia is an increase in the number of cells in an organ/tissue; it may be pathological or physiologically normal.

Endometrial hyperplasia consists of a variety of changes in endometrial glandular and stromal elements. It is characterised by proliferation of endometrial glands resulting in greater gland-to-stroma ratio than in normal endometrium. These glands vary in size and shape and may show cytological atypia.

World Health Organization classification of endometrial hyperplasia
- glandular/stromal architectural pattern
  - simple (cystically dilated glands with occasional outpouching)
  - complex (back to back crowding of glands with minimal intervening stroma)
- presence or absence of nuclear atypia

Risk factors

Endometrial hyperplasia is oestrogen-dependent but its precise role is unknown. Conditions such as polycystic ovarian syndrome, unopposed oestrogen therapy, ovarian tumours (oestrogenic or virilising) and obesity are associated with an increased risk of hyperplasia. Other risk factors are infertility, nulliparity and medical conditions (liver disease, hyperthyroid).

Malignant potential
- Cytological atypia is the most useful predictor of the likelihood of cancer progression.
- Simple hyperplasia without atypia: about 1% will progress to cancer; 80% regress after curettage and other treatment.
- Complex hyperplasia without atypia: 3% progress to cancer.

- Simple hyperplasia with atypia: 8% progress to cancer.
- Complex atypical hyperplasia: 29% progress to carcinoma; up to 25% of women have well-differentiated cancers when hysterectomies are done within 1 month of curettage.

Diagnosis and screening
- common presentations: menorrhagia and abnormal bleeding per vagina
- investigations: ultrasound scan to assess thickness of the endometrium; hysteroscopy and endometrial curettage; endometrial sampling; cytological sample from the cervix and/or vagina (sensitivity is low: 35% for atypical hyperplasia, and 20% for adenomatous hyperplasia)

Management
- oral progesterone: by providing a more complete sloughing of the endometrium, reducing the number of oestrogen receptors on endometrial cells and by affecting the metabolism of oestrogen; when using cyclical therapy, the duration of therapy is important (i.e. at least 12 days per month)
- levonorgestrel-releasing intrauterine system (Mirena)
- stop unopposed oestrogen
- surgical treatment: dilatation and curettage; hysterectomy

Guides to treatment
- treatment dependent on the type/grading of hyperplasia, the age of the woman and her desire for future fertility
- simple hyperplasia: dilatation and curettage, hormone therapy, monitoring with yearly endometrial sampling
- complex hyperplasia: if fertility required, treatment with progesterone and induction of ovulation; if fertility not required, or in the older woman, treatment with progesterone or hysterectomy with or without oophorectomy; if conservative management used, an endometrial sample recommended in 3–6 months
- atypical hyperplasia: if fertility required, treatment with progesterone and induction of ovulation; if fertility not required, or in the older woman, treatment with hysterectomy and oophorectomy; if conservative management used, an endometrial sample recommended in 3 months

Cancer of the uterine corpus

This is the leading cause of genital cancer in developed countries, with a 1% lifetime risk.

Epidemiology and risk factors
- 80% postmenopausal (peak incidence at 61 years); <5% aged under 40 years
- obesity: increased conversion of androstenedione to oestrone in fat (this lowers sex hormone-binding globulin and raises free oestrogen—a three-fold increased risk if the woman is up to 25 kg overweight and ten-fold if the woman is >25 kg overweight)
- medical conditions: hypertension, previous pelvic irradiation, immunodeficiency, diabetes (raises risk by two to eight times)
- hereditary non-polyposis colorectal cancer (HNPCC): 40%–45% risk
- abnormal hormonal status: unopposed oestrogen therapy, raised endogenous oestrogen (e.g. obesity, polycystic ovarian syndrome, oestrogen-producing tumours, use of tamoxifen)

- parity: up to 35% of women with endometrial cancer nulliparous, representing a two-fold risk compared with multiparous women; late menopause also a risk factor

Pathology of uterine cancer
- Adenocarcinoma accounts for 60%–80% of endometrial cancers.
- Adenosquamous malignancies occur in 15%.
- Papillary serous carcinomas are aggressive, with early peritoneal spread.
- Clear cell carcinoma is rare and the prognosis is poor.

Mode of spread of uterine cancer
- direct invasion of the myometrium and cervix
- at the time of diagnosis, at least 10% with extension of disease beyond the uterus
- lymphatic spread: para-aortic and pelvic nodes
- haematogenous spread in later stages: lungs, liver, bone

Clinical presentation
- postmenopausal bleeding in 90% of cases
- intermenstrual bleeding, menorrhagia

Diagnosis and investigations
- endometrial sampling
- examination under anaesthesia, hysteroscopy, curettage
- full blood count, electrolytes, blood sugar levels, liver biochemistry
- chest X-ray
- computed tomography (CT) of abdomen and pelvis to assess for metastatic disease
- CA125 can be useful to predict extrauterine disease once diagnosis of uterine cancer is confirmed

FIGO staging for uterine cancer
- stage 1: tumour confined to the body of the uterus
  - 1A: tumour limited to endometrium
  - 1B: invasion of less than half of the myometrium
  - 1C: invasion of greater than or equal to half of the myometrium
- stage 2: tumour extension to the cervix
  - 2A: endocervical glandular involvement only
  - 2B: cervical stromal invasion
- stage 3: tumour with local spread and/or positive nodes
  - 3A: tumour invades serosa and/or adnexa, and/or positive peritoneal cytology
  - 3B: vaginal metastasis
  - 3C: metastasis to pelvic and/or para-aortic nodes
- stage 4: tumour spread to pelvic viscera and beyond
  - 4A: invasion of bladder and/or bowel mucosa
  - 4B: distant metastasis, intra-abdominal and/or inguinal nodes

In addition, the stage will include the grade of the tumour (grade 1: well-differentiated; grade 2: moderately differentiated; grade 3: poorly differentiated).

Surgical staging assessment
Myometrial invasion
- Survival rates with endometrial invasion only and superficial myometrium invasion are similar.
- There is reduced survival with deep myometrial invasion.

| Table 20.1 Survival rates for uterine cancer according to FIGO stage ||
Stage	5-year survival
1	75%–90%
2	65%–75%
3	30%–40%
4	10%

Adnexal spread
- This is present in 7%–8%, and often microscopic.

Lymph nodes
- Metastases increase with worsening differentiation of the tumour and increasing depth of myometrial invasion.

Survival rates
- The overall 5-year survival of women with uterine cancer is 65%. Survival depends on tumour stage, grade and cell type (the worst being clear-cell).
- Table 20.1 lists survival rates for uterine cancer according to the FIGO stage.

Management of uterine cancer
Screening and prevention
- Positive cervical smear is found in <50%.
- Aspiration endometrial sampling has up to 96% accuracy.
- Protect endometrium with hormone therapy in conditions of unopposed oestrogens.

Stage 1
- About 75% of patients have stage 1 disease. Survival is better with surgery than radiotherapy alone.
- Standard treatment is total abdominal hysterectomy and bilateral salpingo-oophorectomy and peritoneal washings.
- Intraoperative frozen section to assess tumour grade and myometrial invasion to determine whether lymphadenectomy is required.
- Positive nodes are found in 10% and positive peritoneal cytology in 15%.
- Lymphadenectomy may be used as a prognosticator and treatment modifier (radiotherapy if nodes are positive).
- Incidence of vault recurrence rises with worsening tumour grade and increasing myometrial invasion. Postoperative brachytherapy may reduce vault recurrence from 10% to 3%, but has no effect on overall survival.

Stage 2
- Modified radical hysterectomy, bilateral salpingo-oophorectomy and pelvic and para-aortic lymphadenectomy is associated with better survival when compared with simple hysterectomy.
- Pelvic lymph nodes are positive in up to 20% of cases.
- Postoperative adjuvant radiation is individualised and is given if positive lymph nodes.

Stages 3 and 4
- Treatment must be individualised and may include total abdominal hysterectomy, bilateral salpingo-oophorectomy, debulking of macroscopic tumour, preoperative/postoperative chemotherapy and pelvic irradiation, and hormonal therapy.

Recurrent disease
- About 80% of recurrences occur within 2 years of primary therapy.
- It can be locoregional or distant recurrence.
- Treatment is directed to the site of recurrence.
- Two common sites of vaginal recurrence are apex of vault and lower anterior third of the vagina in the retrourethral position.
- Management includes surgery, irradiation, hormone therapy, chemotherapy or combination.

Hormone therapy and chemotherapy
- high-dose progesterone (gives a better response with well-differentiated carcinoma, as there is a reduction in receptor concentration with worsening histological grade; may be used in the treatment of pulmonary metastasis)
- levonorgestrel-releasing intrauterine system (Mirena): suitable for a patient who is unfit for surgery
- anti-oestrogen
- chemotherapy: carboplatin, paclitaxel, doxorubicin, fluorouracil, cyclophosphamide

Uterine sarcomas

Uterine sarcomas are rare and account for about 3% of all uterine cancers. Sarcomas are mesodermal tumours with an overall 5-year survival rate of 30%.

Classification
Leiomyosarcoma
- It accounts for 50% of uterine sarcomas.
- The mean age at diagnosis is 50 years.
- The risk of malignant change in fibroid is <0.5%.
- Survival is better if it arises in a fibroid.
- It is usually intramural and 60% are solitary.
- Presentation: includes vaginal bleeding/discharge, pain, abdominal mass.
- Diagnosis: 10 or more mitotic figures per 10 high-power fields is associated with a 25% 5-year survival rate.
- There is a 95% 5-year survival rate in those with fewer than 10 mitotic figures per 10 high-power fields.
- Spread of the disease is mainly haematogenous; thus surgical staging is not as important.
- Overall 5-year survival rate is 20%.

Endometrial stromal sarcoma
- It accounts for 15%–25% of uterine sarcomas.
- The mean age of diagnosis is 45 years; only a third of patients are postmenopausal.
- It is divided into low-grade and high-grade categories.
- Low-grade is called endometrial stromal sarcoma. They are relatively indolent and late recurrences may occur. Prolonged survival and even cure is possible even after recurrence. They are responsive to hormonal therapy with progesterone after surgery.
- High-grade is now termed endometrial sarcoma. They are aggressive tumours. Prognosis is poor.

Malignant mixed müllerian tumour
- The mean age at diagnosis is 65 years.
- It is a mixture of sarcoma and carcinoma (thus also termed carcinosarcoma).

- Risk factors include increasing age, hypertension, diabetes, obesity and previous pelvic irradiation.
- Prognosis: metastasise early; overall 5-year survival rate is 25%.

Management of uterine sarcomas
Surgery
- Staging: includes laparotomy, total abdominal hysterectomy, bilateral salpingo-oophorectomy.
- Radical hysterectomy has no significant effect on survival.
- Disseminated disease: value of debulking is uncertain.

Radiotherapy
- Leiomyosarcoma is resistant to radiotherapy.
- In malignant mixed müllerian tumours, radiotherapy reduces pelvic recurrence but may not improve survival rates.

Chemotherapy
- The value of chemotherapy has yet to be proven.

Cancer of the fallopian tubes

Primary cancer of the fallopian tube is rare. It accounts for <0.5% of all gynaecological cancers, and only about 1000 cases have been reported. The mean age at diagnosis is 55 years. The only identified risk factor is an inherited mutation in BRCA1 or BRCA2 gene.

Pathology
- Malignancy is mostly due to secondary disease.
- Most primary carcinomas are adenocarcinoma; very rarely there are sarcomas or choriocarcinomas.

Clinical presentation
- There is a classic triad of pelvic pain, pelvic mass and watery vaginal discharge in 15% of patients.
- It is often asymptomatic, but may present with a mass with ascites.
- The most common symptoms are abnormal vaginal bleeding (30%) and vaginal discharge (20%).

Treatment
- similar to that for epithelial ovarian cancer
- surgery: total abdominal hysterectomy, bilateral salpingo-oophorectomy, omentectomy, lymphadenectomy, appendicectomy, peritoneal washings and biopsy
- adjuvant platinum combination chemotherapy
- radiotherapy: may be used in palliative therapy

Five-year survival rate
- overall survival is 56%
- stage 1, 70%; stage 2, 50%; stage 3, 30%; stage 4, 10%

Further reading

Berek JS, Hacker NF (eds) 2005 Practical gynecologic oncology, 4th edn. Philadelphia: Lippincott Williams & Wilkins

Hernandez E 2001 Endometrial adenocarcinoma. Obstetrics and Gynecology Clinics of North America 28:743–757

Marsden DE, Hacker NF 2001 Optimal management of endometrial hyperplasia. Best Practice and Research Clinical Obstetrics and Gynaecology 15:393–405

Chapter 21

Ovarian neoplasms

Amy Tang

Features of malignant versus benign ovarian neoplasms

- Age: in childhood and in older women, there is an increased risk of malignancy.
- Pain: pain can occur in both. Acute pain usually indicates torsion or haemorrhage.
- Rapid growth: suspect malignancy.
- Bilaterality: 75% of malignant disease and 15% of benign lesions are bilateral.
- Consistency: solid, nodular and/or irregular features are suggestive of malignancy.
- Fixation of the mass: suspect malignancy.
- Ascites: ascites is associated with malignancy.
- Leg/vulval oedema, venous obstruction/thrombosis: this is strongly suggestive of malignancy.
- Evidence of distant metastasis: indicates malignancy.

Risk of Malignancy Index (RMI)

RMI is useful to help determine those women with a pelvic ovarian mass who would benefit from direct referral to a tertiary gynaecological oncology unit.

$$RMI = \text{Menopausal status} \left(1 \text{ or } 3\right) \times \text{Ultrasound features} \left(0, 1 \text{ or } 3\right) \times CA125$$

- menopausal status: premenopausal = 1; postmenopausal = 3
- ultrasound features (multiloculated, solid areas, bilateral pathology, ascites, metastases): no features = 0; one feature = 1; more than one feature = 3
  If RMI >=200, there is a high risk of malignancy and the woman should be referred to a gynaecological oncologist.

Screening for ovarian cancer

Screening for ovarian cancer has not been proven to reduce ovarian cancer deaths in the general population. It may have a role in high-risk patients (e.g. a strong family history).
- Bimanual pelvic examination: low-cost, requires no special equipment but not specific or sensitive in the detection of ovarian cancer.
- Ultrasound scan: malignant features include semisolid or cystic areas, thick septa, surface papillary growths, neovascularisation, bilateral masses and/or ascites.

- Cytology: routine cervical cytological tests give abnormal results in 10%–30% of advanced ovarian cancer cases. Peritoneal cytology is not specific or sensitive, and is time-consuming and painful to perform.
- Prophylactic salpingo-oophorectomy: this should be considered in women with a strong family history of ovarian cancer or women who are BRCA carriers; 7% of women with ovarian cancer have had a previous laparotomy; 0.2% of women who have had their ovaries conserved during operations for benign gynaecological disorders develop ovarian cancer.

Tumour markers for ovarian cancer
- Markers are used in diagnosis, prognosis and to detect subclinical disease.
- The four types of potential markers for ovarian cancer are oncodevelopmental markers, carcinoplacental, metabolic and tumour-specific/tumour-associated antigens. None has sufficiently high specificity for screening.
- CA125 tumour-associated antigen is a high molecular weight glycoprotein expressed in coelomic epithelium during embryogenic development; 80% of patients with ovarian carcinoma have levels >35 IU/mL. It is elevated in about 1% of healthy women and also in non-malignant conditions such as endometriosis, inflammation, benign tumours and pregnancy. CA125 levels fall with age. It is a good marker for epithelial carcinoma, except mucinous tumours, but has poor specificity (not useful for screening).
- CA19.9 is usually elevated in mucinous tumours and pancreatic cancers.
- CEA is useful to exclude metastatic bowel primary if patient complains of bowel symptoms.
- The markers may be used in combination to improve specificity and sensitivity.
- False-negative results can occur in early-stage disease.

Ovarian cancer

Epidemiology
There are geographical variations in the incidences of ovarian cancer. The peak incidence by age group occurs in the seventh to eighth decade. Ovarian cancer accounts for up to 35% of all gynaecological cancers.

Risk factors
- nulliparity, infertility
- family history: a woman with a mother or sister with ovarian cancer has a twenty-fold increased risk; increased risk is associated with inherited mutations in the BRCA1 and BRCA2 genes
- previous other cancers: breast, endometrial
- oral contraceptive pill affords protection
- other risk factors: blood group A, Peutz-Jeghers syndrome

Pathology of ovarian cancer
- epithelial tumours: make up 90% of ovarian malignancies
- types of epithelial ovarian cancer: serous, mucinous, endometroid, Brenner, clear-cell
- sex cord stromal tumours: granulosa cell, Sertoli-Leydig cell (androblastoma, arrhenoblastoma), fibroma, sex cord tumours with annular tubules
- germ cell tumours: dysgerminoma, non-dysgerminoma (endodermal sinus tumour, embryonal carcinoma, choriocarcinoma, mature and immature teratomas)
- secondary tumours: Krukenberg (gastrointestinal, especially stomach), breast

Presentation
- Ovarian cancer is often asymptomatic in early disease.
- The woman may present with:
  - abdominal pain, pelvic pressure, frequency of urine
  - abdominal swelling, dyspepsia, back pain
  - constipation, deep venous thrombosis

Examination
- general examination
- assess for lymphadenopathy
- examination of breasts, thyroid, abdomen/liver, ascites
- pelvic and rectal examination

Investigations for ovarian masses
- tumour markers: CA125, CA19.9, CEA
- consider human chorionic gonadotrophin (hCG), alpha-fetoprotein, inhibin, lactate dehydrogenase (LDH) if suspect non-epithelial ovarian tumours
- full blood count, electrolytes, liver biochemistry
- radiology: abdominopelvic ultrasound and/or computed tomography (CT) scan, chest X-ray, colonoscopy

FIGO staging for ovarian cancer
Staging is based on clinical examination, laparotomy, histology and cytology findings.
- stage 1: growth limited to ovaries
  - 1A: growth limited to one ovary, capsule intact, no ascites, negative peritoneal cytology
  - 1B: growth limited to both ovaries, no ascites, no tumour on the external surfaces, capsule intact
  - 1C: tumour either stage 1A or 1B, but with tumour on surface of one or both ovaries; or capsule ruptured; or with ascites present containing malignant cells or with positive peritoneal washings
- stage 2: growth involving one or both ovaries with pelvic extension
  - 2A: extension and/or metastases to the uterus and/or tubes
  - 2B: extension to other pelvic tissues
  - 2C: tumour either stage 2A or 2B, but with tumour on surface of one or both ovaries; or with capsule(s) ruptured; or with ascites present containing malignant cells or with positive peritoneal washings
- stage 3: tumour involving one or both ovaries with peritoneal implants outside the pelvis and/or positive retroperitoneal or inguinal nodes; superficial liver metastasis equals stage 3; tumour is limited to the true pelvis but with histologically proven malignant extension to the small bowel or omentum
  - 3A: tumour grossly limited to the true pelvis with negative nodes, but with histologically confirmed microscopic seeding of abdominal peritoneal surfaces
  - 3B: tumour involving one or both ovaries with histologically confirmed implants of abdominal peritoneal surfaces; none >2 cm in diameter
  - 3C: abdominal implants >2 cm in diameter and/or positive retroperitoneal or inguinal nodes
- stage 4: growth involving one or both ovaries with distant metastases; if pleural effusion present, there must be positive cytology to allot a case to stage 4; parenchymal liver metastasis equals stage 4

Epithelial ovarian tumours
These account for 90% of ovarian cancer.

Five-year survival rates
- stage 1: 80%
- stage 2: 50%
- stage 3: 25%
- stage 4: 10%

Serous tumours
- These are the commonest epithelial tumours, malignant or benign.
- 50% are bilateral and usually unilocular.

Mucinous tumours
- These are large, unilateral multilocular cysts.
- 5%–10% are malignant.
- *Pseudomyxoma peritonei* is a rare complication of perforation and spillage of cyst contents.

Endometrioid tumours
- 20% are associated with endometrial carcinoma.
- They may be associated with endometriosis.
- They account for 15% of ovarian cancers.
- They are usually well-differentiated, with good prognosis.

Clear-cell tumours
- These arise in the cervix, vagina, endometrium, broad ligament and ovaries.
- They may be associated with endometriosis.
- They are large, solid/cystic, unilateral tumours with poor prognosis.

Brenner tumours
- These are usually benign, small and unilateral.

Prognostic factors for epithelial ovarian cancer
- The stage at time of diagnosis is important.
- Cell types:
  - poor prognosis: clear cell and serous tumours
  - moderate prognosis: mucinous
  - good prognosis: endometroid.
- Tumour grade is an important prognostic factor: grade 1, well-differentiated; grade 2, moderately differentiated; grade 3, poorly differentiated.
- The ability to achieve optimal surgical debulking with no residual disease is a major prognostic factor.

Management
Preoperative preparation
- Optimise health if other medical problems are present.
- Admit for bowel preparation and anaesthetic review.
- Employ prophylactic antibiotics and anticoagulation therapy.

Surgical treatment
- vertical abdominal incision
- assessment for free fluid and collection of peritoneal washings
- systematic exploration and biopsy of all intraperitoneal surfaces
- diaphragmatic sampling

- total abdominal hysterectomy and bilateral salpingo-oophorectomy; debulking tumour (primary cytoreduction), preferably to <1 cm to achieve optimal debulking
- omentectomy and appendicectomy
- pelvic and para-aortic node sampling
- the insertion of intraperitoneal port if optimal debulking

Chemotherapy
- used for adjuvant treatment and palliation
- most commonly used agents are combination carboplatin and paclitaxel
- can be given intravenously or intraperitoneally
- used at an earlier stage in cases with poorer prognostic factors, such as poorly differentiated tumours, cyst rupture or ascites
- can be used as neoadjuvant treatment in stage 4 disease or in those patients who are not fit for initial upfront surgery (e.g. recent pulmonary embolism)

Aims of surgery
- to improve tumour response to further therapy
- to delay/prevent inevitable complications, such as gastrointestinal obstruction
- to alter immunological state and immunosuppresion
- to relieve symptoms and to achieve psychological benefit from the removal of a large mass

Sex cord stromal tumours
Stromal cells retain the potential for differentiation into any of the cells/tissues from mesenchymal gonad (i.e. granulosa, theca, Leydig and Sertoli cells).
- Some tumours produce sex steroid hormones:
  - feminising: granulosa and theca cell tumours
  - masculinising: Sertoli-Leydig (androblastoma).

Granulosa cell tumours
- These account for 2% of ovarian tumours and occur at any age.
- These solid tumours are usually unilateral (bilateral in 2%–5%).
- They vary in size, with an average of 10 cm in diameter.
- Rupture or haemorrhage into the tumour may occur.
- They can produce oestrogen and inhibin.
- Histopathology: Call-Exner bodies are granulosa cells arranged around small spaces containing nuclear fragments.
- They are associated with endometrial hyperplasia and even endometrial cancer in 5%–6% of cases.
- They are mostly diagnosed at stage 1 disease, are usually a slow-growing tumour, and late recurrences are not uncommon.

Management
- surgery: if childbearing complete, total abdominal hysterectomy and bilateral salpingo-oophorectomy; if early-stage and the patient still requires fertility, uterine curettage and removal of the affected ovary and fallopian tube
- chemotherapy: for disease beyond the ovary or for late recurrences

Androblastoma
- These are solid tumours with low malignant potential, composed of Sertoli and/or Leydig cells (pure Sertoli cell tumours are rare; Leydig cell tumours are hilus or lipoid cell tumour).
- They present with masculinisation, abdominal pain and menstrual dysfunction.

Fibroma
- This large, firm and lobulated mass consists of fibroblast-like cells.
- It is usually benign; bilateral in 10% of cases.
- It is associated with Meigs' syndrome (ascites and right hydrothorax), which resolves with removal of the tumour.
- If marked atypia and mitosis, it is termed fibrosarcoma; this tumour is very aggressive.

Germ cell tumours
Germ cell tumours are the second largest group of ovarian neoplasms. They occur predominantly in childhood and adolescence. The commonest germ cell tumour in all ages is the mature cystic teratoma/benign dermoid. This is derived from multipotent germ cells (i.e. from primitive germ cells before sexual differentiation occurs).
- Treatment intent is curative with conservation of ovarian function and fertility.
- Tumour markers: alpha-fetoprotein is produced by yolk sac cells; hCG is produced by syncytiotrophoblast.

Dysgerminoma
- This is the commonest malignant germ cell tumour.
- Peak age incidence is 10–30 years, especially in patients with developmentally abnormal gonads.
- It is hormonally inert.
- It is associated with elevated lactate dehydrogenase.
- Rapid growth can occur; most tumours are over 10 cm in diameter at time of diagnosis.
- It is solid, rubbery and bilateral in 15% of cases; most (75%) present in stage 1.

Management
- The tumour is very radiosensitive and chemosensitive.
- Stage 1A: unilateral salpingo-oophorectomy, peritoneal cytology, exploration of abdomen and removal of retroperitoneal lymph nodes, biopsy of contralateral ovary if suspicious. No adjuvant chemotherapy is required.
- All other stages: conservative surgery can be offered, but will need chemotherapy. BEP (bleomycin, etoposide and cisplatin) is recommended.
- Overall 5-year survival rate is over 90%, but prognosis is worse if the tumour is at an advanced stage and other germ cell elements are present.
- Careful follow-up is required, as 15%–20% of tumours recur.
- Consider karyotyping the patient.

Choriocarcinoma
- This is the rarest of the germ cell group. It can be mixed with other germ cell elements.
- It secretes hCG.
- It may present with precocious puberty.
- Choriocarcinoma in the ovary can occur as metastasis from gestational trophoblast disease in the uterus, malignant change in an ovarian ectopic pregnancy or as a primary ovarian germ cell tumour.
- It is highly malignant, with early local and lymphatic spread compared with gestational trophoblast.
- Management comprises combination chemotherapy.

Embryonal carcinoma
- This is the least well-differentiated of the germ cell tumours.
- It can differentiate along somatic line to produce teratoma, or extraembryonal to endodermal sinus or choriocarcinoma.

- It can produce tumour markers such as hCG, alpha-fetoprotein.
- It is highly malignant with early metastasis.
- Management: remove ovary for tissue diagnosis. These tumours are not radio-resistant, but treatment is usually with combination chemotherapy.

Intersex
- Dysgenetic gonad has high malignant potential.
- The commonest tumours are dysgerminoma and gonadoblastoma.
- The greatest risk occurs when associated with the Y chromosome.

Endodermal sinus tumour
- This is a yolk sac tumour with alpha-fetoprotein as the tumour marker.
- The median age at presentation is 18 years.
- It is the most aggressive of germ cell group tumours, with rapid growth.
- Presentation: acute abdomen, a large mass with haemorrhage and necrosis; 50% of patients complain of symptoms for <24 hours, and rarely symptoms are present for >2 weeks.
- Management: radical surgery produces no better results than local tumour removal. Irradiation is not helpful. Combination chemotherapy may be curative. The ideal management is conservative surgery and combination chemotherapy. Alpha-fetoprotein is the marker to gauge the woman's response to treatment and is also used as a marker for recurrence.

Teratoma
All but 1% are cystic, mature teratomas or benign dermoid cysts. Cells are derived from all three germ cell layers of the embryo: the ectoderm, mesoderm and endoderm. Teratomas are often asymptomatic, unilateral, and large at time of diagnosis.

Malignancy
- occurs in solid immature teratomas
- occurs in the first two decades of life
- very rarely found in the postmenopausal woman
- immature teratomas with neurogenic elements have better prognosis
- stage 1A grade 1 immature teratoma can be managed by surgery alone without BEP

Mature cystic teratoma/dermoid cyst
- accounts for 20%–40% of ovarian tumours in pregnancy
- presentation: asymptomatic; torsion in pregnancy or puerperium; rupture, especially with torsion; infection is uncommon; malignant change is found in up to 3% of cases, most commonly squamous cell carcinoma, to be managed by surgery (prognosis depends on the presence of extraovarian disease)

Struma ovarii
- a monodermal teratoma which is usually benign
- usually involves non-functioning thyroid tissue
- treatment: surgery

Carcinoid tumour of the ovary
- a rare monodermal teratoma, usually occurring in older women
- one-third present with the carcinoid syndrome of flushes due to histamine release, diarrhoea, tachycardia, hypertension
- slow-growing and rarely metastasises

- investigation: raised urinary 5-hydroxyindole acetic acid
- treatment: surgical excision.

Borderline (low malignant potential) tumours

Low malignant potential tumours account for 15% of all epithelial ovarian cancers. Up to 20% occur with metastases. Metastases may represent disease of multifocal origin, rather than spread from a single site. The average age at time of diagnosis is the late 40s. About 30% of women are nulliparous.

FIGO and World Health Organization criteria for diagnosis of low malignant potential tumour are the presence of epithelial stratification, cellular atypia, mitotic activity with multilayering and nuclear pleomorphism, but with absence of ovarian stromal invasion.

Pathology
- 80%–95% are serous or mucinous
- 50%–80% are stage 1 at diagnosis
- 8%–35% are stage 3 at diagnosis

Management
- Initial management is similar to that for any patient with a pelvic mass.
- Perform a thorough physical examination.
- Test for tumour markers, renal and liver biochemistry.
- Ultrasound scan and/or CT scan of the pelvis.
- Laparotomy/laparoscopy: staging and debulking as indicated.
- Management of early-stage disease: when fertility is desired and disease is localised, conservative surgery is indicated. This includes unilateral salpingo-oophorectomy and biopsy of the contralateral ovary if suspicious and omental biopsy. In older patients, or if fertility is not required, treatment is with total abdominal hysterectomy/bilateral salpingo-oophorectomy.
- Recurrence in stage 1 disease: if managed by cystectomy alone, this is associated with a 25% recurrence rate; with oophorectomy of the affected ovary alone, a 10% recurrence rate. If total pelvic clearance, the recurrence rate is <5%.
- Management of advanced disease: treatment is similar to that for invasive ovarian cancer (total abdominal hysterectomy, bilateral salpingo-oophorectomy, debulking of tumour deposits, omentectomy, lymphadenectomy and appendicectomy).
- Chemotherapy is not indicated for stage 1. In advanced stages, chemotherapy does not appear to be as effective as in invasive ovarian cancer because the tumour is slow-growing with poor clinical response to chemotherapy or radiotherapy.

Prognostic features
- *Pseudomyxoma peritonei* with mucinous tumours is associated with a poor prognosis.
- Ploidy (DNA analysis by flow cytometry): most tumours are diploid and follow an indolent course. Two-thirds of ovarian cancer are aneuploid, compared with 5%–12% in low malignant potential tumours.

Further reading

Berek S, Hacker N (eds) 2005 Practical gynecologic oncology, 4th edn. Philadelphia: Lippincott Williams & Wilkins

Shafi M, Luesley D, Jordan J (eds) 2001 Handbook of gynaecological oncology. London: Churchill Livingstone

Chapter 22

Premalignant and malignant vulval diseases

Amy Tang

Vulval intraepithelial neoplasia (VIN)

VIN was once classified according to the degree of abnormality into VIN1, VIN2 and VIN3 (or mild, moderate and severe dysplasia). Since there is no evidence to suggest VIN 1 is precancerous, it is now called low-grade VIN, while VIN2 and VIN3 are referred to as high-grade VIN.

Classification
The International Society for the Study of Vulvar Diseases 2004 classifies high-grade VIN:
- The usual type (warty, basaloid and mixed) is related to human papillomavirus (HPV) (mostly 16, 18 and 31), is often multifocal, and it occurs in younger, premenopausal women.
- The differentiated type is non-HPV related, usually unifocal, and is seen in older women with chronic vulvar dystrophy, such as lichen sclerosus or squamous cell hyperplasia.

General
- The incidence of VIN is increasing worldwide, especially in younger women.
- Risk factors are smoking, immunosuppression and HPV infection.
- There are up to 50% with associated cervical or vaginal intraepithelial neoplasia.
- Clinical presentation includes: pruritus, perineal pain, vulval lesion, with 50% asymptomatic.
- Diagnosis is by tissue biopsy after colposcopic examination. The entire lower genital tract and perianal area should be examined.

Treatment
- Treatment should be individualised depending on histology, location and extent of disease.
- The goal of treatment is to prevent development of cancer and to relieve symptoms.
- Surgical treatment is preferable, and this includes wide local excision, skinning vulvectomy and laser ablation.
- Medical treatment is reserved for situations where surgery is not feasible. This includes topical imiquimod cream (Aldara) or 5-fluorouracil (5-FU).
- The response rate for medical therapy has been reported to be 75%.
- The recurrence rate for VIN is about 30%. Therefore, long-term follow-up is necessary.

Paget's diseases of vulva

Paget's disease is an intraepithelial neoplasia. About 10% of patients have invasive Paget's disease, and 4%–8% have an underlying adenocarcinoma.
- It mostly affects postmenopausal white women in their 60s and 70s.
- Symptoms include pruritus and vulvar pain.
- The lesion is well demarcated and has an eczematoid appearance with slightly raised edges.
- Diagnosis is by tissue biopsy.
- Patients should be investigated for synchronous cancer, as 25% may have a non-contiguous cancer involving the breast, rectum, bladder, urethra, cervix or ovary.
- Treatment is by wide local excision, including underlying dermis. Positive margins can be common, as Paget's disease usually extends well beyond the gross lesion.
- Recurrent local recurrences are common and they are treated with surgical excision.

Vulval cancer

Vulval cancer accounts for 3%–5% of all gynaecological cancers.

Aetiology
- There is no clear aetiological agent. Smoking is a risk factor.
- It mainly occurs in postmenopausal women with a long history of vulval irritation/pruritus.
- It is often associated with vulval skin dystrophy; however, dystrophy may be a consequence of irritation and scratching.
- Dystrophies appear to have malignant potential only if there is evidence of atypia.
- Oncogenic HPV infection may be associated.
- Progression of VIN 3 to cancer while not fully established is a high risk.
- There is common association with other squamous intraepithelial lesions of the lower genital tract.

Histopathology of vulval cancer
Squamous cell carcinoma
- the commonest type of vulval cancer (up to 90% of cases)

Melanoma
- the second commonest: up to 5% of cases
- as with melanoma found elsewhere, prognosis is dependent on depth of disease

Bartholin's gland
- up to 1%–3% of vulval cancers
- associated with higher groin node metastases and poorer prognosis than squamous cell cancer due to late diagnosis

Others
- basal cell carcinoma: low propensity for lymph spread
- sarcoma: rare
- invasive Paget's disease: low lymphatic spread
- secondary spread from vagina, ovary, breast, kidney, thyroid and gastrointestinal tract

Presentation and spread of vulval cancer

It usually presents in the seventh decade of life. Often there is significant delay (mean of 10 months) in the diagnosis, as the woman does not seek attention early. Another contributing factor is the failure of adequate assessment.

Presentation
- pruritus and irritation occurring in up to two-thirds of patients; often present for months to years before diagnosis
- mass or ulcer
- bleeding or discharge
- pain
- the most common site of vulval cancer: the labia, on the left more often than on the right; may also present on the clitoris and perineum (in assessment of groin nodes, clinical error occurs in up to 35% of cases)
- biopsy for tissue diagnosis

Spread of vulval cancer
- The major route of spread is local invasion and via the lymphatic system.
- Lymphatic spread usually occurs in an orderly fashion (i.e. to the inguinofemoral nodes, then to the pelvic nodes, and then to the para-aortic nodes).
- About 25% of patients have local spread to the vagina, urethra, anus and rectum.
- Haematogenous spread to distant sites (e.g. lungs, liver and bone) can also occur.

FIGO staging for vulval cancer
- stage 1: lesions ≤2 cm confined to the vulva or perineum; no lymph node metastases
  - 1A: lesions ≤2 cm confined to the vulva or perineum with stromal invasion not >1 mm; no nodal metastases
  - 1B: lesions ≤2 cm confined to the vulva or perineum with stromal invasion >1 mm; no nodal metastases
- stage 2: tumour as stage 1 but >2 cm; no palpable nodes
- stage 3: tumour of any size with adjacent spread to lower urethra and/or vagina or anus and/or unilateral inguinal node involvement
- stage 4
  - 4A: tumour invading any of the following: upper urethra, bladder mucosa, rectal mucosa, pelvic bone and/or bilateral inguinal node involvement
  - 4B: distant metastasis, including pelvic lymph nodes

Up to 70% of patients present in stage 1 and 2 disease (i.e. with no nodal spread). The overall 5-year survival rate is 60%. Women with stage 1 disease have a 90% 5-year survival rate.

Management of vulval cancer
Superficially invasive stage 1a
- Wide local excision is used when <2 cm in diameter, <1 mm invasion, no lymphvascular space involvement, no abnormal nodes clinically.
- The risk of inguinal node involvement is almost zero.

Other early-stage
- For stage 1B disease, risk of inguinal node metastases is >8%. If lesion is unifocal, >1 cm from mid-line, and not located in the anterior portion of labia minora, a wide local excision plus ipsilateral groin node dissection is performed. If positive nodes, then contralateral node dissection or irradiation is indicated.
- For other stage 1B and stage 2 disease, bilateral groin node dissection is performed.

• When two or more microscopically positive inguinal nodes are found, bilateral groin and pelvic radiotherapy is indicated.

Reasons for less radical surgery
• Wound healing is superior with separate incisions, compared with the butterfly incision radical vulvectomy, and results are not inferior.
• Superficial groin node dissection may be sufficient, as metastatic progression along the inguinal node chain occurs in an orderly fashion.
• Surgical node dissection is more a prognostic indicator and treatment modifier than a definitive therapy.
• There is less morbidity with superficial dissections.
• Groin dissection is very important, except in early superficial disease, as there is a high mortality in those who develop recurrence in the undissected groin.

Sentinel lymph node biopsy
• Promising but limited data from observational studies have suggested that this approach incurs less morbidity compared with inguinofemoral dissection, without compromising detection of lymph node metastases.
• Use of a combination of blue dye and radiolabelled colloid yields more accurate results.

Advanced vulval cancer: stages 3 and 4
• Radiotherapy and surgery can be combined.
• It may require pelvic exenteration and radical vulvectomy if the anus, rectum, rectovaginal septum or proximal urethra is involved.
• Irradiation is associated with severe vulval necrosis and poor survival rates in those treated with irradiation alone as primary therapy.

Complications of vulval surgery
• lower extremity lymphoedema 30%
• wound breakdown and infection 30%
• thromboembolism
• haemorrhage
• urinary tract infection
• femoral nerve trauma
• hernia
• osteitis pubis
• lymphocyst
• psychosexual problems

Further reading

Berek JS, Hacker NF (eds) 2005 Practical gynecologic oncology, 4th edn. Philadelphia: Lippincott Williams & Wilkins

Hopkins MP, Nemunaitis-Keller J 2001 Carcinoma of the vulva. Obstetrics and Gynecology Clinics of North America 28:791–804

Sideri M, Jones RW, Wilkinson EJ et al 2005 Squamous vulvar intraepithelial neoplasia: 2004 modified terminology, ISSVD Vulvar Oncology Subcommittee. Journal of Reproductive Medicine 50 (11):807–810

Chapter 23

Vaginal disease

Amy Tang

Benign conditions

Vaginal epithelium changes in different phases of life:
- In the newborn, it is thick with much glycogen due to the maternal oestrogen effect; then, with the withdrawal of oestrogen, the vaginal epithelium atrophies and the basal layer is covered by a thin, cornified epithelium.
- At menarche, the epithelium regenerates.
- At climacteric, the epithelium reverts to its prepubertal state.

Vaginal discharge

Physiological vaginal discharge is a product of vaginal mucosal transudate, cervical mucus and secretions from Bartholin's and Skene's glands. Excess physiological discharge occurs during pregnancy, sexual arousal, at mid-cycle/ovulation, with use of a high-oestrogen oral contraceptive or an intrauterine contraceptive device, and with large cervical ectropion.

Abnormal vaginal discharge may originate from diseases of the vagina, cervix, uterus or fallopian tubes. Causes of abnormal vaginal discharge include infections, foreign body, atrophic vaginitis and neoplasia of the upper and lower genital tract.

History
- colour, consistency, odour and duration of discharge
- blood-stained discharge
- pruritus, pain
- associations with menstrual cycle, coitus
- medical history (e.g. diabetes)
- medications, contraception
- cervical cytology

Examination
- general examination
- genital/pelvic: vulval examination
- speculum: examining vagina and cervix, checking discharge (colour, odour), cervical ectropion, malignancy, cervical cytology, microbiological swabs
- pelvic examination for cervical excitation and palpable masses

Vaginal infections

During the reproductive life, the vaginal pH is <4.5, and this offers some protection against infections.

Trichomonas
- It is a flagellate, about 20 microns in size.
- It presents with vaginal discharge and pruritus.
- Examination reveals a yellow/green frothy discharge, punctate injection of vagina with pH >5.0.
- Treat with metronidazole 400 mg orally three times a day for 7 days or a 2 g dose statim, and treat the partner.

Candida
- It presents with vaginal discharge and vulval pruritus, and curd-like patches which are adherent to the epithelium.
- Predisposing factors include pregnancy, premenstrual period of cycle, glucose intolerance, and the use of the oral contraceptive pill, antibiotics and corticosteroids.
- It may be distinguished as uncomplicated (isolated episodes, albicans species and normal host), and complicated (severe, recurrent, non-albicans *Candida* species, abnormal host).
- Treatment: miconazole, econazole or clotrimazole inserted into the vagina for the short term, or single-dose oral fluconazole. Complicated *Candida* requires longer duration therapy.

Gardnerella vaginalis
- It is also called bacterial vaginosis.
- It is a highly prevalent polymicrobial syndrome.
- The vaginal epithelium is coated with the small bacteria; on microscopy, clue cells are present.
- It is present in up to 40% of women.
- It presents with grey, frothy, offensive discharge and pruritus.
- Treat with metronidazole 400 mg orally three times a day for 7 days or 2 g dose statim, or vaginal clindamycin cream.

Postmenopausal woman
- Atrophy secondary to oestrogen deficiency predisposes to bleeding and secondary infection.
- Perform microbiological swabs and cervical cytology.
- Treat with oestrogen if atrophic.

Other vaginal conditions
Cysts
- Endometriosis: involves pain, dyspareunia, postcoital bleeding.
- Gartner's duct runs lateral and anterolateral, at any level from the cervix to urethra. If it is small, no treatment is required; marsupialise if large.

Fistula
- It occurs between the vagina and gastrointestinal or genitourinary system.
- It may be congenital or acquired.

Vaginal intraepithelial neoplasia (VAIN)

VAIN coexists with cervical intraepithelial neoplasia in 1%–3% of cases. The mean age at diagnosis is 52 years. The cause is unknown, but it may be associated with the human papillomavirus (HPV).

Classification
- VAIN1: low-grade squamous intraepithelial lesion
- VAIN2 and VAIN3: high-grade squamous intraepithelial lesion

There is no adequate study to prove the progression of VAIN to cancer. If the lesion is small, treatment options include an excisional biopsy, topical chemotherapy with imiquimod (Aldara) or 5-fluorouracil (5-FU), laser or cryotherapy.

Vaginal carcinoma

It may be primary or secondary. It usually occurs by direct spread or metastasis from the cervix, uterus, vulva, bladder, rectum or sigmoid colon. It accounts for 1% of female genital tract cancer. Squamous cell cancer presents in the sixth to seventh decade of life.

Histopathology
- Primary disease is usually squamous cell (80%–90%) or adenocarcinoma.
- Clear-cell adenocarcinoma is related to maternal diethylstilboestrol ingestion.
- Rarer tumours include melanoma, sarcoma botryoides, verrucous squamous cell carcinoma and endodermal sinus tumour.

Presentation, site and spread
- It involves postmenopausal bleeding, vaginal discharge, pain and urinary symptoms.
- Diagnosis can be missed if the lesion is small. A Pap smear may detect malignant cells in 20% of cases.
- About 50% occur in the upper vagina, 30% in the lower vagina and 20% in the mid-vagina.
- Posterior-wall tumour is the most common, followed by anterior-wall and lateral-wall; therefore, the most common site is in the posterior upper third, and then anterior lower third of the vagina.
- Spread is by direct extension and via the lymphatic system.

Investigations
- examination under anaesthesia and biopsy
- cystoscopy, sigmoidoscopy
- chest X-ray, ultrasound scan, computed tomography (CT) scan, intravenous pyelogram

FIGO staging for primary cancer of the vagina
This is a clinical (not surgical) staging (same as for cervical cancer).
- stage 1: limited to the vaginal wall
- stage 2: involvement of subvaginal tissue, but not extending to the pelvic wall
  - 2A: subvaginal infiltration, but not to the parametrium
  - 2B: parametrial involvement, but not to the pelvic wall
- stage 3: tumour extending to the pelvic wall
- stage 4: involves mucosa bladder/rectum; extends beyond the true pelvis
  - 4A: spread to adjacent organs and/or direct extension beyond the true pelvis
  - 4B: spread to distant organs

Five-year survival rates
- stage 1: 70%–80%
- stage 2: 30%–45%

- stage 3: 25%
- stage 4: 0%–30%

Management of vaginal cancer
- Therapy is individualised depending on the stage and site of vaginal disease.
- Generally, radiotherapy and/or surgical excision are performed.
- Stage 1 upper vaginal <2 cm lesions can be treated with either surgery (radical hysterectomy, upper vaginectomy, bilateral pelvic lymphadenectomy) or intra-cavitary radiotherapy.
- Less radical surgery may be appropriate as the primary treatment in some forms of vaginal cancer (e.g. basal cell carcinoma).
- Chemoradiation therapy is currently being assessed.

Further reading

Berek S, Hacker N (eds) 2005 Practical gynecologic oncology, 4th edn. Philadelphia: Lippincott Williams & Wilkins

Joura EA 2002 Epidemiology, diagnosis and treatment of vulvar intraepithelial neoplasia. Current Opinion in Obstetrics and Gynecology 14:39–43

Shafi M, Luesley D, Jordan J (eds) 2001 Handbook of gynaecological oncology. London: Churchill Livingstone

Stewart EG 2002 Developments in vulvovaginal care. Current Opinion in Obstetrics and Gynecology 14:483–488

Chapter 24

Benign vulval disease

Neroli Ngenda

Infections

Fungal
Candida albicans
- predisposed groups: newborns, females between puberty and menopause, postmenopausal women on hormone replacement therapy (HRT), women with diabetes mellitus
- symptoms: vulval pruritus, cheesy discharge, dyspareunia
- premenstrual and postcoital exacerbation can occur
- diagnosis: on vaginal swab
- treatment: vaginal imidazoles (e.g. clotrimazole) and, if required, single-dose oral therapy fluconazole; vaginal boric acid may be used
- apply imidazoles and boric acid intravaginally only, not to the vulva
- longer term oral therapy may be required for recurrent candidiasis (e.g. ketoconazole, fluconazole)

Non-albicans yeast infection
- *Candida glabrata, C. krusei, C. parapsilosis, C. guillermondii*
- relatively resistant to imidazoles
- boric acid is used for treatment

Tinea cruris
- It produces a well-demarcated erythematous lesion extending from the labia to the inner aspect of the thigh.
- Diagnosis is via microscopy of scrapings.
- Topical treatment with imidazoles may help; however, oral antifungal treatment is required for cure (e.g. griseofulvin).

Pityriasis versicolor (tinea versicolor)
- caused by *Malassezia furfur*
- may be asymptomatic or cause vulval pruritus
- treatment: topical or oral azoles

Viral
- herpes simplex virus 1 and 2
- human papillomavirus
- molluscum contagiosum

Bacterial
- pyogenic vulval infection (impetigo, folliculitis, abscess, carbuncle, cellulitis), Bartholin's gland infection, chancroid, donovanosis, syphilis, lymphogranuloma venereum

Parasitic

- pediculosis pubis (pubic lice), scabies, worms, trichomoniasis, schistosomiasis, filariasis, hydatid disease

Non-infectious dermatoses

Contact/allergic dermatitis

- may be triggered by local irritants (e.g. perfumes, soaps, fabric softeners, detergents, feminine sprays, urine, pads and panty liners, toilet paper); drugs; topical creams; latex in condoms
- causes vulval pruritus
- examination may reveal vulval erythema and/or swelling; fissuring in the interlabial sulci may occur
- lichenification can occur from scratching
- important to exclude the presence of candidiasis
- important to avoid the trigger and other irritants such as perfumes, soaps, fabric softener, nylon underwear, tight clothing, excessive pad/panty liner use, toilet paper with fragrance
- use aqueous cream or sorbelene to wash the vulva
- zinc, castor oil cream or Vaseline may be useful to protect the skin in cases of urinary incontinence
- topical steroids can assist in resolution

Lichen sclerosus

- can occur at any age, but is most common in postmenopausal women in whom it is a chronic condition
- also can occur in childhood (usually regresses at puberty)
- autoimmune condition
- causes vulval pruritus and eventually decreased clitoral sensation
- in advanced stages can result in dyspareunia due to introital stenosis
- sites of occurrence include the vulva, perineum and perianal area (spares the labia majora and vagina)
- examination includes the vulva and review of the perineum and perianal area
- the skin develops a white appearance; ecchymoses can develop
- the condition alters the vulval architecture resulting in atrophy (resorption of labia minora, phimosis of clitoral hood, introital stenosis, fissuring of the fourchette and/or vestibule during intercourse)
- malignant potential: 1%–4% risk of vulval squamous cell carcinoma (if adequately managed risk is reduced)
- biopsy is used to confirm the diagnosis
- histology reveals homogenised collagen in the upper dermis; basal layer vacuolar degeneration and lymphocytic inflammatory infiltrate; acanthosis of the epidermis
- in established lesions, histology reveals hyperkeratosis, dermal hyalinisation and fibrosis

Management

- Topical steroid therapy can be used for symptoms and to slow the progression of anatomical distortion.
- Treatment starts with potent topical steroids (e.g. betamethasone dipropionate; mometasone furoate 0.1%) and may move to mid-strength topical steroids for maintenance (e.g. betamethasone valerate 0.02%; triamcinolone acetonide).
- Use of topical pimecrolimus may be necessary in cases resistant to topical steroids.

- Vulval care is important: gentle drying of the vulva after washing; cease use of perfumes, deodorants, douches, soaps, fabric softeners, nylon underwear, tight clothing, excessive pad/panty liner use.
- The condition will recur after surgical excision; therefore, vulvectomy has no place.
- Surgery, however, may be necessary to exclude malignancy or to treat introital stenosis.
- Regular follow-up is required due to malignant potential; biopsy any suspicious lesions.

Lichen planus
- Aetiology is uncertain.
- Most cases affect the mucosa of the mouth and gums; 25% of cases have vulval involvement.
- Symptoms include pain, soreness, dyspareunia, discharge and bleeding from lesions.
- It causes epithelial erosions, usually on the medial aspect of the labia minora, extending to a variable degree into the vagina.
- In severe cases, adhesions can cause partial obliteration of the vagina.
- Treatment is with intravaginal steroids or pimecrolimus.
- Oral steroids may be required.
- Lignocaine gel applied prior to intercourse may be helpful.
- Vaginal dilators may be required to help decrease vaginal scarring.

Lichen simplex chronicus (LSC)
- refers to lichenified skin where no other pathology is diagnosed
- causes vulval pruritus especially at night
- skin thickening occurs in response to scratching
- the skin may appear white if moist; fissuring and excoriation may be present
- the condition may have commenced due to a pruritic process (e.g. allergic reactions, fungal infection)
- need to exclude other causes of vulval pruritus to make the diagnosis
- check for iron deficiency, which may be present in LSC
- treatment: topical steroids; behaviour modification (breaking the itch–scratch cycle); eliminate exposure to any irritants
- usually a good resolution if the itch–scratch cycle can be broken

Psoriasis
- autoimmune disease
- causes vulval pruritus
- lesions are erythematous and well demarcated
- no scale is present on vulval lesions
- spares the labia minora, clitoris and vestibule
- can extend to the natal cleft
- look for extragenital lesions to help establish the diagnosis (knees, elbows, scalp)
- treatment: topical steroids

Vulvodynia

- genital dyaesthesia described as pain, burning, stinging and irritation in the absence of visible findings or identified disease of the vulva or vagina
- neuropathic pain: increased concentration of nerve endings in the vestibule have been demonstrated
- can be provoked, unprovoked or mixed/generalised or localised

- may be triggered by: infection (recurrent candidiasis, herpes simplex virus, human papillomavirus), vulval laser or diathermy, trauma, vaginal surgery
- often no apparent trigger
- on examination with a Q-tip swab, one can find tenderness over the vestibular glands and vestibule (which may be erythematous)
- exclusion of candidiasis is imperative; if candidiasis is present, treat with long-term oral antifungals
- a biopsy is only indicated if there is suspicion of other vulval pathology (e.g. lichen sclerosus, vulval intraepithelial neoplasia)
- management involves a multidisciplinary approach: physiotherapy, psychologist (biofeedback), psychosexual counselling, pain management, support groups
- medication for treatment: low-dose amitriptyline or nortriptyline for 3–6 months; explain to patient that not being used as an antidepressant; antiepileptics (e.g. carbamazepine; gabapentin)
- lignocaine gel may be helpful for intercourse
- surgery: rarely indicated, but vestibulectomy may be required for refractory cases

Further reading

Dennerstein G, Scurry J, Brenan J, Allen D 2005 The vulva and vagina manual. Melbourne: Gynederm Publishing

Farage M, Galask R 2006 Vulvar vestibulitis syndrome: a review. National Vulvodynia Association News, USA Winter

Goldstein A 2006 Dermatological diseases of the vulval. National Vulvodynia Association News, USA, Summer

Chapter 25

Gestational trophoblastic disease

Amy Tang

Gestational trophoblastic diseases are disorders in which the normal regulatory mechanisms controlling the behaviour of trophoblastic tissue are lost.

Incidence. Incidence is 1 in 1400 pregnancies.

Hydatidiform mole

Risk factors
- varying between populations
- dietary factors
- maternal age >35 years (complete mole)
- previous molar pregnancy

Complete hydatiform mole
Chromosomes
- Origin is entirely paternal.
- It is usually a 23X duplication, with a haploid sperm fertilising an empty egg and duplicating itself.
- 46XY moles are rare.

Pathology
- no identifiable fetal tissue
- chorionic villi with generalised hydatidiform swelling and diffuse trophoblastic hyperplasia

Partial hydatidiform mole
Chromosomes
- It involves a triploid karyotype, paternal 46XX/XY and maternal 23X (i.e. a normal egg with dispermy).
- If maternal 46XX and paternal 23X or 23Y, the result is a triploid fetus.
- Thus, placental growth is dependent on paternal genetic material.

Pathology
- chorionic villi of varying size with focal hydatidiform swelling, cavitation and trophoblastic hyperplasia

- marked villous scalloping, prominent stromal trophoblastic inclusions
- identifiable fetal tissues

Presentation
- most diagnosed on ultrasound scan
- vaginal bleeding, hyperemesis
- uterus large for dates, theca lutein cysts
- pre-eclampsia, hyperthyroidism

Investigations
- full blood count, blood group and cross-match, quantitative human chorionic gonadotrophin (hCG)
- ultrasound scan of the pelvis, chest X-ray

Management
- suction curettage with oxytocics
- hysterectomy is an option if the woman has completed childbearing
- register in the trophoblastic registry

Follow-up
- involves weekly quantitative serum or 24-hour urinary hCG until normal (usually takes 8–12 weeks); then monthly hCG levels for 12 months (6 months if partial mole)
- contraception is required, and the oral contraceptive pill may be used
- advise to avoid pregnancy for at least 9 months after hCG levels return to normal

Persistent gestational trophoblastic disease

This is a complication for about 20% of women with complete moles and in up to 4% of partial moles. This condition is also known as gestational trophoblastic neoplasia.

Diagnosis and presentation
- plateau or rising hCG levels over 3 weeks after suction curettage
- delayed postevacuation bleeding
- raised hCG longer than 6 months
- evidence of metastatic disease
- presence of histologic choriocarcinoma

Investigations
- Assess risk factors and arrange further work-up: computed tomography (CT) scan of abdomen and pelvis, chest X-ray, quantitative hCG, full blood count, electrolytes, liver biochemistry.
- CT brain scan will also be required if presence of neurological symptoms or if lung/liver metastases are present.

Modified World Health Organization (WHO) scoring system for FIGO 2000 staging
This is used to determine if a patient belongs to a high-risk or low-risk group so the appropriate treatment can be offered. The prognostic factors used to calculate this score include: age, type of antecedent pregnancy, interval from index pregnancy, pretreatment hCG level, largest tumour size including uterus, site and number of

metastases, and presence of previous failed chemotherapy. A score <7 indicates low-risk group and a score of ≥7 indicates high-risk group.

Management

- For low-risk patients, single-agent chemotherapy is the first-line treatment. Cure rate for these patients is almost 100%.
- Methotrexate and folinic acid: 2-weekly courses continuing for two courses after hCG returns to normal.
- About 10% of patients suffer from side effects (especially serositis and mucosal ulceration) and require a change of chemotherapy to actinomycin D every 2 weeks.
- Treatment failure rate is 10%, and this requires second-line therapy: actinomycin D if hCG levels are below 100 IU/L; etoposide, methotrexate, actinomycin D, cyclophosphamide and oncovine (EMACO) if hCG levels are over 100 IU/L. Potential side effects include thrombocytopenia, hepatotoxicity and hair loss.
- Follow up patient with a weekly quantitative hCG until normal, and then monthly for 6–12 months.

High-risk gestational trophoblastic disease

Definition. This is a disease that is not cured by low-risk chemotherapy, or with a histological diagnosis of choriocarcinoma, or with other high-risk features such as metastatic disease in the brain or liver, over 12 months between the antecedent pregnancy and starting therapy and term antecedent pregnancy. WHO scoring =7 or more.

Investigations

- quantitative hCG, full blood count, electrolytes, liver biochemistry
- CT scans of chest, abdomen, pelvis and brain
- lumbar puncture to measure blood-to-cerebrospinal fluid hCG ratio (normally, the ratio is 65:1, but with metastases this is reversed)
- selective angiography of abdomen and pelvic organs if indicated
- histological confirmation not required

Management

- Follow the EMACO regimen.
- If the central nervous system is involved, use EMACO with 1000 mg methotrexate and intrathecal methotrexate 12.5 mg weekly.
- With a single large brain metastasis, seek neurosurgical review for possible removal before chemotherapy.
- Second-line therapy uses high-dose cisplatinum VP-16.

Follow-up

- weekly hCG tests
- four courses of chemotherapy continued after hCG returns to normal
- after chemotherapy, monthly hCG levels required for 2 years, and then 3-monthly levels for 3 years
- advise against pregnancy until hCG levels have been normal for 12 months
- cure in 80% of non-metastatic disease, 50% with metastatic disease
- if central nervous system metastases appear during or after high-risk chemotherapy, survival rate is 0%–20%

Theca lutein cysts

- These are present in 20%–25% of molar pregnancies.
- They are thin-walled benign cysts with an average size of 7 cm.
- They usually reduce in size with decreasing hCG levels.
- Complications include rupture, torsion and bleeding.
- If present after curettage, they are associated with a risk of persisting trophoblastic disease.
- Management of uncomplicated cysts is conservative.

Choriocarcinoma

- This is a malignant tumour of villous trophoblast with anaplastic syncytiotrophoblast and cytotrophoblast.
- It has a tendency to early vascular invasion and widespread dissemination.

Placental site trophoblastic tumour

- the least common form of gestational trophoblastic disease
- shows predominance of cytotrophoblast with little syncytium
- intermediate trophoblasts are present
- hCG levels are often low; human placental lactogen is produced by the tumour
- does not readily respond to standard chemotherapy
- diagnosis: by curettage
- treatment: surgically when disease confined to uterus

Further reading

Hancock BW, Tidy JA 2002 Current management of molar pregnancy. Journal of Reproductive Medicine 47:347–354

Royal College of Obstetricians and Gynaecologists (RCOG) Guidelines and Audit Committee 2009 The management of gestational trophoblastic disease. RCOG Greentop Guideline No. 38, 2nd draft, May. London: RCOG

Shapter AP, McLellan R 2001 Gestational trophoblastic disease. Obstetrics and Gynecology Clinics of North America 28:805–817

Appendix

Objective Structured Clinical Examinations (OSCEs) in gynaecology

Miriam Lee
Amy Mellor

Case 1

Information for candidate
Dear Doctor,

Thank you for seeing Liz, aged 36, in your gynaecology outpatient clinic. She has an 8-month history of hirsutism and irregular menses.

Yours sincerely,

Dr Jones

(General Practitioner)

Encounter 1

'I will play the role of the patient and you the gynaecologist. Please commence.'

Encounter 2

'So Doctor, what did my tests show?' (Results requested from encounter 1 supplied.)

Encounter 3

You are seeing Liz at 6 weeks postlaparotomy, total abdominal hysterectomy–bilateral salpingo-oopherectomy (TAH—BSO) and staging. (Histology report now supplied.)

'Doctor, what happens from here with respect to the cancer? I'm also having terrible hot flushes.'

Investigation results (if requested)
- beta-human chorionic gonadotropin (B-hCG): <2
- CA125: 12
- cortisol: normal
- 170H progesterone: normal
- dehydroepiandrosterone sulfate (DHEAS): normal
- testosterone: >200
- free androgen index: elevated
- prostaglandin E2/progesterone: normal
- luteinising hormone/follicle-stimulating hormone (LH/FSH): normal

Pelvic ultrasound
- 4 cm posterior wall fibroid
- endometrial thickness 6 mm
- normal left ovary
- 8 cm lesion in right adnexae, solid and cystic components
- increased vascularity
- no normal ovarian tissue seen

Histology
- right ovary: Sertoli-Leydig tumour
- normal left ovary, normal uterus
- washings negative, appendix and omental biopsies normal

Information for examiner
Case summary

The candidate plays the role of the gynaecologist in the outpatient clinic. Liz has been referred by her general practitioner with an 8-month history of hirsutism and irregular menses. She has a history of breast cancer, and on examination is found to have an 8 cm adnexal mass. An ultrasound reveals a complex lesion and androgen levels are raised. Gynae–oncology referral is called for, with an explanation of likely management. The patient returns following a TAH–BSO with a diagnosis of stage 1 Sertoli-Leydig tumour. The patient is suffering with hot flushes and a discussion of treatment options on a background of breast cancer is required.

Encounter 1
History
- increased hair growth on abdomen and face last 8/12
- previously regular cycles; now 2–3 days/2–3 months
- no weight gain
- normal Pap smear 1 year ago
- implanon in situ
- G2P2: both spontaneous vaginal delivery (SVD) at term (now aged 12 and 10)
- hypertension: on captopril 1 year
- modified radical mastectomy and chemotherapy 6 years ago for breast cancer
- nil allergies, non-smoker, social alcohol
- sister and aunt also with breast cancer

Examination
- body mass index: 25
- blood pressure: 150/90
- acne, facial and abdominal hirsutism
- palpable mass in right adnexae

Expectations of candidate
- history and examination
- order investigations
- hCG, CA125
- thyroid function tests, prolactin
- testosterone/free androgen index
- DHEAS, 17-OH progesterone, cortisol
- pelvic ultrasound
- organise follow-up

Encounter 2
Expectations of candidate
- explain possible suspicious nature of lesion
- arrange gynae–oncology referral
- staging investigations
- chest X-ray, computed tomography abdomen/pelvis, full blood count, enzyme liver function tests
- explain procedure
- laparoscopy, oophorectomy +/− laparotomy +/− staging +/− TAH–BSO if family complete

Encounter 3
History
- uneventful recovery
- hirsutism resolved
- several hot flushes/day, night sweats

Examination
- looks well
- laparotomy scar well healed
- no masses felt on bimanual

Expectations of candidate
- explain findings
- stage 1: prognosis good
- no adjunctive treatment required
- no hormone replacement therapy, as history of breast cancer; discuss alternatives (e.g. tibolone, venlafaxine)
- discuss referral for breast cancer gene (BRCA) testing
- organise follow-up

Scoring for case 1	
Encounter	**Mark**
Encounter 1	
• History and examination	____ out of 1
• Order investigations	____ out of 2
• Arrange follow-up	____ out of 1
Encounter 2	
• Explain possible diagnoses	____ out of 1
• Gynae–oncology referral	____ out of 1
• Staging investigation	____ out of 1
• Explain surgery	____ out of 1
Encounter 3	
• History and examination	____ out of 1
• Explain findings	____ out of 1
• Adjunctive treatment	____ out of 1
• Hormone replacement therapy	____ out of 2

(Continued)

Scoring for case 1—Cont'd	
Encounter	Mark
• BRCA	____ out of 1
• Follow-up	____ out of 1
Global competence	____ out of 5
TOTAL SCORE	**____ out of 20**

Case 2

Information for candidate

Dear Doctor,

Thank you for seeing Mrs Smith who is a 60-year-old woman with urinary incontinence.

Yours sincerely,

Dr Brown

(General Practitioner)

Encounter 1

'I will play the role of the patient and you the gynaecologist. Please commence.'

Encounter 2

'So Doctor, what do you think the problem is and what are you going to do?'

Encounter 3

Mrs Smith returns for a review 3 months later. She has been to the physiotherapist and has commenced oxybutynin. Mrs Smith tells you that:

- urgency is much improved; triggers resolved
- no urge incontinence
- voids six times during the day and 0–1 times at night
- voided volumes (from urinary diary) increased from an average of 100 mL to 250 mL
- still complains of urinary stress incontinence

'How can you help me doctor?'

Encounter 4

You are seeing Mrs Smith following her urodynamics. Here is the report:

First uroflowmetry
Voided 220 mL, normal flow rate
Residual volume 55 mL

Cystometrogram
Stable bladder, normal capacity
Maximal urethral closure pressure of 63 cm H20
Marked leakage in sitting position due to urodynamic stress incontinence

Second uroflowmetry
Good flow rate, voided to near completion

'So what are you going to do to help me doctor?'

Information for examiner
Case summary

The candidate plays the role of the gynaecologist in the outpatient clinic. Mrs Smith has been referred by her general practitioner with a history of urinary incontinence. She has mixed incontinence. Initial management is conservative with mid-stream specimen of urine (MSU), pelvic floor rehabilitation, reduction of caffeine, and anticholinergics plus topical oestrogen.

Mrs Smith responds well to the treatment of her overactive bladder and returns with ongoing urinary stress incontinence. Urodynamics confirms a stable bladder, urodynamic stress incontinence and no voiding problems.

The candidate is to discuss management options and risks of surgical options.

Encounter 1

History
- worsening urinary incontinence with activity (stress incontinence) over the past 5 years
- urgency
- occasional urge incontinence
- triggers: key in the door, turning on the taps
- daytime frequency/voids = 10
- nocturia = 3
- denies coital incontinence
- no voiding difficulty
- wears incontinence pads regularly
- no known urinary tract infection
- drinks 4–5 cups tea/coffee a day; total fluid intake 1500 mL
- constipation: for many years

Past history
- three vaginal deliveries
- total abdominal hysterectomy (TAH) at aged 42 for menorrhagia
- no glaucoma
- no other medical history

Examination
- body mass index: 25
- blood pressure: 140/80
- mild atrophy, no significant prolapse, no pelvic masses
- small urinary leak on coughing

Encounter 2
- explain that there is a mixed picture; treatment of the overactive bladder is conservative
- MSU
- urinary diary
- pelvic floor rehabilitation with physiotherapist/continence nurse
- reduce tea/coffee and increase water intake
- medication
  - anticholinergics: common side effect is constipation
  - topical oestrogen
- review

Expectations of candidate
- history and examination
- discuss management
- order MSU
- refer to physiotherapist/continence nurse
- organise follow-up

Encounter 3
- for urodynamic assessment

Expectations of candidate
- to explain procedure

Encounter 4
- Urodynamics has confirmed pure urodynamic stress incontinence.
- Mrs Smith has had a trial of conservative management. Surgery is a viable option.
- Management options for urodynamic stress incontinence: vaginal devices or surgery.

Surgical options
- primary procedure: slings, colposuspension
- risks: 15% failure to treat the stress incontinence, voiding difficulty with prolonged catheterisation or clean intermittent self-catheterisation, overactive bladder symptoms, injury to lower urinary tract and pelvic structures
- anaesthetic risks: deep venous thrombosis (DVT), bleeding, infection

Scoring for case 2	
Encounter	**Mark**
Encounter 1	
• Elicit history of mixed incontinence	____out of 2
• Risk factors (e.g. caffeine, constipation)	____out of 1
Encounter 2	
• Explain possible diagnoses	____ out of 2
• Investigation	____ out of 1
• Initial management (e.g. physiotherapy, caffeine)	____ out of 2
• Medical therapy and side effects	____ out of 2
Encounter 3	
• Order urodyamics	____ out of 1
• Explain urodynamics	____ out of 1
Encounter 4	
• Management	____out of 1
• Risks of surgery	____out of 2
Global competence	____ out of 5
TOTAL SCORE	____ **out of 20**

Case 3

Information for candidate
Dear Doctor,

Thank you for seeing Mrs Green who is a 67-year-old woman with symptoms of vaginal prolapse.

Yours sincerely,

Dr Lane

(General Practitioner)

Encounter 1

'I will play the role of the patient and you the gynaecologist. Please commence.'

Encounter 2

'So Doctor, how can you help me and what are you going to do? I do not want to have an operation.'

Encounter 3

Mrs Green returns 2 weeks later. The pessary fell out after a week. During the first week, she had good relief of the prolapse symptoms and was voiding much better.

'How can you help me doctor? What are my options now and can you tell me the risks?'

Information for examiner
Case summary
The candidate plays the role of the gynaecologist in the outpatient clinic. Mrs Green has been referred by her general practitioner with symptoms of vaginal prolapse and voiding dysfunction. Initial management is a mid-stream specimen of urine (MSU), check residual urine (ultrasound, in–out catheter or urodynamics), exclusion of a pelvic mass, pelvic floor rehabilitation and discussion about management, including vaginal pessary.

Mrs Green's voiding difficulty improves temporarily with a pessary, but the pessary fell out and the candidate needs to discuss surgical options, including vault suspension. The candidate is to discuss management options and risks of surgical options.

Encounter 1
History
- worsening vaginal lump over the past 9 months
- needs to reduce the prolapse frequently
- needs to reduce the prolapse to overcome voiding difficulty, no need to reduce to defecate
- urinary frequency, problems initiating voiding, especially as the day progresses
- daytime frequency/voids = 10
- nocturia = 3
- not sexually active at present, husband unwell
- urinary tract infection 6 weeks ago, no recent test
- no constipation
- no per vaginal bleeding

Past history
- four vaginal deliveries
- left inguinal hernia
- tubal ligation
- hypertension controlled

Examination
- body mass index: 28
- blood pressure: 130/85
- atrophy, thickening and cornification of cervix and anterior vaginal wall
- palpable bladder
- no urinary incontinence with prolapse reduced
- prolapse Aa+2, Ba+3, Ap+1, Bp+2, C+5
- significant anterior vaginal wall prolapse, posterior vagina wall prolapse and cervical descent

Encounter 2
- explain that there is a significant prolapse and probable voiding dysfunction
- MSU
- options: pessary, surgery
- patient does not want surgery
- assess voiding function: ultrasound, in–out catheter or urodynamics
- topical oestrogen
- review

Expectations of candidate
- history and examination
- discuss management
- order MSU
- check residual
- organise follow-up

Encounter 3
Pessary has fallen out. Mrs Green was voiding much better with the pessary in situ. There was also reduction in her frequency and no urinary stress incontinence.

Expectations of candidate
- try a bigger or different pessary (e.g. shelf)
- surgery: counselling
  - repair of anterior/posterior and vault suspension; possible uterine conservation
  - may be performed vaginally or abdominally or combination
  - voiding difficult may persist
  - risks of surgery
    - general surgical: anaesthetic, deep venous thrombosis (DVT), infection, bleeding
    - injury to pelvic structures (e.g. bladder/urethra, rectum, ureter)
    - dypspareunia
    - occult urodynamics stress incontinence
    - if sacrospinous colpopexy: buttock pain
    - recurrence of prolapse

Scoring for case 3	
Encounter	Mark
Encounter 1	
• History: elicit voiding difficulty	____ out of 2
• Examination	____ out of 1

(Continued)

Scoring for case 3—Cont'd	
Encounter	**Mark**
Encounter 2	
• Options: pessary and explain follow-up, risk	____ out of 2
• MSU	____ out of 1
• Check residual volume	____ out of 1
• Follow-up	____ out of 1
Encounter 3	
• Option 1: try bigger pessary or shelf pessary	____ out of 1
• Option 2: surgery	____ out of 1
• Types of surgery available	____ out of 2
• Risks of surgery include occult stress incontinence	____ out of 2
• Risk of ongoing voiding difficulty	____ out of 1
Global competence	____ out of 5
TOTAL SCORE	**____ out of 20**

Obstetrics

Chapter 26

Antenatal care

Michael Flynn

Prepregnancy care

Ideally, all couples should seek prepregnancy care. Most couples are not reviewed until after the critical fetal developmental period.

Aims of counselling before conception
- Advise the woman and her partner on general healthcare (e.g. on nutrition/diet/folate, smoking, alcohol and drugs).
- As the oral contraceptive pill may deplete red cell folate, use alternative contraception for 1 month while commencing folic acid.
- Carry out general screening, including rubella and varicella serology, and immunise when required; cervical cytology; blood pressure.
- Assess and advise on the effects of existing disease and its management on the pregnancy, and the effects of pregnancy on the disease. Treat preexisting diseases to minimise the problems that may arise in pregnancy.
- Assess and advise on the problems that may recur from previous pregnancies and deliveries.
- Provide genetic counselling with full genetic history, especially in high-risk racial groups.
- Preconception care often requires a team of obstetricians, physicians, geneticists, dietitians, and specialised educators such as diabetic educators.

Antenatal care

Antenatal clinics act as a screening tool to identify and then manage problems that arise during the pregnancy. As this is also often the first time healthy women are assessed, they may provide information for long-term healthcare.

Aims of antenatal care
- Screen and manage/prevent maternal problems.
- Screen and manage/prevent fetal problems.
- Provide antenatal education regarding general health, nutrition and childbirth.

Booking assessment
- history: age, gravidity, parity
- menstrual history
- problems so far in pregnancy, such as bleeding and nausea
- past obstetric and gynaecological history
- past medical/surgical history
- family and social history
- medication, drugs, alcohol and smoking
- allergies

Examination
- weight, height
- blood pressure, urinalysis
- general: teeth/gums, thyroid, breast, chest, heart, varicose veins
- abdomen: scars, fundal height, masses, pain
- pelvic: cervical cytology if indicated; vaginal examination

Investigations
First visit
- full blood examination
- ABO blood type, Rhesus blood group and antibodies (the antibody screen should be performed at the beginning of every pregnancy)
- rubella immunity (antibody titres may decline, so check at the start of each pregnancy)
- syphilis serology using specific *Treponema* assay (e.g. *T. pallidum* haemaglutination assay (TPHA))
- hepatitis B serology
- urine for culture and sensitivity
- hepatitis C and human immunodeficiency virus (HIV) serology, offered after appropriate counselling
- cervical cytology if no normal smear within the previous 18 months
  Other tests considered but not mandatory include:
- testing for vitamin D deficiency in dark-skinned or veiled women
- screening for haemoglobinopathies (especially if mean corpuscular volume (MCV) or *mean* corpuscular haemoglobin concentration (MCHC) are abnormal)
- varicella serology
- cytomegalovirus (CMV)/toxoplasma serology: recommended only in at-risk women and ideally as prepregnancy test

Discussion of antenatal screening
Antenatal screening for Down syndrome and other fetal aneuploidy should be discussed (*see Ch 27*).

Obstetric ultrasound scan at 18–20 weeks gestation
All women should be offered fetal morphology assessment prior to 20 weeks gestation.

Haemoglobin, platelet count, Rhesus antibody status
- should be reviewed at 28 weeks gestation
- if anaemic, then iron deficiency investigated

Gestational diabetes
Screening is recommended.

Group B streptococcus disease (GBS)
This is the leading cause of neonatal sepsis, which if left untreated would affect 1 in 200 newborns, with intrapartum chemoprophylaxis significantly decreasing infection rates. The decision for prophylaxis comes from either screening via low vagina/anorectal swab at 35–37 weeks gestation or treating via clinical risk factor analysis.

Continuing antenatal visits
- routine antenatal visits every 4 weeks to 28 weeks gestation, then every 2 weeks to 36 weeks gestation, then every week until delivery

- at each visit, assessment of:
  - history of events since previous visit, fetal movements, blood pressure, review of risk factors
  - fundal height, clinical amniotic fluid assessment, fetal heart sounds, and (in the third trimester) fetal lie and presentation
  - discussion of anti-D prophylaxis at 28 and 34 weeks gestation, and at any time of blood loss in a Rhesus-negative woman

Indications for ultrasound scan in antenatal care

- First trimester: vaginal bleeding, abdominal pain, hyperemesis gravidarum, before procedures (e.g. amniocentesis, chorionic villus sampling or cervical suture). Down syndrome screening and definitive diagnosis of multiple pregnancies is offered early in the second trimester.
- Second trimester: at 18–20 weeks to confirm dates, assess fetal morphology and exclude multiple pregnancies; to assess complications of pregnancy, including antepartum haemorrhage, threatened premature labour and preterm prelabour rupture of membranes.
- Third trimester: fundal height small or large for gestation, previous intrauterine growth restriction, multiple pregnancies, antepartum haemorrhage, malpresentation, maternal medical conditions such as diabetes, renal disease, pre-eclampsia. Late pregnancy tests of fetal wellbeing for assessment of the fetoplacental function may be appropriate.

Chapter 27

Antenatal diagnosis of fetal and chromosomal abnormalities

Jackie Chua

In all, 2%–3% of children are born with a significant physical/mental handicap, and a further 3% have mild retardation.

Major malformations are present in 10%–15% of abortions, 50% of stillbirths and 3% of newborns. One-third of malformations are associated with genetic abnormalities. Table 27.1 lists causes of malformation. Multifactorial causes of malformation include neural tube defects, congenital heart defects or cleft lip/palate. The recurrence rate is about 2%–4%.

Indications for prenatal diagnosis

- chromosomal abnormalities: suspected parental carriers, maternal age, previously affected pregnancy, known abnormality in either parent
- metabolic disease
- neural tube defect
- isoimmunisation
- skeletal dysplasia
- all women with a high risk
- fetus with a diagnosable defect

Tests available for antenatal diagnosis

Screening
- maternal age
- first trimester: combined nuchal translucency
- second trimester: triple/quadruple test, morphology test

Diagnosis
- first trimester: chorionic villus sampling
- second trimester: amniocentesis
- other: fetal blood sampling

Table 27.1 Causes of malformation

Cause	Incidence
Single gene defect	9%
Chromosomal defect	6%
Multifactorial	20%
Environmental	5%
Unknown	60%

Genetic counselling

All women who choose to have an antenatal screening test should have access to adequate counselling. Specialist genetic counselling clinics should be available for:
- discussion of abnormal screening tests
- discussion of abnormal ultrasound and karyotype findings
- patients with a family history of genetic disorders
- a specific medical condition of the mother with possible fetal transmission (e.g. human immunodeficiency virus (HIV))
- three or more miscarriages
- consanguinity
- chemical or radiation exposure in pregnancy

Indications for genetic counselling
- previously affected child
- history of genetic condition in family
- consanguinity
- advanced maternal age
- prenatal diagnosis
- physically or mentally handicapped parent

Aims of genetic counselling
- make accurate diagnosis
- provide adequate pedigree information
- explain risks to family
- identify methods of avoiding or decreasing risks
- arrange follow-up
- explain options available: ignore risks, have no more children, adoption, sperm or ovum donation, prenatal diagnosis and selective termination

Indications for chromosome studies
- recurrent abortion
- fetus or infant suggestive of malformation
- fetus or infant with one or more malformations
- fetus over 13 weeks gestation with ambiguous genitalia
- macerated fetus/stillbirth
- severe intrauterine growth restriction
- advanced maternal age

Distribution of chromosomal abnormalities
- first-trimester abortion: 50%–60%
- second-trimester abortion: 35%
- stillbirths: 5%
- live births: 0.5%

After two or more abortions, there is a 5% chance of chromosomal abnormalities in the parents. This rises to 10% with four or more abortions.

Screening

Risk assessment
- low or high risk for aneuploidy
- maternal age: >35 years high risk for aneuploidy

Combined nuchal translucency and biochemical screening
- combined nuchal translucency (ultrasound assessment performed between 11 weeks and 1 day and 13 weeks and 6 days) and biochemical screening (free beta-human chorionic gonadotrophin (HCG) and pregnancy-associated plasma protein A (PAPP-A) combined with maternal age)
- detection rate of 90%, with a false-positive of 5%
- other markers used to increase sensitivity (but not currently used in the Australian risk assessment program) include:
  - presence or absence of nasal bone
  - presence or absence of tricuspid regurgitation
  - presence or absence of ductus venosus A-wave
  - fetal maxillary facial angle
  - biochemical markers may also be used to screen for pre-eclampsia, intrauterine growth restriction and fetal demise

Second-trimester screening
- Screening is performed using alpha-fetoprotein (AFP), unconjugated estriol, free beta-hCG and inhibin A combined with maternal age. Sensitivity is 70%.
- AFP is the principal plasma protein of the fetus in early gestation. It is initially produced in the yolk sac, and then the fetal liver and gut:
  - Fetal AFP: plasma levels peak at 12–13 weeks gestation and fall throughout pregnancy.
  - Maternal serum AFP rises in the second trimester, reaches maximum levels at approximately 30 weeks and then falls.
  - Amniotic fluid AFP parallels levels in the fetal plasma, but in a ratio of 1:200.
  - Raised AFP (>2.0 multiples of the median (MoM)) may be due to neural tube defects, gastrointestinal defects (omphalocele, gastroschisis, oesophageal and duodenal atresia), cystic hygroma, threatened abortion or antepartum haemorrhage, fetal death in utero, multiple pregnancy and advanced gestation.

Ultrasound screening
- There is 50% sensitivity for babies with Down syndrome.
- Nearly all trisomy 13/18 have ultrasound findings.
- Previous soft markers of echogenic focus in the heart, choroid plexus cysts and hypoplasia of the middle phalanx of the fifth finger are not generally used anymore.

Definitive diagnosis tests

- Fluorescent in situ hybridisation (FISH) analysis for trisomy and specific marker genes may give rapid diagnosis.
- Confirmation is from long-term culture karyotypes.
- Free fetal DNA for Rhesus (Rh) cases in the future.

Amniocentesis
- It is usually performed after 16 weeks gestation when the amnion has fused with the chorion.
- Information gained includes chromosomes and DNA analysis, AFP and enzymology.
- Fetal loss is 1 in 200 procedures.
- False-positive results occur in 0.3%, inadequate cell collection in up to 2% of samples, and maternal contamination in 1 of 1000 samples.
- Anti-D prophylaxis is required if the woman is RhD-negative.

Chorionic villus sampling
- It is usually performed at 11–14 weeks gestation. As the sample is directly from the chorion, there is a 1% risk of mosaicism (i.e. the presence of a genetic cell line that is not fetal, but purely placental in origin and therefore a false-positive result). If this occurs, amniocentesis is required for fetal karyotyping.
- An earlier test has the advantage that termination of pregnancy may be performed earlier, possibly operatively rather than induction in comparison with amniocentesis.
- The tissue may be collected transabdominally or transcervically. The risk of fetal loss from the procedure is 1%–2%.
- It has a false-positive rate of 2%, inadequate specimen collection in up to 8%, and maternal contamination in 1%–2%. Up to 4% of cases require follow-up by amniocentesis.
- The oromandibular limb hypogenesis syndrome has been reported with procedures performed at 56–66 days gestation and is probably due to vascular insult in early pregnancy.

Cordocentesis/fetal blood sampling
- collection of fetal blood sample from cord; performed in second and third trimester
- use: fetal karyotype, viral serology, full blood count, blood group, blood gases, metabolic abnormalities and DNA analysis, as well as treatment such as transfusion
- fetal loss of 1%–2%

Chromosomal abnormalities

Translocations
- If the mother has a translocation, there is a 10% recurrence risk.
- If the father has a translocation, there is a 2% recurrence risk.

Reciprocal translocation
If this is demonstrated through an unbalanced translocation in the offspring, the risk of unbalanced translocation in another offspring is 10%–20% for female carriers and 5%–10% for male carriers. If amniocentesis shows a balanced translocation and the parents have normal chromosomes, the child will look normal, but there is a 1 in 8 risk of intellectual handicap, as some genes may be lost during the translocation.

Robertsonian translocation

This involves acrocentric chromosomes (13, 14, 15 21 and 22). The carrier has 45 chromosomes. Be aware of the risk of uniparental disomy with the imprinted chromosomes (i.e. 14 and 15). Of people with Down syndrome, 4% have a parent with a Robertsonian translocation. When the translocation occurs on the same chromosome, the risk of another affected child is 100%.

Trisomies

After one affected fetus, the recurrence risk is 1% plus the risk for maternal age.

Trisomy 21
- Incidence is 1 in 800 live births.
- The only factor related to trisomy 21 is maternal age (see Table 27.2).

The incidence of all chromosomal abnormalities is about twice that of trisomy 21. Women affected by trisomy 21 are often infertile. However, if the woman becomes pregnant, the risk of trisomy 21 to her offspring is 33%, which is less than the expected 50% because of an increased trisomic loss in early pregnancy.

Other genetic syndromes

Fragile X syndrome
- incidence of 1 in 1000 male births; responsible for 25% of male intellectual handicap
- second only to trisomy 21 as a chromosomal cause of mental impairment; 35% of heterozygote females are mentally impaired
- prenatal testing available, though parental karyotype comparison important
- diagnosis by presence of nucleotide triplet repeat and expansion of >220 repeats in males.

Cystic fibrosis

This is an autosomal recessive disorder, with an incidence in Caucasians of 1 in 2500 and a carrier frequency of 1 in 25.

Genetics. The mutant gene is the cystic fibrosis transmembrane conductance regulator, situated on the long arm of chromosome 7 (CFTR gene). In 75% of cases, cystic fibrosis is due to the deletion of a single codon (delta F508 is the most common).

Screening. If one parent has a close relative with cystic fibrosis, then the carrier risk is reduced to a 1 in 99 chance by a negative result in tests for F508 and other common gene deletions. Prenatal diagnosis may be necessary if ultrasound abnormalities are discovered, such as hyperechogenic bowel. Prenatal diagnosis is possible by 12–19

Table 27.2 Risk of trisomy 21	
Maternal age	Risk
20	1 in 2000
25	1 in 1200
30	1 in 700
35	1 in 400
37	1 in 250
40	1 in 100
43	1 in 50

mutation panel, which detects 80% of the most common mutations. The whole CFTR gene can be sequenced (sent to New Zealand).

Muscular dystrophies

Duchenne muscular dystrophy has an incidence of 0.3 in 1000 male births. It is an X-linked recessive disorder with the mutant gene at Xp21. Presentation is one of progressive muscle wasting, with death in the second or third decade of life. Diagnosis is based on the absence of dystrophins on immunoblotting muscle biopsy.

Myotonic dystrophy is an autosomal dominant inheritance with associated abnormalities of mental retardation, cataracts, diabetes, cardiomyopathy and infertility. Pregnancy in an affected woman can increase the severity of disease, causing prolonged labour, uterine atony, postpartum haemorrhage and polyhydramnios.

Phenylketonuria

- Phenylketonuria has an incidence of 1 in 12,000 births. It is an autosomal recessive disorder.
- The pathology is that of an inborn error of metabolism with a deficiency of the enzyme phenylalanine hydroxylase. This enzyme converts phenylalanine to tyrosine. In phenylalanine hydroxylase deficiency, there is a rise in serum phenylalanine levels in children, leading to impaired myelination of the brain and subsequent mental retardation.
- The concentration gradient across the placenta produces fetal levels that are twice maternal levels.

Marfan's syndrome

Marfan's syndrome is an autosomal dominant connective tissue disorder.

Neurofibromatosis

Neurofibromatosis is an autosomal dominant disorder.

Thalassaemia

Alpha-thalassaemia is due to gene deletion. Beta-thalassaemia has more than 40 gene mutations. Both have lethal forms.

Incidence in ethnic and racial groups

Genetic disorders are more common in certain ethnic and racial groups. For example:
- Ashkenazi Jews: Tay-Sachs disease
- African Americans: sickle cell anaemia
- South-East Asians, Greeks, Italians: thalassaemia

Morphology ultrasound assessment

Under defined protocol, assessments are performed typically between 18 and 20 weeks gestation. Common anomalies screened include the following.

Trisomy 21

Detection features include short femur/humerus, cardiovascular lesions such as atrioventricular septal defect, duodenal atresia, hypoplastic nasal bone and growth restriction with polyhydramnios.

Trisomy 18

- The incidence is 1 in 3000.
- Diagnostic features include congenital heart disease, diaphragmatic hernia, omphalocele and growth restriction.

- Choroid plexus cysts are present in 1%–2.5% of normal fetuses (previously associated with trisomy 18, so look at previous screening and other ultrasound features for trisomy 18).

Trisomy 13
- The incidence is 1 in 5000.
- Diagnostic features include congenital heart disease, omphalocele, renal abnormalities and intrauterine growth restriction holoprosencephaly.

Neural tube defects
- includes anencephaly and spina bifida
- detection rate: close to 100%
- incidence: 1 in 650 births
- prevention: 4 mg folic acid per day can reduce the risk of recurrence of neural tube defect from 3.5% to 1%; supplementation with folate should begin 3 months before conception and continue to the end of the first trimester; also helpful for cleft lip and palate
- increased risk of recurrence with a previous history of spina bifida and anencephalics
- diagnosis: uses ultrasound scan—open defect of the spine seen with or without intracranial head signs; maternal serum AFP (false-negative occurs in 12% of anencephalics and 21% of open spina bifida); amniotic fluid AFP (not used any more); ultrasound markers of associated chromosome anomalies

Gastrointestinal anomalies
- include tracheo-oesophageal fistula (causing polyhydramnios and absent stomach)
- omphalocele is a ventral wall with variable degree of herniation of abdominal contents with covering membrane present; can be associated with trisomies
- gastroschisis is a full thickness ventral wall defect, with no membrane present, which can be diagnosed after 12 weeks (after physiological herniation of the bowel has resolved); not usually associated with chromosome abnormalities
- duodenal atresia, on ultrasound scan, has a characteristic double-bubble sign; up to 50% of these fetuses will have other abnormalities and 30% are associated with trisomy 21

Renal tract anomalies
- Those detected on ultrasound scan include renal agenesis resulting in oligohydramnios, congenital polycystic kidneys and renal tract obstruction.
- A common renal finding is renal pelvis dilatation. Postnatal paediatric review is usually recommended.
- Renal function is reflected by liquor volume and is associated with pulmonary hypoplasia.

Cardiac abnormalities
- incidence of 4 in 1000 live births
- complex cardiac defects: paediatric cardiology review recommended as some anomalies have improved outcome with antenatal diagnosis

Dwarfism
- In the heterozygote for achondroplasia, bony abnormalities may not be obvious on ultrasound scan until 24 weeks gestation. It can be non-lethal.
- Bony characteristics for lethal skeletal dysplasias should be looked for, especially if early onset.
- Genetic counselling is recommended.

Cleft lip/palate
- higher incidence in males
- recurrence rate: 4% with one sibling
- simple cleft lip not usually associated with chromosome abnormality but median or bilateral cleft lip and palate can be, especially with trisomy 13

Further reading and resources

Bethune M 2007 Management options for echogenic intracardiac focus and choroid plexus cysts: a review including the Australian Association of Obstetrical and Gynaecological Ultrasonologists consensus statement. Australasian Radiology 51:324–329

Callen PW 2007 Ultrasonography in obstetrics and gynecology. Philadelphia: Elsevier Saunders

Dugoff L, Hobbins JC, Malone FD et al 2005 First-trimester maternal serum PAPP-A and free-beta subunit human chorionic gonodatropin concentrations and nuchal translucency are associated with obstetric complications: a population-based screening study (the FASTER Trial). American Journal of Obstetrics and Gynecology 191 (4):1446–1451

Nicolaides KH 2003 Screening for chromosomal defects. Ultrasound in Obstetrics and Gynecology 21:313–321

Nuchal Translucency Ultrasound, Education and Monitoring Program: www.nuchaltrans.edu.au/index.shtml

Nyberg DA, McGahan JP, Pretorius DH, Pilu G 2003 Imaging of fetal anomalies. Philadelphia: Lippincott Williams & Wilkins

Wald NJ, Rodeck C, Hackshaw AK, Rudnicka A 2004 SURUSS in perspective. BJOG: an International Journal of Obstetrics and Gynaecology 111:521–531

Chapter 28

Assessing fetal wellbeing

Jackie Chua

The method used in the assessment of fetal wellbeing depends on:
- level of risk to the fetus
  - low-risk pregnancy
  - high-risk pregnancy
- antenatal or intrapartum monitoring

In a fetus with low-risk status, screening only fetal movements has been shown to identify the fetus at risk of intrauterine death.

Tests available for assessing fetal wellbeing

- fetal movement, including kick charts
- cardiotocography (CTG)
- biophysical assessment
- amniotic fluid volume assessment
- growth
- Doppler flow studies
- fetal scalp pH or lactate

Fetal movement
Antepartum stillbirths account for 50% of the perinatal mortality rate. In late antepartum intrauterine fetal death, 60% occur at less than 37 weeks gestation and 2% at gestation over 42 weeks.

Fetal movement in late pregnancy
- Activity of individual fetuses varies, with only 1% of quiet phases lasting over 45 minutes.
- The perception of fetal movement varies between different women. There is reduced activity in fetuses with malformations.
- There appears to be no advantage to formal counting compared with informal inquiry at antenatal clinic.
- Fetal movement assessment should be used as a screening test to prompt other investigations.

High-risk pregnancies, including hypertensive disorders, vascular diseases, thyroid disease, diabetes, isoimmunisation, multiple pregnancies, as well as reduced fetal movements, vaginal bleeding and prolonged pregnancy, should have regular assessment, including umbilical artery Doppler recordings, fetal growth measurement, amniotic fluid volume, as well as CTG and biophysical profile score.

Cardiotocography (CTG)

A CTG is considered normal when the fetal baseline heart rate is between 120 and 160 beats/minute, the variability of heart rate is between 5 and 25 beats/minute, there are two or more accelerations in a 10-minute period and there are no baseline decelerations. An acceleration of fetal heart rate is a rise in heart rate of ≥15 beats/minute and lasting for 15 seconds or more.

Non-stress test (NST) is a reactive CTG where there are two accelerations exceeding 15 beats/minute amplitude and 15-second duration in 20 minutes.

Some factors that need to be taken into consideration when interpreting a CTG are the gestational age, drugs administered to the mother, the speed of the paper (usually at 1 cm/minute), maternal positioning and fetal abnormalities (e.g. complete heart block).

The variability represents fetal reserve and is an indicator of central, cerebral and myocardial oxygenation. If the period of unreactivity lasts longer than 40 minutes, this is considered a suspicious CTG. If the resting phase is over 120 minutes in duration, the positive predictive value for fetal morbidity/mortality is up to 85%.

False-positive rates of CTG in prediction of fetal hypoxia are up to 20%–40%. False-negative rates are 0.3/1000 for stillbirth and 7/1000 for hypoxia or acidosis. About 10%–15% of CTG recordings are unsatisfactory for interpretation.

Vibroacoustic stimulation has been shown to shorten testing time and the incidence of a non-reassuring CTG in term fetuses. Positive result elicits an acceleration after application.

Biophysical assessment

Biophysical assessment involves the following five parameters with a score of 0 or 2 for each:

- CTG
- fetal breathing movement >30 seconds in 30 minutes
- fetal movements of at least three in 30 minutes
- fetal tone considered normal if prompt return to flexion after extension of limbs/trunk
- amniotic fluid volume: more than one pool of >2 cm in two planes

Table 28.1 lists perinatal mortality rates for biophysical assessment scores.

- false-positive rate 50%
- not shown to improve outcome in high-risk pregnancies
- however, normal biophysical assessment has a good negative predictive value and tends to be reflective of the normal Doppler readings

Amniotic fluid volume assessment

- amniotic fluid volume is a reflection of fetal wellbeing or placental health
- different methods of measurement: amniotic fluid index (AFI), deepest vertical pocket (DVP)

Table 28.1 Biophysical assessment: perinatal mortality rates	
Score	Perinatal mortality rate
8–10/10	<1 in 1000 (false-negative 0.9/1000)
6/10	>90 in 1000
4/10	60–600 in 1000

- decreased liquor volume is associated with increased perinatal mortality and increased risk of operative delivery
- should be used in conjunction with other methods

Growth
- In high-risk pregnancies, estimated fetal weight can help identify the small-for-gestational-age pregnancies.
- Customised growth charts for ethnicity have been proposed.

Doppler flow studies
- low-risk pregnancies: not shown to reduce mortality or morbidity
- high-risk pregnancies:
  - fetal umbilical artery Doppler monitoring reduces perinatal morbidity and mortality
  - also can decrease inductions
  - the risk increases with the worsening of Doppler flow
  - resistance index (RI) thought to be best predictor of outcome
  - other blood vessels have been investigated for prediction of adverse pregnancy outcomes, such as uterine artery Doppler, but not currently used routinely
  - mainly helpful in timing of delivery

Fetal scalp pH or lactate
- Test in labour when the membranes have ruptured.
- The pH is proportional to pCO_2 and lactic acid.
- In the first stage of labour, the mean fetal scalp pH is 7.33.
- A pH >7.25 is regarded as normal.
- A pH of 7.20–7.25 is an equivocal result; repeat in 1 hour.
- A pH <7.20 indicates acidosis; delivery should be undertaken immediately.

Other methods of assessment in labour are fetal pulse oximetry and fetal scalp lactate testing. A lactate reading >4.2 mmol/L may be more sensitive then scalp pH for adverse outcome.

Further reading

Bricker L, Neilson JP 2000 Routine Doppler ultrasound in pregnancy. Cochrane Database of Systematic Reviews. Issue 2. Art. No. CD001450. DOI: 10.1002/14651858

Devoe LD 2008 Antenatal fetal assessment: contraction stress test, nonstress test, vibroacoustic stimulation, amniotic fluid volume, biophysical profile, and modified biophysical profile—an overview. Seminars in Perinatology 32:247–252

East CE, Leader LR, Colditz PB et al 2006 Intrapartum fetal scalp lactate sampling for fetal assessment in the presence of a non-reassuring fetal heart rate trace. Cochrane Database of Systematic Reviews, Issue 4. Art. No. CD006174. DOI: 10.1002/14651858

Gribbin C, James D 2004 Assessing fetal health. Best Practice and Research Clinical Obstetrics and Gynaecology 18 (3):411–424

Lalor JG, Fawole B, Alfirevic Z, Devane D 2008 Biophysical profile for fetal assessment in high risk pregnancies. Cochrane Database of Systematic Reviews. Issue 1. Art. No. CD000038. DOI: 10.1002/14651858

Nabhan AF, Abdelmoula YA 2008 Amniotic fluid index versus single deepest vertical pocket as a screening test for preventing adverse pregnancy outcome. Cochrane Database of Systematic Reviews. Issue 3. Art. No. CD006593. DOI: 10.1002/14651858

Tan KH, Smyth RMD 2001 Fetal vibroacoustic stimulation for facilitation of tests of fetal wellbeing. Cochrane Database of Systematic Reviews. Issue 1. Art. No. CD002963. DOI: 10.1002/14651858

Chapter 29

Drugs and drugs of abuse in pregnancy

Justin Nasser

The decision on whether to prescribe a drug to pregnant women must take into account the risk of the therapy and the risk of withholding the treatment. This requires a thorough up-to-date understanding of the drug and its risk/benefit ratio in pregnancy, as well as knowledge about the pharmacokinetics of the drug in pregnancy and the accurate assessment of the gestational age at the time of possible in utero exposure.

During the period from fertilisation to implantation, the pregnancy is relatively immune from teratogenic effects from medications, as the fetomaternal circulation has not developed. The period of organogenesis (17–70 days postconception) is when the embryo is most susceptible to teratogens. After this period, the risk of structural defects abates, but the fetus may be affected by anomalies in the functional development of organs and systems.

Teratogens

A teratogen is an agent that acts to irreversibly alter the growth, structure or function of a developing embryo or fetus. Recognised teratogens include:
- viruses (e.g. rubella, cytomegalovirus)
- environmental factors (e.g. hyperthermia, irradiation)
- chemicals (e.g. mercury)
- therapeutic/recreational drugs

Information on the teratogenic effect of specific medications is not always readily available, as few therapies have been specifically tested for safety and efficacy in human pregnancies. Current methods to assess teratogenic risk rely on pregnancy registries and case-control surveillance studies which have inherent shortcomings in design.

Information about the potential teratogenic risk of medications can be sourced from the Australian Government Therapeutic Goods Administration (see Box 29.1) and online databases (see Box 29.2).

Drug pharmacokinetics and pregnancy

Drug pharmacokinetics is affected by the complex changes that occur in maternal, fetal and placental physiology during pregnancy.

Box 29.1 **Australian categorisation of drugs in pregnancy**

Category A
These are drugs which have been taken by a large number of pregnant women and women of childbearing age without any proven increase in the frequency of malformations or other direct or indirect harmful effects on the fetus having been observed.

Category B
These are drugs which have been taken by only a limited number of pregnant women and women of childbearing age without an increase in the frequency of malformations or other direct or indirect harmful effects on the human fetus having been observed.
- B1: studies in animals have not shown evidence of an increased occurrence of fetal damage.
- B2: studies in animals are inadequate or may be lacking, but available data show no evidence of an increased occurrence of fetal damage.
- B3: studies in animals have shown evidence of an increased occurrence of fetal damage, the significance of which is considered uncertain in humans.

Category C
These are drugs which, owing to their pharmacological effects, have caused or may be suspected of causing harmful effects on the human fetus or neonate without causing malformations. These effects may be reversible.

Category D
These are drugs that have caused, are suspected to have caused or may be expected to cause, an increased incidence of human fetal malformations or irreversible damage. These drugs may also have adverse pharmacological effects.

Category X
These are drugs which have such a high risk of causing permanent damage to the fetus that they should not be used in pregnancy or when there is a possibility of pregnancy.

Box 29.2 **Examples of databases on teratogenic information**

- Organisation of Teratogen Information Services: www.otispregnancy.org
- Reproductive Toxicology Centre: www.reprotox.org
- European Network Teratology Information Services: www.entis-org.com
- Teratogen Information System: http://depts.washington.edu/terisweb/

Drug absorption
- Reduction in intestinal motility results in a 30%–50% increase in gastric and intestinal emptying time.
- Reduced gastric acid secretions result in an increase in gastric pH.
- Nausea and vomiting may affect the ability of a drug to be absorbed.
- Increased cardiac output, respiratory rate, tidal volumes and pulmonary blood flow influence absorption of inhalational agents.

Drug distribution
- Plasma volume increases by 50%, resulting in a decrease in peak serum concentration of many drugs.

- Body fat is increased in pregnancy, creating a larger volume of distribution for lipophilic substances.

Protein binding
- Plasma volume increases at a greater rate than albumin production, resulting in a physiologic dilutional hypoalbuminaemia.
- Maternal and placental hormones occupy available binding sites on proteins, thereby decreasing the ability to bind drugs.
- The net effect of a decreased binding capacity is an increase in the unbound ('free') pharmacologically active drug fraction.

Drug elimination
- Glomerular filtration rate increases by 50% in pregnancy, resulting in increased renal clearance of drugs.
- Pregnancy hormones have a variable effect on hepatic microsomal enzymes and biliary excretion, resulting in altered drug metabolism.

Placental–fetal compartment
- Unbound, non-ionised, lipid soluble molecules have a greater ability to cross the placental barrier.
- Fetal albumin concentrations increase as pregnancy advances, and fetal plasma proteins show variable binding affinities for different drugs.
- Fetal and placental drug metabolism occurs.
  Subsequently, embryonic/fetal exposure to maternally ingested drugs is complex, and the effect is dependent on the specific drug properties and gestational age at the time of exposure.

Specific drugs in pregnancy

Anticonvulsants
- Aim for monotherapy (at higher dose if necessary) if possible.
- Supplemental folic acid reduces the risk of associated congenital abnormalities.

Carbamazepine
- often considered drug of choice because of relatively low teratogenic effects
- associated with neural tube defects

Phenytoin
- associated with fetal hydantoin syndrome: intrauterine growth restriction (IUGR), microcephaly, digital/nail hypoplasia, cleft lip/palate, low nasal bridge, rib/heart/genitourinary anomalies

Valproic acid
- associated with neural tube defects (1%–2%) and cardiac anomalies

Antibiotics
- the most commonly prescribed drugs in pregnancy

Penicillins/cephalosporins
- clearance increased and, therefore, higher dose required to achieve similar antimicrobial concentrations
- reassuring large clinical experience

Tetracycline
- may cause discolouration of adult teeth

Nitrofurantoin
- little teratogenic risk
- associated with haemolytic reactions in those with glucose-6-phosphate dehydrogenase deficiency

Sulfonamides
- displaces bilirubin from carrier protein and may increase risk of neonatal jaundice if used late in third trimester

Doxycycline
- little teratogenic risk

Metronidazole
- little teratogenic risk

Azithromycin
- little teratogenic risk

Methotrexate
- Exposure in first trimester is associated with craniofacial, skeletal, cardiopulmonary and gastrointestinal abnormalities, and developmental delay.
- Exposure later in pregnancy appears to be safe.

Warfarin
- a recognised teratogen
- warfarin embryopathy: nasal hypoplasia, microphthalmia, limb hypoplasia, IUGR, central nervous system (CNS) abnormalities, deafness, developmental delay and neurologic dysfunction
- associated with intrauterine fetal death (IUFD) and stillbirth
- compatible with breastfeeding, as does not enter breast milk to significant degree

Lithium
- associated with small increased risk of cardiac anomalies
- associated with fetal and neonatal cardiac arrhythmias, hypoglycaemia, nephrogenic diabetes insipidus, polyhydramnios and preterm delivery

Retinoids
- can affect multiple organ systems, including CNS, cardiovascular and endocrine

Angiotensin-converting enzyme (ACE) inhibitors
- Exposure in first trimester is associated with risk of heart and CNS abnormalities.
- Exposure in later pregnancy is associated with renal failure, oligohydramnios, aortic arch obstructive malformations, patent ductus arteriosus and IUFD.

Selective serotonin reuptake inhibitors (SSRIs)
- There is a small increase in the risk of cardiac defects (especially paroxetine).
- Sertraline is associated with an increased risk of omphalocele.
- Paroxetine is associated with the risk of anencephaly, craniosynostosis and omphalocele.

- Exposure late in pregnancy is associated with transient neonatal complications, including jitteriness, transient tachypnoea of newborn, weak cry and poor tone.

Drugs of abuse in pregnancy

Alcohol
- Alcohol and its metabolites cross the placenta and are directly toxic to the fetus.
- Minimum safe exposure levels are uncertain.
- Fetal alcohol syndrome is associated with neurological impairment, microcephaly, long philtrum, thin upper lip, flattening of maxilla, microphthalmia, hypotonia and IUGR.

Cigarette smoking
- Smoking is associated with spontaneous abortion, IUGR, low birth weight, preterm delivery, premature rupture of membranes, placenta praevia and placental abruption.
- These complications contribute to an increased perinatal mortality rate in smokers.
- Effects are dose related.
- Mothers who smoke are more likely to use illicit drugs concurrently.

Cocaine
- Cocaine use results in vasoconstriction, tachycardia, hypertension and an increase in circulating catecholamines.
- It is associated with an increased risk of spontaneous abortion, IUGR, prematurity and placental abruption.
- Teratogenic effects are uncertain.
- Beta-blockers should not be used to control maternal blood pressure because the resultant unopposed alpha-adrenergic stimulation can lead to coronary vasoconstriction and end-organ ischaemia.

Cannabis
- Cannabis is the most common drug of abuse in pregnancy.
- Cannabis use does not appear to be an independent risk factor for adverse pregnancy outcomes.
- Cigarettes, alcohol and other illicit drug use are common.

Amphetamines
- High quality information on the effect in pregnancy is lacking.
- Amphetamines are associated with abruption and preterm delivery.

Lysergic acid diethylamide (LSD)
- There are isolated reports of amniotic bands with LSD use in pregnancy.

Glue/petrol
- Long-term toluene inhalation is associated with cerebellar degeneration and cortical atrophy.
- Infants have an increased risk of neurodevelopmental problems, including spastic quadriplegia and lead poisoning.

Opiates
- Opiate abuse is associated with a two to five times increased risk of perinatal mortality.

- Many of the maternal risks are similar to those that occur in the non-pregnant state: infection, vasculitis, nutritional deficiencies and psychosocial difficulties. Pregnancy-specific complications include pre-eclampsia, antepartum haemorrhage and puerperal morbidity.
- Fetal problems include microcephaly, IUGR, prematurity, malpresentation and passage of meconium.
- Neonatal problems include those associated with prematurity, opiate withdrawal ('neonatal abstinence syndrome'), postnatal growth deficiency, microcephaly, neurobehavioural deficits and sudden infant death syndrome.
- The time of onset of neonatal opiate withdrawal depends on the half-life of the drug: heroine and morphine 48 hours; methadone 72 hours.

Management of opiate abuse in pregnancy
- methadone stabilisation preferred
- acute withdrawal avoided
- regular antenatal care, preferably at multidisciplinary specialised clinics
- screen for blood-borne viruses and sexually transmitted diseases
- serial ultrasound assessment of fetal growth and wellbeing
- antenatal paediatric assessment regarding neonatal withdrawal and social circumstances/safety
- avoid narcotics for pain relief if possible
- continuous cardiotocograph monitoring in labour (may show reduced variability)
- avoid opioid antagonists as may precipitate acute withdrawal

References

Buhimschi C, Weiner C 2009 Medications in pregnancy and lactation. Part 1: teratology. Obstetrics and Gynecology 113:166–188

Buhimschi C, Weiner C 2009 Medications in pregnancy and lactation. Part 2: drugs with minimal or unknown human teratogenic effect. Obstetrics and Gynecology 113:417–432

Loebststein R, Koren G 2002 Clinical relevance of therapeutic drug monitoring during pregnancy. Therapeutic Drug Monitoring 24:15–22

Chapter 30

Infections in pregnancy

Michael Flynn

Urinary tract infection

Asymptomatic bacteriuria
- Incidence is 2%–10% in pregnancy. This is similar prevalence to non-pregnant women.
- If untreated, 15%–45% will develop symptomatic infection.
- Treatment can prevent 70%–80% of urinary tract infections and pyelonephritis.
- Diagnosis: a single voided specimen urine culture can detect 80% of asymptomatic carriers.
- About 75%–90% of urinary tract infections in pregnancy are due to *Escherichia coli*.
- Treatment: amoxycillin or cephalosporin are safe in pregnancy.
- Prevention: screening mid-stream urine (MSU) is performed as first-visit screen.
- Bacteriuria is associated with increased risk of preterm birth, low birth weight and increased perinatal mortality, and treatment has been shown to decrease these risks.

Acute symptomatic urinary tract infection
- Acute cystitis occurs in about 1% of pregnancies, especially in the second trimester. Pyelonephritis occurs in 1%–2% of pregnancies, in which 7% of women will suffer from bacteraemia and 1% septic shock.
- Possible reasons for increased pyelonephritis in pregnancy include anatomic changes to the urinary tract, and possible immunosuppression.

Management
- Rehydrate.
- Diagnose from MSU specimens and blood cultures.
- Antibiotics are given intravenously if the patient is systemically unwell.
- Lower temperature (paracetamol).
- Assess the fetus.
- There is a recurrence of 10%–15%; therefore, test urine regularly.

Relapses and reinfection
- *Relapse* means recurrence of infection by the same organism, and *reinfection* is due to a different strain of bacteria after successful eradication.
- Relapse or reinfection occurs in 10%–15% of treated urinary tract infections.

Management
- Treat the current infection.
- Prophylaxis uses oral nitrofurantoin 50 mg daily or cephalothin 500 mg daily for duration of pregnancy.
- Intravenous pyelogram is required after delivery.

Syphilis

Incidence. Incidence in Australia is 2 in 1000.

Screening
- This should be performed with a specific *Treponena pallidum* assay (e.g. *T. pallidum* haemagglutination assay (TPHA) or *T. pallidum* particle assay or syphilis enzyme immunoassay (EIA)).
- Syphilis may be transmitted to the fetus in the second trimester, with the following consequences:
  - premature delivery in 20%
  - intrauterine fetal death (IUFD) in 20%
  - subclinical infection in 20%
  - congenital infection in 40%

Clinical syndromes
Primary syphilis
- Incubation period is 10–90 days with an average of 21 days.
- It presents as a painless genital sore; then in the third to sixth week lymphadenopathy occurs, and serology is positive in 25% of cases.

Secondary syphilis
- Bilateral symmetrical papulosquamous eruption appears 2 weeks to 6 months after primary lesion. *T. pallidum* is present in lymph nodes and condyloma lata.

Latent syphilis
- This covers early syphilis (duration <4 years) and late syphilis (duration >4 years). It is non-infectious except in pregnancy.

Tertiary syphilis
- Neurological and vascular lesions are present.
  In pregnancy, the fetus is 'safe' under 18 weeks gestation because it cannot mount an immunological attack and cause tissue damage and inflammation. Congenital syphilis is associated with intrauterine growth restriction (IUGR), café-au-lait spots, bullous rash, saddle nose, nasal congestion, hepatosplenomegaly, notched teeth, osteochronditis and corneal scarring. Congenital syphilis may also be asymptomatic.

Management of syphilis
- Early syphilis (primary, secondary or latent of <12 months): treat with benzathine penicillin 2.4 million units intramuscularly weekly for 2 weeks, or erythromycin 500 mg four times a day for 15 days.
- Late syphilis (incubation >12 months): treat with intramuscular benzathine penicillin 2.4 million units weekly for 3 weeks, or erythromycin 500 mg four times a day for 30 days.
- Check for other sexually transmitted diseases, and treat the partner.

Toxoplasmosis

- *Toxoplasma gondii* is an obligate intracellular organism. The birth prevalence is 0.23 in 1000 births to non-immune mothers. The rate of maternal infection is 1.6 in 1000.

- The risk of transmission rises with increasing gestational age. However, the fetus is more severely affected if infected before 20 weeks gestation, and is usually asymptomatic if infected in the third trimester.
- Congenital toxoplasmosis can result in microcephalus, hydrocephalus, seizures, reduced intellect, chorioretinitis, cataract, hepatitis and pneumonitis.
- Primary infection is rare in pregnancy in Australia.
- Selective testing is recommended only for those women at increased risk and, preferentially, this testing is prior to pregnancy. Symptoms of acute toxoplasmosis include malaise, fever and cervical lymphadenopathy.
- Immunoglobulin M (IgM) is not a reliable marker of recent infection.
- If IgG-positive and IgM-positive and symptoms suggestive of infection, then repeat and check IgG titres and IgG avidity (suggestive of infection within 3 months).
- If the above is suggestive of recent acute maternal toxoplasmosis, then treatment depends on gestational age.
- Consider treatment with sulfadoxine and pyrimethamine and folic acid or spiramycin.
- Ultrasound and amniocentesis help with diagnosis.

Rubella

- The incubation period is 14–21 days; then a rash develops which lasts 2–7 days.
- Fewer than 5% of women are not immune to rubella at antenatal clinic screening.

Possible outcomes of maternal rubella infection
- no effect on the fetus
- placental infection only
- placental/fetal infection causing asymptomatic infection but affecting organs
- death of fetus (abortion, IUFD)
- congenital rubella syndrome (bilateral cataracts, IUGR, congenital heart disease, especially patent ductus arteriosus, sensorineural deafness and microphthalmia)

Risk to fetus of maternal infection
- At <8 weeks gestation, up to 85% of the fetuses are infected and all infected fetuses will develop complications such as cardiac, eye, ear and neurological defects.
- At <12 weeks gestation, 50%–80% of fetuses are infected, and of these 65%–85% have clinical defects.
- Between 13 and 16 weeks gestation, 30% of fetuses are infected and one-third suffer sensorineural deafness.
- At >16 weeks gestation, 10% of fetuses are infected, with rare clinical manifestations.

Diagnosis of maternal rubella
- four-fold rise in IgG titres
- rubella-specific IgM antibody (false-positives occur with rheumatic factor)
- reinfection: low IgM and rapid rise in IgG
- reinfection occurring more often with vaccination (80%) than with natural immunity (3.4%)

Diagnosis of intrauterine/congenital rubella
- rubella polymerase chain reaction (PCR), culture and fetal IgM can be performed following chorionic villus sampling, amniocentesis of fetal blood sampling
- virus isolated from infant's pharynx, urine and cerebrospinal fluid in the first 3 months of life

- IgM rubella-specific antibody present in cord blood
- persistence of rubella antibodies after 6 months

Vaccination

It is advisable not to vaccinate during or within 3 months of pregnancy. However, if vaccination occurs in pregnancy or 3 months before pregnancy, the risk to the fetus is negligible. Rubella vaccination affords protection in 95% of cases. The vaccine consists of attenuated virus given subcutaneously.

Hepatitis B

The incubation period ranges from 50 to 180 days.

Hepatitis B virus (HBV)
- The infective particle consists of two shells, the outer surface antigen (HBsAg) and the inner core (HBcAg).
- The organism cannot be cultured, and diagnosis is dependent on the presence of serological markers of antigen and antibody to the viral particle.
- The surface antigen (HBsAg) is the first to appear and is present throughout the acute infective stage until the presence of surface antibody (anti-HBs), which signals recovery and immunity.
- The hepatitis Be antigen (HBeAg) is a soluble protein derived from the core. It is detected in the acute phase of the infection and continues to be present as long as viral replication persists. This represents high infectivity.
- Chronic carriers of hepatitis B have HBsAg in their blood for more than 6 months.

Factors in perinatal transmission
The major risk to the neonate is vertical transmission, mostly at the time of delivery:
- About 85%–90% of infants will develop hepatitis B if their mothers are HBeAg-positive.
- Fewer than 5% of infants will be infected if the mother is anti-HBe-positive.
- Intrauterine transmission occurs in only 3%–8% of infants of HBeAg-positive mothers.

Prevention of hepatitis B
- Hepatitis B immunoglobulin and vaccine has 94% efficacy in preventing perinatal transmission.
- Hepatitis B immunoglobulin alone has an efficacy of 71%, while hepatitis B vaccine alone has 75% efficacy.
- Therefore, to prevent transmission to the newborn, it is necessary to give the baby 0.5 mL hepatitis B immunoglobulin (intramuscularly) at delivery and hepatitis B vaccine within 1 week of delivery and to repeat at 1 and 6 months.
- There is no evidence that caesarean section reduces the perinatal transmission of hepatitis B.
- With vaccine and immunoglobulin given, breastfeeding poses no additional risk of vertical transmission.

Hepatitis C

- Screen at first antenatal visit, especially if from high-risk group (intravenous drug use, high-risk ethnic groups, tattoos).

- Vertical transmission is 6% if the hepatitis C virus is ribonucleic acid (RNA)-positive. Risk is proportional to RNA load.
- There is no clear evidence of mode of delivery and reduction of perinatal transmission.
- Decreased use of internal monitoring devices may reduce risk of vertical transmission.
- Hepatitis C virus has been found in breast milk, although studies have not shown a higher risk of vertical transmission during breastfeeding.

Human immunodeficiency virus (HIV) and pregnancy

Transmission to the neonate
- Transplacental: data from termination of pregnancies at 16–24 weeks gestation show that up to 66% of fetuses are infected.
- Labour and delivery: transmission occurs when the neonate is exposed to infected blood.
- Postpartum transmission: occurs through breastfeeding. In industrialised countries, HIV-infected mothers are advised not to breastfeed.

Managing HIV in pregnancy
- Adopt an appropriate multidisciplinary approach with adequate counselling.
- At the first visit, perform the routine screening tests plus those for *Toxoplasma*, cytomegalovirus, tuberculosis, *Cryptococcus* and *Candida*.
- Cervical cytology and colposcopy are essential.
- Review immune status with CD4 lymphocyte count and viral RNA copy number.
- Avoid invasive testing (amniocentesis, chorionic villus sampling, cordocentesis).
- Studies in 1994 confirmed that antiretroviral therapy in pregnant women from the second trimester and continued in infants for 6 weeks after birth reduces transmission from 25% to 8%. Antenatal administration of zidovudine plus intravenous loading dose just predelivery and neonatal oral administration for 6 weeks is preferred protocol.
- In 1999, studies confirmed that elective caesarean section reduces transmission by 50%–80%.
- The risk of transmission through breastfeeding is thought to be 16%.
- The risk of transmission is minimised when there are undetectable viral copy numbers and rupture of membranes <4 hours.
- These strategies will minimise mother-to-infant transmission.
- Ultrasound assessment of growth and wellbeing is appropriate in the third trimester.
- Elective caesarean section is at 38 weeks.

Cytomegalovirus

Cytomegalovirus (CMV) is a herpes virus and the commonest cause of intrauterine infection. Primary infection occurs in 1 in 300 pregnancies, with fetal infection occurring in 40% of these, and 10% of infected fetuses having congenital problems.

Most primary infections are asymptomatic, but suspect in viral illness with atypical lymphocytes which is monospot-negative.

Fetal complications
These include IUFD, IUGR, hepa-tosplenomegaly, central nervous system complications and neonatal jaundice. The major long-term effect is neurosensory deafness.

Diagnosis
- If IgM-positive, then repeat 2–4 weeks later and check IgG avidity.
- IgM can remain positive for up to 2 years after infection.
- Direct viral detection can be via CMV fluorescence antibody, CMV isolation or PCR of maternal fluids.
- Once primary infection is confirmed, fetal diagnosis can be via amniocentesis or fetal blood sampling. However, positive results do not predict any degree of fetal damage.

Pathogenesis of fetal complications
- This includes placental infection.
- Fetal infection causes cytolysis with areas of focal necrosis and healing by fibrosis and calcification. The risk of fetal infection from primary maternal infection is 40%–50%, but the severity of fetal damage is variable and unpredictable.
- Of infants exposed to CMV in utero, 95% may be asymptomatic at birth. Of these, 5% may develop long-term sequelae (sensorineural deafness, epilepsy or learning disability).
- The 5% of exposed neonates who are symptomatic at birth are usually affected by a primary infection. The prognosis is almost invariably associated with long-term defects.

Antenatal advice
- A woman with primary infection during pregnancy has about a 4% risk of delivering a baby with a CMV-related disorder. Half of these cases are restricted to hearing loss.
- All pregnant women should be advised about simple infection control mechanisms to reduce transmission risk (e.g. hand-washing after nappy changes and contact with respiratory secretions in children under age 2).
- There is no therapy that alters the disease course; therefore, counselling and support are required.
- The risk of transmission is equal throughout the pregnancy; however, an adverse neurological outcome is more frequent in the first half of pregnancy.

Listeriosis

Listeria is a small, non-sporing, gram-positive rod-shaped bacterium. Those infected may present with malaise, headache, fever, diarrhoea and abdominal pain.

Bacteriological investigations include blood and urine cultures, and cervical swab culture. Amniocentesis with Gram stain and culture is definitive diagnosis.

Complications of listeriosis in pregnancy
- fetal: IUFD and premature labour; mortality rate if untreated is 40% in the second and third trimesters
- neonatal: microabscesses in liver, lungs, adrenals and central nervous system; treatment of maternal listeriosis is with amoxycillin, gentamicin and delivery dependent on gestation

Varicella zoster

It is known as chickenpox in the primary infection and as shingles with reactivation of the infection. Up to 4% of pregnant women are not immune. The incubation period lasts 14–18 days. The contagious period lasts 7 days after the rash disappears.

Infection in early pregnancy
Abnormalities in the fetus occur in 1%–2% of cases, especially if infection has occurred between 8 and 21 weeks gestation. Effects on the fetus include microcephaly, convulsions, mental retardation and limb abnormalities.

Infection in late pregnancy
In late pregnancy, the severity of perinatal infection is dependent on timing before delivery. Up to 5 days before delivery, maternal IgG is protective and neonatal infection is usually mild. If infection occurs 5 days before or after delivery, there is a risk of severe neonatal varicella infection, with a 30% mortality rate.

Management
- Establish the diagnosis by serology.
- Isolate the woman.
- If zoster rash appears over 7 days before labour and the vesicles have crusted, the risk of transmission is negligible.
- If zoster rash appears within 5 days of delivery, then zoster immunoglobulin for the neonate should be considered.
- Prepregnancy screening should include zoster serology.

Exposure in pregnancy
- if seronegative and the exposure is <96 hours, then passive immunisation with varicella zosta immunoglobulin

Group B streptococcus

This is the leading cause of early-onset neonatal sepsis. Colonisation of the vagina occurs in up to 20% of women at some stage during pregnancy. The reservoir of group B streptococcus (GBS) also occurs in the gastrointestinal tract. This recolonises the genital tract after treatment, so there is no need to treat the asymptomatic woman unless in labour.

Neonatal sepsis occurs with an incidence of 3 in 1000, although 1%–2% of infants will be colonised at birth.

Management
- Antepartum treatment is relatively ineffective because the gastrointestinal tract is the primary reservoir.
- Intrapartum antibiotics are used in the prevention of neonatal sepsis; also to reduce maternal morbidity. This has led to a 7% decline in the incidence of GBS disease. Guidelines for prevention suggest either a risk-based or screening approach to identify those patients requiring intrapartum antibiotics. It is probable that screening has a more protective approach than the risk-based approach.
- Screening is via low vaginal or anorectal swab between 35 and 37 weeks.
- Clinical risk factors include <37 weeks gestation, rupture of membranes >18 hours, maternal fever >38°C.
- All women with a previously affected GBS child or GBS bacteriuria in pregnancy should be treated intrapartum.
- Intrapartum treatment with a penicillin antibiotic is used in those with a positive antenatal culture and in high-risk groups. If penicillin allergy, then use erythromycin or clindamycin.

Herpes simplex

- Incidence of newborn infection is rare (1 in 10,000 to 1 in 40,000).
- Up to 60% of neonates with herpes infection do not have associated maternal history or signs of herpes at the time of delivery. Primary genital herpes is more likely to cause severe infection and neonatal symptoms than recurrent infection.
- Congenital or transplacental spread is rare and is associated with primary infection.
- Vertical transmission at time of vaginal delivery may occur in up to 40%–50% of deliveries from women with primary infection, and in up to 3%–8% with recurrent infection.

Risk factors for intrapartum infection
- maternal primary infection
- multiple lesions
- premature delivery
- premature rupture of membranes

Management
- If lesions are present and membranes have been ruptured for <4 hours, a caesarean section reduces the risk of transmission, particularly in primary infections in women who are herpes simplex antibody negative.
- Acyclovir shortens the duration of viral shedding, especially during the primary attack.

Further reading

Australasian Society for Infectious Diseases (ASID) 2002 Management of perinatal infections. Sydney: ASID

Barnick CGW, Cardozo L 1991 The lower urinary tract in pregnancy, labour and the puerperium. In: Progress in obstetrics and gynaecology, Vol. 9. London: Churchill Livingstone, pp 195–206

Doherty R 2001 Preventing transmission of HIV from mothers to babies in Australia. Medical Journal of Australia 174:433–434

Gilbert G 2002 Infections in pregnant women. Medical Journal of Australia 176:229–236

MacFarlane Burnet Institute 2008 Information for obstetricians: blood borne viruses and pregnancy. Melbourne: MacFarlane Burnet Institute

Mijch AM, Clezy K, Furrier V 1996 Women with HIV. Medical Journal of Australia 164:668–671

Walpole IR, Hogden N, Bower C 1991 Congenital toxoplasmosis: a large survey in Western Australia. Medical Journal of Australia 154:720–724

Chapter 31

Red cell isoimmunisation

Michael Flynn

Perinatal mortality rate

Perinatal mortality due to Rhesus D (RhD) isoimmunisation before the use of prophylaxis was 15 in 1000, or 4% of perinatal deaths. Today, the perinatal mortality rate from RhD isoimmunisation is 0.54 in 10,000, or 0.3%. The reduced perinatal mortality is due to anti-D immunoglobulin prophylaxis and the fall in numbers of large families.

A third of women who become isoimmunised have no demonstrable antibodies at the first antenatal visit, so investigations for antibodies must be repeated during pregnancy in RhD-negative women.

There is a correlation between the time of first antibody detection and the severity of haemolytic disease of the newborn. The earlier the antibodies are present during the pregnancy, the higher the risk of fetal/neonatal problems. If an antibody is present in pregnancy, serial monitoring of antibody levels is required.

Prevention of RhD isoimmunisation

The aim is to provide passive immunisation at times of risk of fetomaternal transfusion. If no prophylaxis is given, 1% of RhD-negative women will develop anti-D antibodies by the end of the first pregnancy and a further 3%–5% have detectable antibodies 6 months after delivery. About 90% of sensitisations can be prevented. 100 IU anti-D immunoglobulin is able to neutralise 2 mL fetal blood. This is given within 72 hours of fetomaternal transfusion for maximum effect. In an RhD-negative woman with no anti-D antibodies present, anti-D prophylaxis is indicated in the following cases:

- Sensitising events in the first trimester (including miscarriage, ectopic pregnancy, termination of pregnancy, chorionic villus sampling) require 250 IU intramuscular RhD immunoglobulin for single pregnancy and 625 IU for multiple pregnancy.
- Events in the second and third trimester (e.g. amniocentesis, cordocentesis, abdominal trauma sufficient to cause fetomaternal haemorrhage, external cephalic version or antepartum haemorrhage) require 625 IU injection of anti-D.
- There is routine administration of 625 IU at 28 and 34 weeks gestation in addition to doses given for sensitising events.
- Postpartum administration of 600 IU is necessary within 72 hours.
- With this prophylaxis regimen, antibody formation rate is reduced to 0.2%.

Contraindications for anti-D prophylaxis
- RhD-positive or Du-positive individual
- RhD-negative or Du-negative individual previously sensitised to RhD

Prevention of postpartum isoimmunisation
- With anti-D prophylaxis, only 0.2% are sensitised.
- In 0.5% of deliveries, a fetomaternal haemorrhage of over 30 mL occurs.
- There is an increased risk with manual removal of the placenta and caesarean sections.

Screening
- All pregnant women have a red cell antibody screen in the first trimester and, when negative, again at around 28–30 weeks gestation.
- When RhD antibody is present, screen the partner's blood to detect the likelihood of the fetus carrying D antigen. If the partner is RhD-negative, the fetus will be unaffected.

Antenatal management of Rhesus isoimmunisation

Aims
- Identify the severely affected fetus.
- Correct anaemia by transfusion.
- Deliver the fetus when mature.

Determination of fetal Rhesus type
- If the fetal Rhesus type is RhD-negative, then there is no antenatal risk and fetal and maternal monitoring is not required.
- Determine paternal Rhesus type and zygosity, as if homozygous RhD-positive then 100% of babies are at risk, but if heterozygous only 50% are affected.
- Amniocentesis: polymerase chain reaction (PCR) testing on amniocytes to determine fetal blood group is used, although there is up to 1.5% false-negative rate.
- Free fetal DNA: flow cytometry of maternal blood for fetal cells, which are then blood typed, is used. Meta-analysis is reporting 99% accuracy.

Antibody levels
- The first investigation is an assessment of the amount of antibody in maternal circulation.
- Levels may be given as a titre or quantitative value.
- Further investigations are required when the antibody titre is 1:64 or at any time when titres are increased by two dilutions (e.g. a rise from a titre of 1:4 to 1:32).

Antibody quantification
- When levels are lower than 4 IU/mL, the fetus is minimally affected, and fewer than 5% then require an exchange transfusion.
- Levels of 4–8 IU/mL indicate moderate disease, and delivery is advised by 38 weeks gestation.
- Levels >10 IU/mL suggest the risk of severe disease in the fetus. Management is by further assessment of the fetus and delivery by 36 weeks gestation.
- Repeat maternal serum testing every 2 weeks.
- This is for first affected pregnancies. Pregnancies after this involve a greater severity of fetal neonatal haemolytic disease.

Assessment of the fetal anaemia
- Severe anaemia seen as hydrops is not seen until fetal haemoglobin is <40 g/L.
- Middle cerebral artery peak systolic velocity is used as the best non-invasive tool to predict fetal anaemia.

- The anaemic fetus preserves brain oxygenation by increasing cerebral flow.
- Sensitivity if use >1.5 multiples of the median for gestational age of measurement of flow for prediction of moderate to severe anaemia was 100%.
- Screening interval appears to be 1–2 weeks.
- Amniocentesis and measurement of amniotic fluid bilirubin as indirect assessment of severity of fetal anaemia was previously first-choice investigation; however, similar sensitivity and specificity to middle cerebral artery flows has led to decreased use of this invasive procedure.

Fetal blood sampling
- Information available includes fetal blood group, haemoglobin, total bilirubin, platelet count and haematocrit. These are the only direct assessments of the severity of disease.
- Fetal loss rate from the procedure is 1%–2%.
- The procedure can provoke marked rises in maternal antibody levels, as there is a 50%–70% risk of fetomaternal haemorrhage.
- Intrauterine transfusion with O negative is indicated if haematocrit is <2 standard deviations for gestational age and the fetus is immature.
- The second transfusion takes place 2 weeks after the first, as the rate of decrease in haematocrit after the first transfusion is unpredictable. The rate of fall in haematocrit is 0.5%–2% per day.
- Donor blood is not susceptible to destruction; thus, the time interval between transfusions tends to increase.
- Suppression of fetal erythropoiesis occurs after two to three transfusions.

Neonatal management
- Arrange delivery at appropriate time (after 34 weeks gestation if requiring intervention).
- At delivery, collect cord blood for fetal haemoglobin, blood group, direct Coombs' test and bilirubin concentration.
- Exchange transfusion is required if the fetal haemoglobin is <100 g/L.
- Measure bilirubin concentration every 6 hours for the first 48 hours. Be aware of the risk of chronic hypoplastic anaemia.

Other red cell antibodies

There are about 700 red cell antibodies, but only a few cause severe haemolytic disease of the newborn. Many antibodies (A, P(I), Le(a), M, I) produce an immunoglobulin M (IgM) response only, which cannot cross the placenta, so they are of no significance in pregnancy. Some red cell antigens are poorly developed on fetal red cells, so antibodies (Lu(b), Y+(a)), even if IgG produced and crosses the placenta, have no adverse affect. Antibodies known to stimulate haemolytic disease of the newborn include:
- anti-Kell
- anti-c (less commonly anti-C)
- anti-E (less commonly anti-e)
- anti-Fya and anti-Fyb
- anti-Ra and anti-Rb

In Western countries, these have a higher frequency than D alloimmunisation and may be due to unmatched blood transfusions.

Anti-Kell
Over 90% of the population is Kell-negative. Most Kell antibodies develop because of incompatible transfusion. There appears to be a poor correlation between the antibody titre and the effect on the fetus or neonate. Anti-Kell severity can change rapidly due

to the antibodies' ability to suppress erythropoiesis. Ultrasound assessment of fetal liver size is useful.

Management
The management of all red cell antibodies is similar in principle to Rhesus disease, including paternal genotype, serial titres, assessment of fetal anaemia and early delivery.

ABO incompatibility
- This mostly occurs when the mother is group O and the baby A or B. It occurs in 15% of pregnancies, but only 1 in 30 show mild jaundice, 1 in 150 mild anaemia, and 1 in 3000 require exchange transfusion.
- ABO incompatibility can occur in the first pregnancy, with no tendency to increase in severity with subsequent pregnancies.

Further reading

Moise KJ 2008 The usefulness of middle cerebral artery Doppler assessment in the treatment of the fetus at risk for anemia. American Journal of Obstetrics and Gynecology 198:161

Oepekes D, Seaward PG, Frank PHA et al 2006 Doppler ultrasonography versus amniocentesis to predict fetal anemia. New England Journal of Medicine 355:156–164

Chapter 32

Antepartum haemorrhage

Michael Flynn

Definition. Antepartum haemorrhage is bleeding from the genital tract in the period from 20 weeks gestation to the birth of the baby.

Incidence. It occurs in 3% of pregnancies of >28 weeks gestation and 5% of pregnancies of >20 weeks gestation.

Aetiology

- placenta praevia
- placental abruption
- marginal bleed
- vasa praevia
- uterine rupture
- local causes: cervix, vagina

The source is almost entirely maternal in origin.

Placenta praevia

Incidence. Incidence is about 1%, rising with frequency of previous caesarean section.

Presentation. The placenta is attached to the lower segment of the uterus and/or covering the cervix. The presentation is usually that of a painless antepartum haemorrhage with a high presenting part. The absence of contractions and pain makes diagnosis more likely.

Routine second-trimester ultrasound will diagnose low-lying and placenta praevia.

Classification

- complete or grade 4 placenta praevia where placenta completely centrally covers the os
- marginal or grade 3 placenta praevia where the os is covered by the placenta edge
- marginal or grade 1 and 2 where the placenta is near but does not cover the os

The diagnosis is usually made in the third trimester. At the second trimester morphology assessment, a low-grade placenta praevia will be termed a 'low lying placenta' for complete assessment in the third trimester. Diagnosis of normal placental site is >5 cm from the cervical os.

Risk factors
- increased number of caesarean sections
- increased parity

Management
If asymptomatic and diagnosed at morphology scan, management is confirmation of diagnosis in the third trimester and planning elective caesarean section.
- It may involve resuscitation of the mother, fetal assessment and delivery (dependent on the amount of bleeding, continuation of bleeding and fetal maturity).
- Pregnancy may need to be prolonged to decrease prematurity and lower perinatal mortality.
- Insert intravenous line, and cross-match for blood.
- Confirm the diagnosis with an ultrasound scan.
- Use expectant management if preterm and the blood loss is small.
- Order serial growth scans to exclude intrauterine growth restriction (IUGR).
- Admit the patient and plan for her to remain in hospital until delivery by caesarean section if it is a major grade praevia.
- Use steroid prophylaxis for lung maturity if the fetus is premature.
- Iron supplementation is useful.
- Use anti-D prophylaxis if the mother is Rhesus D-negative.
- Perform caesarean section if a large bleed has occurred and is continuing.
- Watch for postpartum haemorrhage, and counsel regarding possible hysterectomy.
- Avoid digital examination and intercourse in the third trimester.

Placenta percreta

Invasion of the placenta to within the myometrium should be suspected in previous cases of placenta praevia. This is especially so in the case of placenta praevia and previous caesarean section where the rate of placenta acreta is 5%. As there is a significant risk of major haemorrhage, delivery via caesarean section should be well planned with blood products available and counselling of the possibility of hysterectomy.

Placental abruption

Incidence. Incidence is 1%.
   Definition. Abruption is haemorrhage from decidual detachment of a normally situated placenta. The woman presents with abdominal pain, tense and tender uterus, which is large for dates, and hypovolaemic shock that may be out of proportion with visible bleeding.

Risk factors
- hypertension
- increased parity
- poor nutrition
- previous abruption (after one abruption the recurrence risk is 5%–15% and after two the risk is 25%)
- trauma, external cephalic version
- sudden reduction in uterine volume (e.g. after delivery of the first twin)

Differential diagnosis
- placenta praevia
- uterine rupture
- degeneration of fibroid
- rectus sheath haematoma
- acute polyhydramnios
- acute surgical conditions

Complications of placental abruption
- coagulopathy (abruption is the commonest obstetric cause of coagulopathy: 10% of abruptions demonstrate significant changes in coagulation profiles; there is a reduction in platelets and fibrinogen, increased fibrin degradation products and prothrombin time; fibrin degradation products inhibit myometrial activity, increase the risk of postpartum haemorrhage and may have cardiotoxic effects)
- postpartum haemorrhage
- renal failure
- acute tubular necrosis from hypovolaemia and disseminated intravascular coagulopathy
- perinatal mortality of 119 in 1000 births complicated by abruption

Management
- Resuscitate and restore circulatory volume to prevent renal shutdown and to clear fibrin degradation products.
- Cross-match for blood and, if indicated, platelets and fresh frozen plasma. Check full blood count, coagulation profile, renal function and electrolytes and liver biochemistry.
- Monitor urine output.
- Perform fetal assessment and delivery.

Vasa praevia

This is associated with the rupture of fetal vessels. It is often associated with velamentous insertion of the cord, with vessels present within the fetal membranes.

Diagnosis
Vasa praevia must be included in the differential diagnosis of intrapartum vaginal bleeding, and is associated with an ominous cardiotocography pattern. Diagnosis can occur in the antenatal period with transvaginal ultrasound and colour Doppler assessment of vessels across the top of the cervical os. In the presence of blood loss and ominous fetal heart rate, although theoretical tests (Apts) are available, vasa praevia may result in fetal anaemia and death. Hence, emergency delivery is indicated.

Local causes
These include cervicitis, polyps, ectropion and cervical cancer.

Further reading

Morgan K, Arulkumaran S 2003 Antepartum haemorrhage. Current Opinion in Obstetrics and Gynaecology 13:81–87
Scott JC 1988 Antepartum haemorrhage. In: Whitfield CR (ed), Dewhurst's textbook of obstetrics and gynaecology for postgraduates. Oxford: Blackwell Scientific Publishers

Chapter 33

Fetal complications in later pregnancy

Jackie Chua
Michael Flynn

Intrauterine fetal death (IUFD)

Definition. IUFD is the delivery of a live fetus with no signs of life after 20 weeks. The intrauterine diagnosis is via the absence of fetal heart sounds and fetal movements. Signs of longer duration demise include Spalding's sign (overlapping skull bones on X-ray) or Robert's sign (gas in the fetal cardiovascular system). About 50% of all IUFDs occur at over 37 weeks gestation.

Aetiology
Aetiology varies with gestational age and between developed and non-developed countries. Within developed countries, near-term the aetiologies include:
- unexplained
- intrauterine growth restriction (IUGR)
- placental abruption
- infection
- chromosomal and congenital anomalies

Complications
- infections, especially with rupture of membranes
- maternal distress
- coagulopathy and disseminated intravascular coagulopathy

Coagulopathy and disseminated intravascular coagulopathy
This can occur when gestation is over 14 weeks, and generally when the fetus has been dead for over 4 weeks. There is a slow reduction in fibrinogen of about 500 mg/L per week, which is unlikely to be associated with bleeding tendency until levels are lower than 1 g/L. The coagulopathy is due to fibrinogen consumption with release of thromboplastins from retained products of conception. There may also be raised fibrin degradation products, prothrombin time and activated partial thromboplastin time with a reduction in platelets. Disseminated intravascular coagulopathy occurs in one-third of patients with IUFD for over 4 weeks. Spontaneous labour occurs in 80% of cases within 2 weeks, with only 10% undelivered after 3 weeks.

Investigations
- photograph of the fetus
- X-ray/magnetic resonance imaging (MRI)

182

- cytogenetics: blood, skin, placenta/amnion
- autopsy
- bacteriology: swabs of the fetus and placenta
- maternal: blood group and antibodies, full blood count, Kleihauer test, antiphospholipid antibodies, HbA1c, *Toxoplasma,* cytomegalovirus and rubella serology, thyroid function

Delivery of the dead fetus
Prostaglandins
Prostaglandin pessaries or gel
- Give prostaglandin E_2 analogue 1–2 mg via gel or sustained release, as in term induction of labour.
- Contraindications include hypersensitivity to prostaglandin and induction of labour at term.
- Cautious use is required with the concomitant use of oxytocin after previous uterine surgery and in patients with obstructive airways disease.

Vaginal
Misoprostol (prostaglandin E_1 analogue)
- This appears to be effective in induction of IUFD. The possibility of uterine rupture with previous caesarean section is noted.
- It is the method of choice with dose decreasing from mid-trimester to late-third trimester.

Oxytocin
- If the cervix is favourable, artificial rupture of membranes may be performed to reduce induction to delivery interval without a significant rise in infection rates.

Caesarean section
- Indications include major placenta praevia, severe cephalopelvic disproportion, previous classical caesarean section or more than two previous caesarean sections, the presence of uterine rupture or transverse lie and unsuccessful version.

Intrauterine growth restriction (IUGR)

Definition. IUGR is where the estimated birth weight is less than the tenth percentile for gestational age (but some neonates with IUGR will be heavier). The clinical relevance of IUGR is a four-fold rise in intrauterine fetal death, greater risk of birth hypoxia, neonatal complications and impaired neurodevelopment. The majority of term IUGRs have no morbidity or mortality.

Causes
- idiopathic, racial
- uteroplacental insufficiency as a result of pre-eclampsia, or abruption
- chromosomal abnormalities
- structural/anatomical abnormalities
- infections
- maternal causes (e.g. smoking, drugs, alcohol, nutrition)
- multiple pregnancies

Screening
- Clinical assessment alone detects fewer than 50% of cases. This includes abdominal palpation and symphysial fundal height, which has a sensitivity of 60%–74% and a false-positive rate of 55%.

Diagnosis
- Abdominal circumference and estimated fetal weight by ultrasound are the most accurate diagnostic measurements to predict growth retardation. Ultrasound scan measuring abdominal circumference in the third trimester can detect 85% of IUGRs.
- There used to be differentiation between symmetrical and asymmetrical IUGR, but it is not generally used any more as an indicator for chromosome type of growth restriction.
- IUGR and polyhydramnios can be an indication for chromosome abnormality.

Management
- ultrasound
  - biometry and estimated fetal weight +/–10%
  - Doppler: monitoring umbilical artery Doppler for brain sparing then decompensation type of parameters
    - other blood vessels looked at include middle cerebral artery, ductus venosus and umbilical vein
    - uterine artery for presence or absence of a notch in the waveform may indicate high risk for placental insufficiency in first and second trimester
  - amniotic fluid index: decreases
- biophysical profile: late signs
- cardiotocography (CTG): late signs
- delivery
  - timing difficult
  - Growth Restriction Intervention Trial (GRIT) trial: no difference in total perinatal deaths between immediate versus delayed delivery group and both had similar 2-year neurological outcomes
  - Doppler best indicator for delivery after 29 weeks with ductus venosus a good predictor of intact survival
  - Cochrane for high-risk and low-risk pregnancies and Doppler surveillance found no benefit with an increased intervention rate

Disorders of amniotic fluid volume

- amniotic fluid homeostasis: fetal urine production and swallowing, secretions and transfer across membranes

Screening
- abdominal palpation
- increased abdominal girth and difficulty feeling fetal parts
- smaller than expected

Diagnosis
- ultrasound
- subjective assessment
- objective assessment

- amniotic fluid index
- deepest vertical pocket (twins)

Polyhydramnios
Risk factors
- fetal abnormalities (neural tube defects, gastrointestinal defects limiting swallowing of liquor)
- hydrops fetalis
- multiple pregnancy, especially monozygotic twins
- maternal diabetes
- idiopathic

Complications of polyhydramnios
- preterm rupture of membranes
- premature labour
- unstable lie and fetal malpresentation
- cord prolapse
- postpartum haemorrhage, placental abruption
- maternal discomfort

Management
- ultrasound examination of fetus and assessment of amount of liquor
- glucose tolerance test
- indomethacin: risk of premature closure of ductus arteriosus
- close monitoring in high-risk unit with possible amnio reduction

Oligohydramnios
Factors associated with reduced amniotic fluid volume
- placental insufficiency and IUGR
- iatrogenic
- fetal abnormalities (renal or renal tract abnormalities)
- premature rupture of membranes
- post-term pregnancy

Complications of oligohydramnios
- cord compression and fetal distress
- increased perinatal morbidity and mortality
- postural/musculoskeletal deformities
- pulmonary hypoplasia, especially if early onset or prolonged

Management
- ultrasound examination of fetus for anomalies
- assessment of fetal wellbeing
- assessment for rupture of membranes

Further reading

Baschat AA, Galan HL, Bhides A et al 2006 Doppler and biophysical assessment in growth restricted fetuses: distribution of test results. Ultrasound in Obstetrics and Gynecology 27:41–47
Bricker I, Neilson JP, Dowswell T 2008 Routine ultrasound in late pregnancy (after 24 weeks' gestation). Cochrane Database of Systematic Reviews. Issue 4. Art. No. CD001451. DOI: 10.1002/14651858

GRIT Study Group 2004 Wellbeing at 2 years of age in the Growth Restriction Intervention Trial (GRIT): multicentre randomized controlled trial. Lancet 364:513–520

Grivell RM, Wong L, Bhatia V 2009 Regimens of fetal surveillance for impaired fetal growth. Cochrane Database of Systematic Reviews. Issue 1. Art. No. CD007113. DOI: 10.1002/14651858

Kinzler WL, Vintzileos AM 2008 Fetal growth restriction: a modern approach. Current Opinion in Obstetrics and Gynecology 20:125–131

Lalor JG, Fawole B, Alfirevic Z, Devane D 2008 Biophysical profile for fetal assessment in high risk pregnancies. Cochrane Database of Systematic Reviews. Issue 1. Art. No.: CD000038. DOI: 10.1002/14651858

Chapter 34

Breech presentation

Michael Flynn

Incidence. There is an increase in incidence with decreasing gestation. At 20–25 weeks gestation, 30%–40% of fetuses are breech, and at 32 weeks gestation the incidence is 15%, while at term 2%–4% of fetuses are in the breech presentation.

Types

- frank/extended at knee: 65% of breech presentations
- complete/flexed at knee: 10% of breech presentations
- footling: 25% of breech presentations

Risk factors

Fetal and maternal risk factors are listed in Table 34.1.

External cephalic version
Spontaneous changes in fetal polarity are reduced with increasing gestation. The likelihood of spontaneous version at 32 weeks is about 55%, compared with 25% at 36 weeks. The risks of external cephalic version include tocolytic side effects, placental abruption, cord accidents and premature labour.

The absolute contraindications to external cephalic version include multiple pregnancy, antepartum haemorrhage, placenta praevia, rupture of membranes, labour and fetal abnormalities. Relative contraindications include previous caesarean section, intrauterine growth restriction (IUGR) and oligohydramnios. Tocolysis improves success of external version. Anti-D is required in women who are Rhesus-negative. The success rate is 50%–90%, but there appears to be no significant decrease in overall caesarean section rates.

Management of breech presentation

Diagnosis
- Perform a clinical examination.
- If remote from term, document and observe.
- If after 36 weeks gestation, perform an ultrasound scan to confirm diagnosis; assess fetal anatomy, position of legs and estimated weight; assess amniotic fluid volume.

Term Breech Trial
This randomised multicentre trial compared the policy of elective caesarean section with vaginal birth for selected breech deliveries. The results were:
- no difference in maternal morbidity or mortality in both treatment arms

Table 34.1 Risk factors for breech presentation	
Fetal	**Maternal**
Prematurity	Past history
Multiple pregnancy	Primigravida
Abnormality	Uterine abnormalities
Intrauterine fetal death	Pelvic tumour
Raised or lowered amniotic fluid volume	Contracted pelvis
Placenta praevia	Drugs: anticonvulsants, drugs of abuse
Reduced growth or activity	Idiopathic

- statistically significant increase in perinatal/neonatal morbidity in planned vaginal birth group compared with elective caesarean section

The best method of delivering breech singleton is the planned caesarean section.

Delivery of the breech presentation diagnosed in late labour

- The common method is assisted breech delivery.
- Lithotomy position: clean the perineum and drape.
- Catheterise the bladder.
- Employ analgesia.
- Perform episiotomy.

Breech born by maternal expulsive efforts up to the umbilicus

After the knees have delivered, flex the knees by pressing on the popliteal fossa to deliver the legs. Place a warm cloth over the breech and with the next contraction place hands on the baby's pelvis and pull down towards the floor until the anterior shoulder is delivered. The anterior arm is delivered by hooking a finger onto the cubital fossa and pulling the arm down over the baby's abdomen.

Lovset's manoeuvre

Rotating the posterior shoulder to the anterior allows the other arm to be delivered in the same manner as the first. The head is delivered by various ways, including forceps, the Mauriceau-Smellie-Veit manoeuvre, the Wigand-Martin manoeuvre of suprapubic pressure and lateral rotation of head in pelvis, or the Bracht manoeuvre of grasping feet and placing the body onto the maternal abdomen with the symphysis acting as fulcrum.

Possible hazards in vaginal delivery

- occipital bone trauma during vaginal breech delivery from the impact on the maternal pubis
- intra/periventricular injury, secondary haemorrhage or ischaemia (avoiding vaginal delivery does not necessarily prevent intracranial haemorrhage)
- bruising resulting in jaundice
- trauma to internal organs, with the accoucheur placing hands over the baby's abdomen rather than the pelvis
- entrapment of the head, especially in the woman who commences active pushing before the second stage or with a footling breech

Preterm breech presentation

- If not in labour, there is no benefit from external version prior to 37 weeks gestation.
- Term Breech Trial findings may not be applicable to preterm.
- Studies published are all retrospective, and individual decision making is therefore appropriate.
- They are mostly handled by caesarean section.

Further reading

Hannah ME, Hannah WJ, Hewson SA et al (for the Term Breech Trial Collaborative Group) 2000 Planned caesarean section versus planned vaginal birth for breech presentation at term: a randomised multicenter trial. Lancet 356:1375-1383

Hofmeyr GJ, Kulier R 1996 External cephalic version for breech presentation at term. Cochrane Database of Systematic Reviews. Issue 1. Art. No.: CD000083. DOI: 10.1002/14651858

Chapter 35

Multiple pregnancy

Jackie Chua
Michael Flynn

This is considered a high-risk pregnancy because of the increased maternal and perinatal risks.

Incidence. Incidence varies with geographical location. The incidence from spontaneous conception is about 1.25% of births, from clomiphene-induced ovulation 7%, and from assisted reproductive techniques up to 10%–20%. Monozygotic twinning has an incidence of 3.5 in 1000 deliveries.

Mechanism of twinning

Dizygotic twins
- Dizygotic twins are always DCDA (dichorionic diamniotic) and account for 70% of twin pregnancies. This occurs as a result of duplication of the normal process of conception, with separate chorions, amnions and placental circulations.
- The geographic variation in the incidence of twin pregnancies is due to differences in dizygotic twinning.
- The risks for dizygotic twinning include older maternal age (>35 years), past history and family history of twinning.

Monozygotic twins
- Monozygotic twins account for 30% of twin pregnancies.
- Monozygotic twinning is determined by the timing at which splitting of the blastocyst occurs:
  - before 3 days after fertilisation (about 30%): DCDA
    — results in separate chorion, amnion and placental circulation
  - between 4 and 8 days after fertilisation (about 70%): MCDA (monochorionic diamniotic)
    — results in a single common placenta but two amnions and one chorionic membrane
  - after 8 days (about 1%): MCMA (monochorionic monoamniotic)
    — common amnion, chorion and placenta
  - after 13 days (rare): conjoined twins

Diagnosis of chorionicity and amnionicity

- in first trimester, high accuracy rates for chorionicity and amnionicity: determined by number of gestational sacs present, number of fetal heart beats or crown rump length (CRL) seen, or number of yolk sacs or amnions seen

- in second trimester, less accurate: determined by gender, number of placentas, dividing membrane, membrane thickness, presence or absence of the 'twin peak sign'

Prenatal diagnosis

- must know chorionicity
- monozygotic pregnancies have similar risk to singleton pregnancies: one risk for the pregnancy
  - rare: postzygotic non-disjunction
- dizygotic pregnancies
  - each fetus has individual risk
- first trimester screening applicable with or without the biochemistry
- second trimester screening inaccurate as analytes are increased due to number of fetuses
- invasive testing: chorionic villus sampling and amniocentesis
- multifetal reduction in specialised centres for anomalies or reduction of fetal numbers

Complications of twin pregnancy

General
- increased miscarriage rate: vanishing twin
- increased perinatal mortality rate: five to seven times of singleton pregnancies
  - death of one DCDA twin associated with preterm delivery
  - death of one MC twin has risk of hypotensive blood transfusion and 25% risk of neurological damage to the surviving twin
- fetal abnormalities: higher incidence of cardiac and central nervous system malformations
- intrauterine growth restriction (IUGR)
- premature delivery: in up to 45% of twins, compared with 5%–6% of singleton births
- postpartum haemorrhage
- pre-eclampsia: three to five times the risk associated with singleton births; tends to be more severe

Specific: monochorionic twinning
Twin-to-twin transfusion syndrome (TTTS)
- 15% incidence
- requires arterial to venous anastomosis, which is unbalanced, and one of the fetuses, the donor, starts to transfuse the other twin, the recipient
- associated with velamentous cord insertion

Staging (Quintero)
- stage 1: polyhydramnios (deepest vertical pocket of amniotic fluid >8 cm) in one twin and oligohydramnios (deepest vertical pocket of amniotic fluid <2 cm) in the other with bladder seen in the donor
- stage 2: polyhydramnios and oligohydramnios present with no bladder seen in the donor
- stage 3: abnormal Dopplers
  - donor: absent end diastolic flow or reversed in the umbilical artery
  - recipient: abnormal venous Dopplers

- stage 4: fetal hydrops
- stage 5: fetal demise of one or both twins

Management
- termination of pregnancy
- conservative: 90% mortality rate
- cord occlusion/ligation
- serial amnioreduction
- laser coagulopathy: best treatment outcome with decreased morbidity

Selective intrauterine growth restriction (sIUGR)
- 15% incidence
- one twin is small for gestational age where the other twin is growing normally
- associated with increased risk of fetal demise and risk of neurological sequelae
- three classifications

Twin reversed arterial perfusion sequence (TRAP) or acardiac twinning
- 1% of monozygotic pregnancies
- associated with chromosomal abnormalities, arterial to arterial anastomosis
- leads to major deformities/fetal demise in the recipient twin and possible heart failure in the donor twin

Antenatal management of twin pregnancy

Diagnosis
- Multiple pregnancy is a differential diagnosis if the fundal height is greater than dates and is associated with hyperemesis.
- Diagnosis is confirmed by ultrasound scan.

Antenatal care
- More frequent visits are advisable because of raised maternal and fetal risks.
- Weekly visits between antenatal visits and ultrasound assessment from about 30 weeks gestation are appropriate. Advise regarding employment, rest and iron supplementation.

Ultrasound role
- determining zygosity
- look for fetal abnormality
- assess growth and wellbeing: increased fetal surveillance with serial scans
- treatment: laser therapy

Prevention of premature labour
- Twins are five times more likely to be preterm than singletons.
- Delivery prior to 32 weeks is more likely with monochorionic twins.
- No studies have shown that routine hospitalisation, cervical suture or tocolysis increase pregnancy length.

Delivery of twins

- In 70% of cases, the first twin is a cephalic presentation, and both twins are cephalic in 40%.
- Common practice is delivery at 37–38 weeks, as there is increased risk of stillbirth.

Indications for elective caesarean section
- malpresentation of the first twin
- monoamniotic twins
- other obstetric indications, such as placenta praevia

Vaginal delivery
- Vaginal delivery is probably appropriate for cephalic/cephalic presentation with normal growth and wellbeing.
- Evidence is unclear on method of delivery when the second twin is breech.
- Both twins are continuously monitored during labour.
- Epidural anaesthesia is recommended.
- Augmentation and induction of labour is acceptable in the absence of any obstetric contraindications.
- The third stage requires active management because of the risk of postpartum haemorrhage.

Twin with single intrauterine fetal death

The incidence of antepartum death of one twin is 3%–4%. The outcome of the surviving twin is related to whether the twins are monochorionic or dichorionic. In monochorionic twins there is a high rate of vascular communication between the twins and a risk of significant twin-to-twin transfusion. Neurological abnormalities in the surviving twin result from thromboplastins released from the dead fetus, which can cause thrombotic occlusion of cerebral vessels. Fetal magnetic resonance imaging (MRI) is helpful.

Triplet pregnancy

Incidence. Triplet pregnancies have a wide geographical variation, with an increased incidence in Africa. In Western countries, the incidence is 1 in 6400. For clomiphene-induced pregnancies, the incidence is 5 in 1000 and for assisted reproductive techniques 3%–4%.

Complications of triplet pregnancy
- maternal: anaemia, pre-eclampsia, antepartum haemorrhage
- fetal: premature labour, with up to 80% delivering before 37 weeks gestation; IUGR; malpresentation; increased perinatal mortality rate (five times that of singleton)
- reduction to twin or singleton pregnancy reduces morbidity and mortality rates

Delivery
The perinatal mortality rate rises as the time interval between deliveries lengthens. This may be due to progressive fetal anoxia with changes in uteroplacental haemodynamics. As a result, caesarean section is indicated. The risk of postpartum haemorrhage is heightened.

Further reading

Evans MI, Ciorica D, Britt DW, Fletcher JC 2005 Update on selective reduction. Prenatal Diagnosis 25:807–813

Gratacos E, Lewi L, Munoz B et al 2007 A classification system for selective intrauterine growth restriction in monochorionic pregnancies according to umbilical artery Doppler flow in the smaller twin. Ultrasound in Obstetrics and Gynecology 30:28–34

Pharoah POD, Adi Y 2000 Consequences of in utero death in a twin pregnancy. Lancet 355:1597–1602

Quintero RA, Morales WJ, Allen MH et al 1999 Staging of twin–twin transfusion syndrome. Journal of Perinatology 19 (8):550–555

Roberts D, Gates S, Kilby M, Neilson JP 2008 Interventions for twin–twin transfusion syndrome: a Cochrane review. Ultrasound in Obstetrics and Gynecology 31:701–711

Senat M-V, Deprest J, Boulvain M et al 2004 Endoscopic laser surgery versus serial amnioreduction for severe twin-to-twin transfusion syndrome. New England Journal of Medicine 351:136–144

Wald NJ, Rish S 2005 Prenatal screening for Down syndrome and neural tube defects in twin pregnancies. Prenatal Diagnosis 25:740–745

Chapter 36

Preterm prelabour rupture of membranes

Justin Nasser

Definitions. Prelabour (premature) rupture of membranes (PROM) refers to membrane rupture before the onset of uterine contractions irrespective of gestational age. Preterm prelabour rupture of membranes (PPROM) refers to membrane rupture before the onset of uterine contractions in a pregnancy that is <37 completed weeks of gestation.

    Incidence. PROM occurs in 10% of all pregnancies. PPROM occurs in 3% of pregnancies and is responsible for, or associated with, approximately one-third of preterm births.

Aetiology of PPROM

- The pathogenesis of PPROM is poorly understood and in the majority of cases the exact aetiology is unknown.
- There are multiple possible aetiologies that probably share a common final pathway leading to membrane rupture. Such factors include those leading to membrane stretch, membrane degradation, uterine contractility, local inflammation, and increased susceptibility to ascending genital tract infection.

Risk factors of PPROM

- past history of PPROM/preterm delivery
- urogenital tract infection/colonisation
- antepartum haemorrhage
- cigarette smoking
- past history of cervical surgery
- amniocentesis in current pregnancy
- cervical length ≤25 mm
- positive fetal fibronectin (fFN)
- connective tissue disorders
- nutritional deficiencies
- lean maternal body mass
- multiple pregnancy/polyhydramnios

    Most cases of PPROM occur in women without risk factors and there is currently no reliable way of predicting and preventing PPROM.

Clinical significance of PPROM

Both mother and fetus are at risk from complications associated with PPROM.

Maternal risks
- those associated with infection, including chorioamnionitis, endometritis and septicaemia
  - risk of intrauterine infection increases with duration of membrane rupture
  - clinical signs indicating chorioamnionitis include maternal pyrexia, tachycardia, leucocytosis, uterine tenderness, offensive vaginal discharge and fetal tachycardia
- those associated with operative delivery, which is more likely in the setting of PPROM

Fetal risks
- preterm delivery
  - most cases of PPROM will deliver within 1 week after membrane rupture; however, latency increases with decreasing gestational age
  - morbidities associated with preterm delivery: hyaline membrane disease, intraventricular haemorrhage, periventricular leukomalacia and other neurologic sequelae, infection (e.g. sepsis, pneumonia, meningitis), necrotising enterocolitis and retinopathy of prematurity; rates vary with gestational age and are increased by the presence of chorioamnionitis
- pulmonary hypoplasia: hydrostatic pressure from amniotic fluid is essential to lung development and maturation in the mid-second trimester; loss of amniotic fluid at this stage of development can irreversibly arrest lung development and result in pulmonary hypoplasia; associated with significant neonatal mortality regardless of gestational age at birth
- musculoskeletal/facial deformities: due to the reduction in amniotic fluid and restriction of fetal movement
- malpresentation
- placental abruption
- umbilical cord complications (e.g. compression, prolapse)

Diagnosis

In the majority of cases, the diagnosis can be confidently made based on a history of fluid loss per vagina and direct visualisation of amniotic fluid in the posterior fornix by sterile speculum examination. If amniotic fluid is not immediately visible, fluid leakage through the internal os can be provoked by the Valsalva manoeuvre or coughing. Repeat speculum examination after a period of recumbency may assist the diagnosis.

A number of ancilliary tests with varying degrees of sensitivity/specificity and false-positive/false-negative rates can be used to assist in the diagnosis. These include:
- nitrazine test
- ferning/arborisation
- AmniSure test
- other biochemical tests (fFN, alopha-fetoprotein (AFP), diamino-oxydase, prolactin, human chorionic gonadotrophin (hCG))
- ultrasound assessment of amniotic fluid volume
- intra-amniotic indigo carmine with passage of blue fluid per vagina

Other causes of fluid loss include leucorrhoea, urinary incontinence, vaginitis, cervicitis, mucus show, semen and vaginal douches.

Management of PPROM

The management of PPROM is determined by several factors, including:
- gestational age
- available obstetric and neonatal services
- presence/absence of maternal/fetal infection
- presence/absence of labour and/or cervical changes
- fetal presentation
- assessments of fetal wellbeing

These factors need to be considered in each case and a decision made as to whether conservative or aggressive management is most appropriate.

Delivery is indicated when the risk to the fetus of complications of prematurity are outweighed by the risks to the mother/fetus of complications of PPROM.

Initial management
- The initial management involves confirming the diagnosis by history and clinical examination. At the time of sterile speculum examination, endocervical swabs (*Chlamydia*, gonorrhoea) and ano-vaginal swabs (group B streptococcus) should be collected.
- Digital examinations should be avoided unless delivery is anticipated.
- Generally, expeditious delivery is indicated if labour is advanced, or in the presence of non-reassuring fetal status and/or infective complications, regardless of gestational age. In the absence of these conditions, subsequent management is dependent on the gestational age at time of PPROM and the subsequent presence or absence of conditions necessitating delivery.

PPROM: 34–37 weeks
- The risk of serious neonatal complications with delivery after 34 weeks is low.
- There is no significant improvement in neonatal outcomes and an apparent increased risk of chorioamnionitis with expectant management in PPROM after 34 weeks.
- Current evidence suggests that delivery should be expedited to reduce the risk of associated complications when PPROM occurs near term.

PPROM: 24–33 weeks
- PPROM remote from term is generally managed in hospital due to a short latency period and high complication rate/intervention rate.
- Some studies have demonstrated favourable outcomes and cost savings with home management of selected cases after an initial period (48–72 hours) of hospital admission.
- In the absence of complications, ongoing observation, administration of corticosteroids and adjuvant antibiotics (see below), and serial monitoring, is indicated, with consideration for delivery occurring at 34 weeks.

PPROM: <23 completed weeks
- Good quality data to guide management in previable PPROM are sparse.
- Perinatal mortality is high and decreases with advancing gestation.
- More than half are delivered within 1 week of PPROM, either as a result of spontaneous labour or induced labour due to maternal/fetal indications.
- Induction of labour is achieved with either high-dose oxytocin or by vaginal/oral prostaglandins.
- After conservative management, approximately one-quarter will remain pregnant 1 month after membrane rupture. These women should be monitored for signs necessitating delivery.

- Depending on specific circumstances, outpatient management may be appropriate.
- Serial ultrasound assessments should occur to evaluate liquor volume and fetal growth. Ultrasound assessment of lung volumes (direct and indirect) is useful in predicting pulmonary hypoplasia.
- Persistent oligohydramnios following PPROM is associated with poorer outcomes regardless of gestational age at delivery.
- PPROM following amniocentesis is associated with more favourable outcomes.
- If the pregnancy reaches a stage where resuscitation of the newborn is planned, consideration should be given for in utero transfer to an institution with appropriate facilities for emergency delivery and neonatal intensive care.

Antenatal corticosteroids
- Antenatal corticosteroids significantly reduce the risks of respiratory distress syndrome, intraventricular haemorrhage and necrotising enterocolitis, without increasing the risks of maternal or neonatal infections in women with PPROM.
- The maximum benefit is in those fetuses between 28 and 32 weeks gestation.
- Data on the benefit of repeat weekly doses of corticosteroids, or administration of rescue steroids remote from initial course in women with PPROM who remain undelivered, are conflicting.

Adjuvant antibiotics
- Antibiotic therapy in women with PPROM is used in an attempt to treat/prevent ascending infection in order to prolong the latency period and reduce gestational-age-dependent morbidity and neonatal infections.
- Current data support erythromycin 250 mg orally four times daily for 10 days or until delivery following diagnosis of PPROM.
- The use of extended spectrum amoxycillin-clavulanic acid is associated with an increased risk of necrotising enterocolitis and is not recommended.
- Intrapartum antibiotics for group B streptococcus prophylaxis, and antibiotic therapy for chorioamnionitis/sepsis, should be considered in addition to the above regimen.

Tocolysis
- The benefit of tocolytic therapy in the setting of PPROM is unclear and is not routinely recommended. It is contraindicated in the presence of chorioamnionitis.
- As in the setting of preterm labour with intact membranes, tocolysis may have a role in delaying delivery in order to obtain maximum benefit of corticosteroids and allow in utero transfer to an appropriate facility for delivery.

Emerging therapies
- Various agents (gelatine sponge, platelets, cryoprecipitate, fibrin) have been used to form a cervical plug/act as a membrane sealant.
- Amnioinfusion has been used in an attempt to replace amniotic fluid.
- Current data are insufficient to recommend their implementation into routine practice.

Further reading

Canavan T, Simhan H, Caratis S 2004 An evidence-based approach to the evaluation and treatment of premature rupture of membranes: part I. Obstetrical and Gynecological Survey 59(9):669–677

Canavan T, Simhan H, Caratis S 2004 An evidence-based approach to the evaluation and treatment of premature rupture of membranes: part II. Obstetrical and Gynecological Survey 59(9):678–689

Kenyon S, Boulvain M, Neilson JP 2003 Antibiotics for preterm rupture of membranes. Cochrane Database of Systematic Reviews. Issue 2. Art. No.: CD001058. DOI: 10.1002/14651858

Mercer BM 2004 Preterm premature rupture of membranes: diagnosis and management. Clinics in Perinatology 31:765–782

Morris J, Roberts C, Crowther C et al 2006 Protocol for immediate delivery versus expectant care of women with preterm prelabour rupture of membranes close to term (PPROMT) Trial [ISRCTN44485060]. BMC Pregnancy and Childbirth 6:9

Royal Australian and New Zealand College of Obstetricians and Gynaecologists (RACOG) 2006 Preterm premature rupture of membranes. Guideline No. 44, November. Melbourne: RACOG

Waters TP, Mercer BM 2009 The management of preterm premature rupture of membranes near the limit of fetal viability. American Journal of Obstetrics and Gynecology 201(3):230–240

Chapter 37

Preterm labour

Justin Nasser

Definition. Preterm or premature labour is the onset of regular painful uterine contractions accompanied by effacement and dilatation of the cervix after 20 weeks and before 37 completed weeks of pregnancy.

Incidence: Preterm labour occurs in 5%–10% of all deliveries.

Common complications in premature infants include respiratory distress syndrome, intraventricular haemorrhage, bronchopulmonary dysplasia, patent ductus arteriosus, necrotising enterocolitis, sepsis, apnoea and retinopathy of prematurity.

The frequency of major morbidity rises as gestational age decreases.

Ongoing advances in neonatal medicine have resulted in dramatically improved outcomes for preterm infants; however, there remains significant risk of long-term morbidity, such as cerebral palsy, developmental delay, visual and hearing impairment, and chronic lung disease.

Significance

- Prematurity is the cause of 75% of perinatal deaths and a major determinant of short-term and long-term morbidity in infants and children.
- Two-thirds of the perinatal deaths occur in the 30%–40% of preterm infants who are delivered prior to 32 weeks gestation.

Aetiology

Preterm labour may be classified as *spontaneous* or *indicated*.

Spontaneous preterm labour
- Spontaneous preterm labour occurs in the absence of overt maternal or fetal conditions necessitating delivery. It commonly occurs in the absence of an obvious cause, or may follow preterm premature rupture of the membranes or related diagnoses such as incompetent cervix.
- Risk factors associated with spontaneous preterm labour include a history of previous preterm birth, multiple pregnancy, polyhydramnios, urogenital tract infection, previous cervical surgery, uterine anomalies, periodontal disease, bleeding in the second trimester, extremes of age, smoking, low prepregnancy weight and pregnancies achieved through assisted reproductive technologies.
- Most women who deliver preterm have no apparent risk factors.

Indicated preterm labour

- Indicated preterm labour occurs when conditions exist that create undue risk to the mother, the fetus, or both, should the pregnancy continue, and a clinical decision is made to expedite delivery. In these situations, the labour may be induced or the delivery achieved by caesarean section.
- The most common diagnoses that precede an indicated preterm birth are pre-eclampsia, fetal distress, intrauterine growth restriction, placental abruption and fetal demise.

Prevention of preterm labour

Many interventions aimed at reducing the incidence of preterm labour have been implemented and assessed, including:
- supplemental progesterone
- cervical cerclage
- detection and treatment of asymptomatic bacteriuria
- detection and treatment of bacterial vaginosis
- smoking cessation
- nutritional supplementation

None of these have shown consistent benefit. In fact, the incidence of preterm labour appears to be rising. The lack of success in preventing preterm labour can be attributed to:
- the current incomplete understanding of the physiology of normal parturition
- the current incomplete understanding of the pathogenesis of preterm labour
- the poor sensitivity and positive predictive value of currently available screening tests

Because of the difficulties of predicting and preventing preterm labour, the main goal of management is in early diagnosis of those at true risk of delivery, and implementation of therapies aimed at optimising perinatal outcomes.

Diagnosis of preterm labour

The clinical diagnosis of preterm labour is often unreliable, with up to 50% of women with signs and symptoms suggestive of preterm labour not progressing to preterm delivery.

A number of ancillary tests have been developed in an attempt to identify both asymptomatic and symptomatic women who are truly likely to deliver prematurely. The most clinically useful of these tests are:
- cervical length and morphology assessment by transvaginal ultrasound
- fetal fibronectin (fFN) detection in cervicovaginal secretions

Cervical length and morphology

- Well-defined, reproducible changes in the appearance of the cervix by transvaginal ultrasound occur as labour progresses.
- The cervix undergoes progressive shortening and widening along the endocervical canal commencing at the internal os ('funnelling').
- The initial changes are almost always asymptomatic and not identified by digital vaginal examination.
- A cervical length of <2.5 cm at 16–24 weeks gestation is a strong predictor of preterm birth when used as a screening test in both low-risk and high-risk women. The shorter the cervical length and the earlier in pregnancy that the shortening occurs, the greater the likelihood of preterm birth.

- In symptomatic women, a cervical length of >3 cm is likely to exclude the diagnosis of preterm labour.

Fetal fibronectin (fFN)
- fFN is a glycoprotein 'glue' that binds chorion to decidua.
- Disruption of the maternal fetal interface causes release of fFN into the cervicovaginal secretions.
- In a normal pregnancy, fFN should be almost undetectable in vaginal secretions from 22–35 weeks.
- The presence of fFN in the cervicovaginal secretions is a predictor of preterm birth; however, its clinical utility is in its negative predictive value, as <1% of women with a negative test will deliver within 1 week.

The use of both fFN and cervical sonography may increase the utility of these tests in assessing at-risk women.

Management of preterm labour

Because of the lack of success in predicting and preventing preterm labour, the aim of management is largely to reduce the likelihood and impact of prematurity-related sequelae. Three interventions have been shown to reduce perinatal morbidity and mortality in women who deliver preterm:
- in utero transfer to a facility with appropriate neonatal facilities
- administration of corticosteroids to the mother to facilitate fetal lung maturation and reduce complications of prematurity
- administration of antibiotics to prevent neonatal group B streptococcus infection

In the setting of preterm labour, tocolytic therapy aims to delay delivery in order to facilitate corticosteroid administration and in utero transfer to an appropriate facility for delivery.

There are a number of therapeutic agents that can suppress uterine muscle activity, but all have potential adverse side effects. Current evidence suggests that:
- Calcium channel blockers (e.g. nifedipine) or an oxytocin antagonist (atosiban) can delay delivery for 2–7 days with minimal side effects.
- Beta-agonists (e.g. ritodrine, terbutaline, salbutamol) are effective at delaying delivery for 48 hours, but are associated with greater side effects.
- Magnesium sulfate is an ineffective tocolytic.
- The benefit of cyclo-oxygenase inhibitors (e.g. indomethacin) is uncertain.

Much of the improvement in perinatal morbidity and mortality associated with prematurity is due to the advances in neonatal management.

Further reading

Grimes-Dennis J, Berghella V 2007 Cervical length and prediction of preterm delivery. Current Opinion in Obstetrics and Gynecology 19:191–195

Goldenberg RL, Culhane JF, Iams JD, Romero R 2008 Preterm birth 1. Epidemiology and causes of preterm birth. Lancet 371:75–84

Iams J 2003 Prediction and early detection of preterm labour. Obstetrics and Gynecology 101:402–412

Iams JD, Romero R, Culhane JF, Goldenberg RL 2008 Preterm birth 2. Primary, secondary, and tertiary interventions to reduce the morbidity and mortality of preterm birth. Lancet 371:164–175

Vidaeff AC, Ramin SM 2009 Management strategies for the prevention of preterm birth. Part I: update on progesterone supplementation. Current Opinion in Obstetrics and Gynecology 21:480–484

Vidaeff AC, Ramin SM 2009 Management strategies for the prevention of preterm birth. Part II: update on cervical cerclage. Current Opinion in Obstetrics and Gynecology 21:485–490

Chapter 38

Induction of labour

Michael Flynn

Assessing the cervix

The cervix remains closed because of its rigidity due to the collagen fibres that make up the bulk of cervical stroma. Cervical connective tissue consists mainly of collagen and a matrix of large proteoglycan molecules.

Cervical changes are due to:
- changes in proteoglycan
- collagen degradation
- increased vascularity
- accumulation of interstitial fluid

A uniform means of assessing the cervix is the Bishop's score (see Table 38.1). The Bishop's score assesses the favourability of the cervix for induction of labour by assigning points to each of the five cervical features and adding these points. With a low score (0–3), there is a high risk of a failed induction, resulting in caesarean section (>20%), compared with a score of 8 or more, where the failed induction rate is <3%. With a high score, the cervix is said to be 'ripe'.

Mechanism of labour

The exact mechanism of labour is still unknown, although it is thought that the production of fetal cortisol increases placental oestrogen and prostaglandin production, and sensitises the myometrium to oxytocin. Other factors such as progesterone, relaxin and prostacycline dominate early in pregnancy to inhibit contractility. Prostaglandin E_2 and F_2-alpha are synthesised by the decidua and amnion, and may sensitise the myometrium to oxytocin.

Induction of labour

Uterine rupture can occur with any agent that enhances uterine tone. The sensitivity of the myometrium to prostaglandin and oxytocin rises as gestation increases. However, the myometrium is relatively insensitive to oxytocin before term.

Cervical favourability (Bishop's score) is an indicator of the myometrial sensitivity to oxytocin. Prostaglandin may augment the action of oxytocin and lead to uterine rupture.

Indications
- prolonged pregnancy (the Canadian Multicenter Post-Term Pregnancy Trial compared induction of labour and conservative management in uncomplicated pregnancies >41 weeks gestation: the results showed lower caesarean section rates in the induction-of-labour group, with both groups showing similar perinatal mortality and neonatal morbidity rates)
- hypertensive disorders of pregnancy

Table 38.1 The Bishop's score

Cervical feature	Bishop's score			
	0	1	2	3
Dilatation	<1 cm	1–2 cm	3–4 cm	>4 cm
Length	4 cm	2–4 cm	1–2 cm	<1 cm
Consistency	Firm	Medium	Soft	
Position	Posterior	Central	Anterior	
Station	3	2	1,0	>+1

Table 38.2 Contraindications for induction of labour

Absolute	Relative
Absolute cephalopelvic disproportion	Antepartum haemorrhage
Presumed fetal distress	Grand multiparity
Placenta praevia	Previous caesarean section
Vasa praevia	Overdistended uterus
Abnormal presentation	Face or breech presentation
Previous classical caesarean section	History of rapid labour
Invasive carcinoma of cervix	
Cord presentation	

- premature rupture of membranes
- intrauterine fetal death
- diabetes
- intrauterine growth restriction
- antepartum haemorrhage
- isoimmunisation
- unstable lie
- maternal diseases

Contraindications
Table 38.2 lists contraindications for induction of labour.

Techniques of induction

Surgical
'Sweeping' of the membranes
- Women who undergo daily sweeping of membranes for 3 consecutive days appear more likely to go into labour than controls.

Amniotomy
- This method of surgically rupturing the forewaters with an amnihook or other instrument is often used in combination with oxytocin.
- Risks include cord prolapse, intrauterine infection (especially with an increased induction-to-delivery interval) and an increased incidence of cardiotocograph abnormalities.

Medical

Oxytocin

- In vivo, oxytocin is synthesised in the paraventricular nucleus of the hypothalamus and is transported to the posterior pituitary gland. It is released as a free peptide in response to suckling/nipple stimulation, genital stimulation and stretching of the cervix. Increased sensitivity of the myometrium occurs with increasing gestational age.
- Although regimens vary, the required oxytocin dose to provide adequate uterine action is usually between 4 and 16 milliunits per minute. As the physiological dose is individualised, low doses are used initially with close monitoring of contractions, uterine relaxation and progress.
- Complications include water retention, hyponatraemia, uterine hyperstimulation and rupture, and neonatal hyperbilirubinaemia.
- Compared with amniotomy alone, the combined use of amniotomy and oxytocin infusion increases the likelihood of delivery within 24 hours, and lowers the risk of operative delivery and of postpartum haemorrhage.

Prostaglandin

The favourability of the cervix is the best available predictor of a successful induction of labour. At present, the most effective method of cervical ripening is the use of local prostaglandins. When comparing local prostaglandin induction with amniotomy/oxytocin induction, prostaglandin is associated with a decrease in length of labour, lower caesarean section rates (by reducing the number of failed inductions), and fewer Apgar scores (at 1 minute) below 4.

Types of prostaglandin agents

Prostaglandin E_2 is used for cervical ripening for induction of labour. It is manufactured in a triactin-based gel with 1 or 2 mg dinoprostone in each unit dose of 3 g (2.5 mL). A slow-release delivery system vaginal insert is also available.

Actions of prostaglandins

These soften and efface the cervix by a combination of reducing the collagen concentration and changing the glycosaminoglycan composition and hydration.

Other effects

Prostaglandin E_2 produces vasodilatation and 30% increased cardiac output. It relaxes bronchial and gastrointestinal smooth muscle.

Contraindications of prostaglandin E_2

These include grand multiparity, rupture of membranes, high presenting part, past uterine surgery, cephalopelvic disproportion, abnormal cardiotocograph, malpresentation and unexplained vaginal bleeding.

Side effects of prostaglandins

These include uterine hyperstimulation (<1%), irritation of the vagina, nausea, vomiting, diarrhoea, pyrexia, broncho-constriction, hypertension, blurred vision, facial flush and vasovagal reaction.

Augmentation of labour

Aims

- accelerate progress of labour
- reduce operative vaginal delivery rates
- lower caesarean section rates

- lower the need for analgesia
- reduce the psychological impact associated with slow labour
- primary role of augmentation is to reduce the rate of dysfunctional labour in primigravid women, which may occur in up to 40% of cases

Methods
- Environment: the presence of a support person may reduce the length of labour.
- Ambulation: this reduces the need for oxytocic augmentation.
- Increase uterine contractility: amniotomy, oxytocin (50% of those diagnosed with slow labour will progress equally with or without oxytocin; 95% of primigravidas in labour with oxytocin augmentation will deliver within 12 hours).

Considerations in augmentation
The differential diagnosis of slow progress in labour includes:
- reduced uterine contractility
- increased resistance in soft tissues (relative disproportion, including malpresentation)
- absolute cephalopelvic disproportion
  To differentiate between these mechanisms, adequate uterine contractility is required and oxytocics are suggested.

Further reading

Bishop EH 1964 Pelvic scoring for elective induction. Obstetrics and Gynecology 24:266
Grant JM 1993 Sweeping the membranes in prolonged pregnancy. British Journal of Obstetrics and Gynaecology 100:889–890
Hannah M, Hannah WJ, Hellmann J et al 1992 Induction of labor as compared with serial antenatal monitoring in post-term pregnancy: a randomized controlled trial. Canadian Multicenter Post-Term Pregnancy Trial Group. New England Journal of Medicine 326 (24):1587–1592

Chapter 39

Malpresentation and malposition

Michael Flynn

Stages of labour

Labour is divided into three stages:
- The **first stage** commences with painful contractions, which dilate and efface the cervix. This stage ends with full dilatation of the cervix, and is further divided into the latent and active stage. The active stage begins at full effacement of the cervix.
- The **second stage** begins at full dilatation and ends with the delivery of the baby.
- The **third stage** ends when the placenta is delivered.

At term, about 95% of fetuses are cephalic in presentation. Of these, up to 95% will deliver in the occipito-anterior position. Malpresentations and malpositions increase the maternal risks of prolonged labour, infection, obstructed labour, tissue necrosis resulting in vesico/rectovaginal fistulas, and deep venous thrombosis. Fetal risks of malpresentation and malposition are cord prolapse, traumatic delivery and hypoxia.

Occipito-posterior position

The fetal head usually engages in the lateral position, and in 80% of cases it rotates anteriorly. About 20% of fetuses are in the occipito-posterior position in early labour (usually occiput to the right). With increasing flexion in labour, there is a tendency for the fetal head to rotate when it reaches the pelvic floor.

Risk factors for persistent occipito-posterior position
- anterior placenta
- anthropoid or android pelvis, where the pelvic brim is longer in the anterior–posterior diameter than in the transverse
- inefficient uterine contractions

Diagnosis
The occipital bone is the only bone that is overridden by its neighbours. When the diamond-shaped anterior fontanelle can be palpated on vaginal examination, this indicates deflexion of the fetal head.

The maternal abdomen appears flat below the umbilicus, and fetal limbs can be palpated anteriorly on the maternal abdomen.

Characteristics of labour
- The woman complains of backache.
- There is a tendency for incoordinate uterine action and prolonged labour.
- There is early distension of the perineum and dilatation of the anus, while the fetal head is high in the birth canal.

Management
- Slow progress in the first stage of labour often requires oxytocin augmentation.
- In the second stage, adequate uterine contractions are required for rotation of the fetal head on the pelvic floor. Occasionally, the fetus will spontaneously deliver in the occipito-posterior position.
- An instrumental delivery may be indicated for a prolonged second stage. Vacuum extraction, using the posterior cup position, will encourage flexion and rotation of the fetal head to correct the relative disproportion. Kielland's rotational forceps may also be used.
- Delivery by caesarean section is indicated if the station of the head is above the ischial spines.

Face presentation

Risk factors
- Fetal factors include anencephaly, cystic hygroma, goitre, prematurity and multiple pregnancy.
- Maternal factors include bicornuate uterus and pelvic tumours.

Diagnosis
Most are diagnosed in labour just before delivery. Up to 75% are in the mento-anterior position. The landmarks at vaginal examination are the mouth, jaw, nose, malar and orbits. The mouth and maxilla form a triangle.

Management
Aim for a vaginal delivery, especially if the baby is in the mento-anterior position. However, if the baby is in the mento-posterior position and there is failure to rotate, the baby cannot be delivered vaginally and caesarean section is required.

Brow presentation

Incidence. Incidence is about 1 in 1000 deliveries.

Risk factors
- fetal: as with face presentation
- maternal: contracted pelvis

Diagnosis
- Vaginal examination: this includes palpation of the anterior fontanelle and orbital ridges.
- Labour in the brow presentation is often prolonged and obstructed.

Management
- No treatment is necessary if diagnosed in early labour and progress of labour is adequate. The baby may deflex to a face presentation or flex to a vertex presentation.
- Perform caesarean section if there is delay in labour or disproportion.
- Instrumental delivery may be attempted if the cervix is fully dilated and there is no clinical evidence of cephalopelvic disproportion.

Transverse and oblique lie

Incidence. Incidence is about 1 in 300 deliveries.

Risk factors
- fetal: prematurity, multiple pregnancy, polyhydramnios, fetal death and placenta praevia
- maternal: multiparity, contracted pelvis, pelvic tumours and abnormal uterine shape

Diagnosis
- Uterus is small for dates; there is no fetal pole in fundus or pelvis.
- Confirm the diagnosis by ultrasound examination.

Labour
- It is often incoordinate and obstructed.
- Uterine rupture may occur and there is a risk of cord prolapse in 10%–15% of cases.

Management
- If the unstable lie persists over 37 weeks, admit the woman to hospital and await labour. If the unstable lie persists after 38 weeks or labour commences, caesarean section is indicated.
- Internal version of the fetus may result in uterine rupture, and this is indicated only for a second twin.

Cord prolapse and presentation

Incidence. Incidence is about 1 in 200–300 deliveries.

Risk factors
- poorly applied presenting part
- fetal: prematurity, long umbilical cord, low-lying placenta
- maternal: multiparity
- iatrogenic: operative manoeuvres, including artificial rupture of membranes and forceps delivery

Management
- Advise the woman to present as soon as possible when membranes rupture, especially women with risk factors.
- When a cord presentation is diagnosed, the presenting part must be pushed away from the cord to avoid cord compression, and immediate delivery of the baby is required.

Diameters of presenting parts

- occipito-anterior = suboccipito-bregmatic = 9.5 cm
- occipito-posterior = occipito-frontal = 11 cm
- face presentation = submento-bregmatic = 9.5 cm
- brow presentation = mento-vertical = 14 cm

Further reading

Ritchie JK 1998 Malpositions of the occiput and malpresentations. In: Dewhurst's textbook of obstetrics and gynaecology for postgraduates. Oxford: Blackwell Scientific

Chapter 40

Operative delivery

Michael Flynn

Caesarean section

Caesarean section births constitute approximately one-quarter of births in many countries. Although now a relatively safe procedure, emergency caesarean section carries an increased risk of maternal mortality and morbidity.

Indications for caesarean section
Elective
- repeat caesarian section
- abnormal fetal lie
- malpresentation: breech, twins
- placenta praevia
- maternal conditions, including pre-eclampsia, diabetes, neurological disease

Emergency
- presumed fetal distress
- failure to progress

Risk of uterine rupture with labour after caesarean section
Classical caesarean section
The overall risk of rupture after a classical caesarean section is about 6%, with 2% scar dehiscence before labour.

Lower segment caesarean section
There is a 0.3% risk of dehiscence overall, increasing to 0.7% with labour and 0.1% at elective caesarean section.

Trial of vaginal delivery after lower segment caesarean section
Up to 40% of women undergo a repeat caesarean section after one lower segment caesarean section for a non-recurring cause. The risks and benefits of repeat caesarean section and trial of vaginal delivery require consideration when deciding on the mode of delivery.

Risks of caesarean section
Maternal risks
- higher overall maternal mortality rate compared with vaginal delivery, although comparable rates with elective caesarean section
- higher febrile morbidity
- increased blood loss
- anaesthetic risks
- increased risk of deep venous thrombosis

Neonatal risks
- increased risk of respiratory distress secondary to retained lung fluid
- birth trauma

Factors to consider in deciding the mode of delivery
- Number of previous lower segment caesarean sections: only small numbers have been reported regarding trial of vaginal delivery after two caesarean sections.
- Indications for the first caesarean section: the vaginal delivery rates are lowest when the initial indication was for failure to progress.
- Previous vaginal delivery: if the woman has had a previous vaginal delivery, there is a greater likelihood of delivering vaginally again.
- Vaginal delivery can be achieved in up to 75% of trials of labour. There is a tendency for higher vaginal delivery rates if oxytocin is used for augmentation and longer labour is allowed. The use of oxytocin remains controversial.

Symptoms and signs of uterine rupture
- acute continuous abdominal pain
- acute fetal distress
- reduction in contractions
- vaginal bleeding

Complications of caesarean section
Haemorrhage
- Haemorrhage accounts for 6% of maternal deaths associated with caesarean section.
- There are higher risks with placenta praevia, placental abruption, atonic uterus, multiparity and prolonged labour.

Urinary tract
- The risk of bladder injury at caesarean section is lower than 1%.
- This is higher in emergency caesarean sections for prolonged obstructed labour or repeat caesarean section with the bladder adherent to the lower segment.
- Ureteric injuries are very uncommon.

Anaesthetic complications
- Regional anaesthesia is a safer alternative to general anaesthesia.
- Anaesthetic complications include supine hypotension and Mendelson's acid aspiration syndrome.

Infections
- Wound infections occur in 1%–9% of caesarean sections. There is a higher risk of infection with premature rupture of membranes and prolonged labour.
- Endometritis: there is a 10–20 times higher risk of endometritis after caesarean section compared with vaginal delivery. The higher risk is associated with increased length of labour and chorioamnionitis. The common pathogens include group B streptococcus, *Escherichia coli* and anaerobes.
- Chest infections are complications for 10% of patients after abdominal surgery. High-risk factors for chest infection include obesity, general anaesthetic, smoking and upper respiratory tract infection.
- Urinary tract infection: there is a 2% risk of urinary tract infection with single catheterisation.

- Antibiotic prophylaxis, given after the clamping of the umbilical cord, has been shown to decrease the risk of postoperative febrile morbidity. This is irrespective of whether the caesarean section was emergency or elective. The choice of antibiotics includes broad-spectrum penicillins and early-generation cephalosporin.
- Thromboembolism accounts for 17% of deaths after caesarean section. The recurrence risk after one episode of deep venous thrombosis is 12%.

Indications for classical caesarean section
- absence of the lower uterine segment (this may occur with extreme prematurity, placenta praevia, or fibroids obscuring the lower segment)
- transverse lie or shoulder presentation
- presence of a uterine constriction ring
- large abnormal baby
- caesarean hysterectomy (commonly for tumours of the cervix)
- conjoint twins

Instrumental delivery

This includes the forceps and vacuum extractor. The indications and prerequisites are similar for both.

Indications
- failure to progress in the second stage
- malposition of the fetal head
- fetal distress during the second stage
- maternal conditions, including pre-eclampsia, neurological conditions and cardiorespiratory diseases

Prerequisites for instrumental delivery
- an indication for the use of instruments
- suitable presenting part
- fully dilated cervix
- membranes ruptured
- clinical assessment not suggestive of absolute cephalopelvic disproportion
- station of presenting part below the ischial spines
- no fetal head palpable abdominally
- position of fetal head (must be known)
- adequate uterine contractions
- empty bladder
- adequate analgesia

Forceps
Types of forceps
- outlet forceps: Wrigley's forceps
- non-rotational: Neville Barnes' forceps
- rotational: Kielland's forceps

Complications
- maternal: genital tract soft tissue injury, increased incidence of episiotomy, bladder and rectal injury
- fetal: facial soft tissue damage, intracranial haemorrhage

Vacuum extractor
Complications
- maternal: genital tract injury
- fetal: swelling on the scalp produced by the vacuum cup (the chignon), which disappears over 1–2 days; scalp markings and abrasions; cephalohaematoma (a collection of blood under the periosteum) in up to 6% of babies delivered with vacuum extraction; subgaleal haemorrhage

Perineal lacerations

Lacerations can occur anywhere along the birth canal, including the uterus, cervix, vagina and perineum.
- **First-degree** perineal laceration means tearing of the skin of the perineum and mucous membrane of the vagina.
- **Second-degree** laceration involves the skin and musculature of the perineum. It can involve the external anal sphincter.
- **Third-degree** laceration involves at least the anal mucosa.

The centrepoint of the perineum is the perineal body. The muscles that blend into this point are the external anal sphincter, levator ani, transverse perineal muscles and bulbocavernosus. The anal sphincter consists of the internal and external layers. The internal sphincter is circular and is situated in the upper two-thirds of the anal canal. The external sphincter consists of three layers. In perineal lacerations, the deep layer is important, as it plays a major role in the continence of flatus and faeces.

Repair of perineal trauma
Up to 70% of women are likely to require perineal repair.

Technique
- The vaginal skin may be repaired with continuous or interrupted sutures.
- The perineal skin closure may be subcuticular or interrupted.
- Comparing the two techniques, studies have shown no difference in the long-term complaints of pain or dyspareunia. However, there appears to be a significant advantage in the reduction of pain, in the short term, when using subcuticular sutures.

Choice of suture
Reports comparing polyglycolic acid and chromic catgut show a definite reduction of pain in the short term when using polyglycolic acid, although no long-term differences were found. Therefore, it appears that the optimal choice in the repair of perineal trauma is the use of polyglycolic acid sutures and subcuticular sutures to the skin.

Episiotomy
Tissues cut by an episiotomy include:
- vaginal epithelium and perineal skin
- bulbocavernosus muscle
- transverse perineal muscles: superficial and deep
- occasionally, the external anal sphincter and levator ani

Therefore, an episiotomy is at least a second-degree perineal laceration.

Indications for episiotomy
- vaginal breech deliveries
- in fetal distress, to expedite delivery

- past history of pelvic floor repair or third-degree tear
- imminent perineal tear
- instrumental delivery

Types of episiotomy
- mid-line
- mediolateral
- J-shaped

Repair of an episiotomy
This has three stages:
- The initial stage of repair commences at the apex of the vaginal laceration. The laceration is repaired down towards the fourchette.
- The second stage consists of repairing the deep muscles of the pelvic floor.
- The final stage is to repair the superficial perineal muscles and skin.
  If the anal sphincters are involved, both ends need to be isolated and repaired.

Further reading

Enkin M, Keirse M, Chalmers I 2000 A guide to effective care in pregnancy and childbirth. Oxford: Oxford University Press

O'Grady JP, Gimovsky M 1992 Instrumental delivery: a lost art? Progress in obstetrics and gynaecology, Vol. 10. London: Churchill Livingstone, pp 183–211

Spong CY, Landon MB, Gilbert S et al 2007 Risk of uterine rupture and adverse perinatal outcome at term after cesarean delivery. Obstetrics and Gynecology 110:801–807

Vacca A 2003 Handbook of vacuum extraction in obstetric practice. London: Edward Arnold

Chapter 41

Pain relief in labour

Michael Flynn

About two-thirds of women in labour consider the pain very severe and intolerable. There is a need for antenatal preparation, with balanced information and opportunity to discuss options of analgesia.

Pain in labour

Causes
- dilatation of the cervix
- contraction and distension of uterus
- distension of the vagina and perineum
- pressure on other organs and lumbosacral plexus

Sensory pathways
- Mild pain of early uterine contractions is conducted through T11–T12.
- When the pain becomes more intense, the pathway is T10–L1.
- The cervix is also supplied by T10–L1.
- Pain in the second stage is conducted via sacral segment S2–S5.

Analgesia in labour

Non-pharmacological methods
- position/postural changes
- warm or cold packs
- massage
- hydrotherapy
- transcutaneous electrical nerve stimulation (TENS), the electrodes being placed paravertebrally at T10–L1 and S2–S4 (uses the gate control theory of pain)
- hypnotherapy
- breathing techniques

Pharmacological methods
- Inhalational agents: nitrous oxide is simple and safe.
- Systemic opioid analgesia: pethidine has a more rapid onset (20–30 minutes, with peak effects at 1 hour) of action than morphine because of its higher lipid solubility. Neonatal depression can occur when administered 2–3 hours before delivery. Side effects include nausea, vomiting and reduced gastric motility.
- Regional anaesthesia: lumbar epidural is the most effective and reliable form of pain relief in labour. The local anaesthetic may be delivered by intermittent boluses or constant infusion.

Advantages of lumbar epidural
- The mother remains conscious, is able to maintain airways, and can participate in the birth.
- There is minimal or no fetal/neonatal depression with higher Apgar scores than those associated with narcotic analgesia.
- It may optimise uteroplacental blood flow and avoid increasing maternal/fetal acidosis and a further rise in maternal catecholamines.
- Better postpartum analgesia top-up pain relief is possible.
- It does not affect rates of caesarean section or obstetric intervention, though it may prolong the second stage.

Disadvantages of lumbar epidural
- It is not always successful in providing analgesia.
- There may be hypotension from reduced peripheral vascular resistance. This is a result of sympathetic blockade with decreased vasoconstriction and increased venous pooling. The blockade also produces a secondary tachycardia. Hypotension is managed with intravenous fluids and ephedrine 5–10 mg intravenously.

Complications of lumbar epidural
- **Local anaesthesia toxicity**. Central nervous system effects of circumoral numbness, restlessness, visual changes, confusion and convulsion, and arrhythmia and hypotension, are managed by ensuring adequate airway/ventilation, assessing cardiorespiratory status and treating convulsions.
- **Massive subarachnoid injection of local anaesthetic**. This is avoided by applying a small test dose. The complications, including hypotension, nausea, coma, fixed dilated pupils, phrenic nerve paralysis and ventilatory failure, are managed by providing ventilatory support, assessing cardiovascular status and giving intravenous fluids (maintain these until the anaesthetic wears off).
- **Dural puncture**. This occurs in about 1% of patients. The majority of these develop symptoms, especially positional headache. The most effective treatment is autologous blood patch, but there is a risk of infection.
- **Anaphylactic reactions**. Allergic and anaphylaxis reaction may occur as with any other pharmacological agents.

Paracervical block
- Relieves contraction pain in up to 80% of cases.

Spinal analgesia
- advantages: rapid onset, a dense block, and minimal risk of toxicity
- disadvantages: hypotension

Chapter 42

Labour ward emergencies

Michael Flynn

Up to 5% of deliveries have postpartum complications.

Unconscious patient

Management
- first aid: left lateral position, clear airway, oxygen, intubation if required, assessing pulse, respiration, blood pressure, colour and fetal heart rate
- intravenous line, collecting blood for full blood count, electrolytes, blood sugar level, blood group and hold, coagulation profile, liver and renal function tests
- monitoring electrocardiograph, pulse, blood pressure, fetal heart rate
- treatment of the cause

Main causes
- supine hypotension
- epilepsy
- eclampsia

Other causes
- neurological: epilepsy, tumour, subarachnoid haemorrhage, local anaesthesia toxicity, total spinal anaesthesia (inadvertent massive subarachnoid dose of local anaesthesia)
- vascular: blood loss, myocardial infarction, hypertensive encephalopathy, thromboembolism and pulmonary embolus
- respiratory: amniotic fluid embolism
- endocrine: hyper/hypoglycaemia, addisonian crisis
- infective causes
- drugs

Postpartum haemorrhage

Primary postpartum haemorrhage
Primary postpartum haemorrhage is the loss of more than 500 mL blood within 24 hours of delivery. The incidence is 1%–5%.

In maternal mortality statistics in Australia, haemorrhage has been a major factor of direct maternal deaths. In these, postpartum haemorrhage was a significant contributor.

Causes
- retained products of conception, retained placenta
- uterine atony (most common cause)
- soft-tissue laceration
- coagulation defect
- uterine rupture

Risk factors
- retained placenta
- grand multiparity with increased fibrous tissue and reduced muscular tissue in the uterus
- antepartum haemorrhage
- overdistension of the uterus with conditions such as polyhydramnios and multiple pregnancy
- large placental site (associated with multiple pregnancy, molar pregnancy)
- past history of postpartum haemorrhage or haemorrhagic disorders
- fibroid uterus (especially intramural)
- prolonged labour
- chorioamnionitis
- tocolytic agents, halogenated anaesthetic agents
- 20% occurring in the absence of risk factors

Management
- Prevention: routine use of oxytocin and an active management of the third stage can reduce postpartum haemorrhage by 40%.
- Resuscitation: the immediate danger is inadequate circulation, not reduced oxygen-carrying capacity. Therefore, restore circulatory volume with intravenous fluids and cross-match blood.
- Haemostasis: if coagulation or platelet count are abnormal, treat with fresh frozen plasma and platelets.
- Fundal massage can be used.

Medical treatment for atonic uterus
This involves an intravenous oxytocin bolus of initially 10 IU or ergometrine 250–500 μg. If haemorrhage is not controlled by simple methods, the woman requires a formal examination and exploration under anaesthesia. The genital tract is assessed for tears, retained products of conception and uterine rupture. If uterine atony continues after these causes are excluded, further medical treatment includes the use of rectal misoprostol, which may be effective in increasing uterine tone. Doses of up to 800 mg are used and maternal pyrexia should be monitored.

Surgical management of continuing postpartum haemorrhage
Uterine artery ligation has minimal complications and reduces the pulse pressure by 60%–70% to allow endogenous haemostatic mechanisms to control bleeding.

Internal iliac artery ligation
This is usually bilateral.

Uterine compression sutures
B-Lynch sutures used to compress the uterus are often effective.

Recombinant activated factor VIIa
This has been used effectively in uncontrolled bleeding.

Hysterectomy

Hysterectomy may be needed for persistent atony, morbidly adherent placenta or uterine rupture. If it is not due to placenta praevia, a subtotal hysterectomy may be the operation of choice, as there is a higher maternal mortality with total hysterectomy.

Secondary postpartum haemorrhage

Definition. Secondary postpartum haemorrhage is fresh bleeding from the genital tract after the first 24 hours but before 6 weeks postpartum. It is most common in the second week.

Causes
- infection
- retained products of conception
- placental site subinvolution

Investigation
- This includes abdominal and vaginal examination to confirm involution of the uterus and closed external cervical os.
- Vaginal microbiological examination is used, and ultrasound examination, to exclude retained products.

Management
- antibiotics: suitable empirical cover for mixed genital flora, including amoxycillin/ potassium clavulanate 500 mg every 8 hours
- evacuation of retained products
- uterotonic agents, including oxytocinon and misoprostol

Summary of management of severe obstetric haemorrhage
- prompt restoration of circulatory volume
- accurate diagnosis of cause
- appropriate treatment to stop bleeding early

Amniotic fluid embolism

Incidence. Incidence is about 1 in 80,000. Previously, there was up to 85% maternal mortality and 40% fetal mortality. It presents with respiratory distress, and cardiovascular collapse. Of those who survive the first hour, 40% will develop a coagulopathy.

Pathophysiology

Amniotic fluid embolism can occur in any trimester and is due to changes in the normal anatomical relationship between the membranes, placenta and uterine wall, with disruption of the integrity of the uterine blood vessels.

In the maternal circulation, the amniotic fluid/debris is deposited in the lungs and causes pulmonary vasoconstriction, which is probably due to an anaphylactic-type reaction to the amniotic fluid/debris. Severe hypoxia occurs with acute left-sided heart failure; disseminated intravascular coagulopathy may also occur.

Risk factors
- hypertonic uterine action
- caesarean section
- polyhydramnios
- precipitate labour

- advanced maternal age
- grand multiparity

Presentation and diagnosis
- There is sudden collapse after rupture of membranes in labour with dyspnoea, pink frothy sputum and cyanosis, leading to shock and apnoea. Convulsions occur in 10%–20% of cases.
- The diagnosis is confirmed by finding fetal squames in the sputum or blood from central venous line, or at postmortem during examination of the maternal lungs when fetal squames and debris are present.

Management
- securing airways and ventilating
- treating cardiovascular collapse
- central venous line
- acute left ventricular failure: digoxin
- vasopressins: dopamine/dobutamine
- correcting coagulopathy
- treating metabolic/electrolyte abnormalities
- watching for infection
- intensive care

Thromboembolism and pulmonary embolism

(*See Ch 47 for further details.*)

Clinical presentation of pulmonary embolism
- anxiety, tachycardia
- shortness of breath, apnoea, cyanosis and unconsciousness
- possible retrosternal chest pain, haemoptysis, pleural friction rub and a split-second heart sound

Emergency management
- resuscitate
- secure airway, oxygen, ventilate if necessary
- anticoagulate with standard or low-molecular-weight heparin
- surgery: employ embolectomy if the embolus is in the proximal part of the main pulmonary artery; if in inferior vena cava, insert umbrella filter

Prophylaxis
- in patients with a past history of deep venous thrombosis, obese patients and/or those who have an operative delivery (*see Ch 47*)

Regional anaesthesia toxicity

Incidence. Incidence is up to 1 in 1000. Increased susceptibility in the pregnant woman is due to:
- increased blood flow to the spinal cord
- reduced epidural space because of distended vessels
- a rise in pressure in the epidural space with uterine contractions

Presentation
- Signs and symptoms may occur almost immediately and within up to 20 minutes of administering local anaesthesia.
- Patient complains of metallic taste, tinnitus, confusion and disorientation.
- Respiratory muscle paralysis and cardiac arrest may occur.

Management
- prevention
- intubation and ventilation
- fluid resuscitation

Eclampsia

(*See Ch 45 for further details on eclampsia/pre-eclampsia.*)
    Incidence. Incidence is up to 1 in 1500.

Presentation
- Presentation includes hypertension, hyperreflexia and clonus, headache, visual changes and seizures.
- 20% of patients with eclampsia have diastolic blood pressure <90 mmHg, urine dipstick test results of <2+ protein and normal reflexes.
- Up to 40% have no significant oedema.
- 70% of deaths are due to intracerebral haemorrhage.
- Three serious complications of eclampsia are cerebrovascular injury, pulmonary oedema and coagulopathy.

Management
- secure airway; ventilate if necessary
- stop seizure and prevent recurrence
- control blood pressure
- diagnose and correct coagulopathy
- prevent pulmonary oedema; maintain strict fluid balance

Inverted uterus

An inverted uterus occurs when the fundus of the uterus descends through the uterine body, cervix and vagina.

Presentation
- includes pain, bleeding
- a vaginal lump after placental delivery
- suspect uterine inversion if the cardiovascular shock is out of proportion to blood loss after delivery (due to a vasovagal response to visceral stimulation)

Risk factors
- overzealous cord traction
- fundal implantation site
- uterine atony
- short cord
- previous inversion: recurrence rate of up to 33%

Management
- resuscitation
- digital replacement, leaving placenta attached
- manual replacement with the aid of tocolytic agents
- O'Sullivan hydrostatic method
- operative procedures of manual removal of placenta and uterine exploration

Shoulder dystocia

Incidence. Incidence is 0.2%–0.4%.

Risk factors
- excess maternal weight gain
- association with gestational diabetes, with estimated fetal weight >4000 g
- unexplained intrauterine fetal death
- high maternal birthweight
- postdates: a 20% incidence of macrosomia with infants delivered at 42 weeks compared with 12% delivered at 40 weeks
- intrapartum risks: 45% diagnosed with failure to progress and prolonged second stage

Management
- Do not pull hard, as this will increase impaction.
- Obtain adequate assistance, including an anaesthetist, paediatrician and nursing staff.
- Episiotomy is required.

Mild shoulder dystocia
- Suprapubic pressure will force the shoulder into the oblique diameter of the pelvis.
- Wood's manoeuvre: this involves a screwing motion by exerting pressure on the anterior surface of the posterior shoulder at the deltopectoral triangle.

Moderate shoulder dystocia
- Hibbard manoeuvre: press firmly against the head, jaw and upper neck, and direct the head towards the rectum. With surapubic pressure, the anterior shoulder is released.
- Delivery of the posterior arm proceeds by placing the hand in the vagina and applying pressure in the antecubital space to flex the baby's arm.

Severe dystocia
- McRobert's manoeuvre: involves sharp flexion of the mother's thighs against her abdomen. This serves to straighten the sacrum relative to the lumbar spine and cause superior rotation of the symphysis. This may free the impacted shoulder.

Chapter 43

Maternal mortality

Vivienne O'Connor

Maternal age is an important risk factor for both obstetric and perinatal outcomes. Adverse outcomes are more likely to occur in younger and older mothers. More Aboriginal or Torres Strait Islander mothers have their babies at a younger age compared with non-Indigenous mothers. One in five (19.5%) Aboriginal or Torres Strait Islander mothers is a teenager, compared with 3.5% of non-Indigenous mothers.

Background facts

Every day 1500 women die from pregnancy-related or childbirth-related conditions in the world. Most deaths occur in developing countries and are avoidable. Worldwide, 13 developing countries account for 70% of all maternal deaths. A woman living in sub-Saharan Africa has a 1 in 16 chance of dying in pregnancy or childbirth. This compares with a 1 in 2800 risk for a woman from a developed region.

The World Health Organization estimates that more than 80% of maternal deaths could be prevented through actions that have been proven to be effective and affordable, including: access to voluntary family planning to ensure that births are spaced properly, skilled attendance at delivery, aseptic birth environments, identification of maternal/fetal/neonatal complications, and minimal delay in reaching a medical facility or in receiving good quality/emergency obstetric care.

In Australia, in the triennium 2003–05, there were 65 maternal deaths (29 direct and 36 indirect) and 34 incidental deaths (see Table 43.1). There were no deaths from termination of pregnancy procedures. Over the past five trienniums, the maternal mortality rates for Indigenous women were between two and five times the maternal mortality rates for non-Indigenous women.

Definitions

The World Health Organization definition of maternal mortality is the death of a woman while pregnant or within 42 days of the termination of pregnancy, irrespective of the duration and site of the pregnancy, from any cause related to or aggravated by pregnancy or its management, but not from accidental or incidental causes. It also includes deaths from assisted reproduction technologies where pregnancy has not occurred, but not from incidental causes. In most Australian states and territories, incidental deaths are included in the definition.

Table 43.1 Australian triennium 2003–05 (65 deaths)			
Causes and numbers of direct maternal deaths		**Causes and numbers of indirect maternal deaths**	
Amniotic fluid embolism	8	Cardiac conditions	10
Hypertensive disease	5	Psychiatric causes (including suicide)	6
Thrombosis and thromboembolism	5	Non-obstetric haemorrhage (e.g. ruptured cerebral aneurysm)	5
Obstetric haemorrhage	4	Other	15
Other	7		
Total	29		36

Classifications

Direct maternal deaths
These result from obstetric complications of pregnancy, labour and puerperium (i.e. as a direct complication of pregnancy itself), from interventions, omissions, incorrect treatment or from a chain of events resulting from any of these.

Indirect obstetric deaths
These result from pre-existing disease or disease that develops during pregnancy that is not due to a direct obstetric cause, but may have been aggravated by physiological changes in pregnancy. Common examples are complications of cardiovascular disease, renal disease and diabetes.

Incidental deaths
These are due to conditions during pregnancy where the pregnancy is unlikely to have contributed significantly to death. Examples include road accidents, homicide and malignancies.

Maternal mortality ratio
This means deaths per 100,000 confinements (including both live and stillbirths). This compares to international standards of deaths per 100,000 live births. The maternal mortality ratio in Western countries is approximately 6–10 per 100,000 (8.4 in Australia: 7.9 for non-Indigenous women and 21.5 for Indigenous women).

Contributing factors in those who died from haemorrhage were the failure to recognise the continuation and/or extent of the haemorrhage, delay in undertaking surgical treatment to arrest haemorrhage, and delay in blood transfusion.

In those with pre-eclampsia, intracerebral bleeding was the major cause of death. The reporting data in Australia can be improved. This includes variation in reporting, in referral for coronial investigation and quality of data on Indigenous status.

Reducing maternal mortality and morbidity

Increasing use of modern contraceptives have made and can continue to make an important contribution to reducing maternal mortality in the developing world by preventing high-risk, high-parity births.

It is estimated that for every maternal death in Australia, there are approximately 80 incidences of severe maternal morbidity, including haemorrhage, uterine rupture, renal failure and eclampsia.

Further reading

Callister LC 2005 Global maternal mortality: contributing factors and strategies for change. MCN: American Journal of Maternal / Child Nursing 30:184–192

Laws P, Sullivan EA 2009 Australia's mothers and babies 2007. Perinatal Statistics Series No. 23. Cat. No. PER 48. AIHW National Perinatal Statistics Unit. Available at: www.preru.unsw.edu.au/PRERUWeb.nsf/page/AIHW+National+Perinatal+Statistics+Unit

Lewis G (ed) 2008 The Confidential Enquiry into Maternal and Child Health (CEMACH). Saving mothers' lives: reviewing maternal deaths to make motherhood safer 2003–05. The seventh report on confidential enquiries into maternal death in the United Kingdom. London: Royal Society of Medicine Press

Stover J, Ross J 2009 How increased contraceptive use has reduced maternal mortality. Maternal Child Health Journal. Available at: www.springerlink.com/content/x182m5012uk6157m/

Sullivan EA, Hall B, King JF 2008 Maternal deaths in Australia 2003–05. Maternal Deaths Series No. 3 Cat. No. PER 42. AIHW National Perinatal Statistics Unit. Available at: www.preru.unsw.edu.au/PRERUWeb.nsf/page/AIHW+National+Perinatal+Statistics+Unit

World Health Organization (WHO) 2003 Maternal deaths disproportionately high in developing countries. Available at: www.who.int/mediacentre/news/releases/2003/pr77/en/index.html

World Health Organization (WHO) 2007 Maternal mortality in 2005: estimates developed by WHO, UNICEF, UNFPA and the World Bank. Available at: www.who.int/mediacentre/news/releases/2003/pr77/en/index.htmlGeneva: WHO

Chapter 44

Perinatal mortality, birth asphyxia and cerebral palsy

Vivienne O'Connor

Background facts for live-born babies

- In 2007, 92.1% of live-born babies had a birthweight in the range of 2500–4499 g. The average birthweight of live-born babies in Australia in 2007 was 3374 g. For singletons, the mean gestational age was 38.9 weeks, compared with 35.3 weeks for twins and 31.3 weeks for triplets.
- 8.1% were preterm (<37 weeks gestation), compared with 7.3% in 1997. The mean gestational age for all preterm births was 33.2 weeks. 13.7% of babies of Aboriginal and Torres Strait Islander mothers were born preterm.
- 6.2% of live-born babies were of low birthweight (<2500 g). A baby may be small due to being born early (preterm), or may be small for its gestational age (intrauterine growth restriction). Low birthweight babies have a greater risk of poor health and dying, require a longer period of hospitalisation after birth, and are more likely to develop significant disabilities. The proportion of low birthweight in live-born babies of Aboriginal and Torres Strait Islander mothers was 12.5%, twice that of babies of non-Indigenous mothers (5.9%).
- 14.5% of live-born babies were admitted to a special care nursery or neonatal intensive care unit.

There are different definitions in Australia for reporting and registering perinatal deaths. The National Perinatal Data Collection (NPDC) uses a definition of perinatal deaths that includes all fetal and neonatal deaths of at least 400 g birthweight or at least 20 weeks gestation.

Definitions

- **Birth rate**. This is the number of live births per 1000 of the estimated mean population.
- **Intrauterine fetal death (IUFD)**. This is death of a fetus in utero after 20 weeks gestation or at birth weighing at least 400 g.
- **Intrapartum death**. This is fetal death during labour. If a baby is born without signs of life, but also without maceration, there is a strong presumption that

death occurred during labour. There are exceptions in both directions, which require judgment on the timing of death in relation to the presumed onset of labour.

- **Stillbirth (fetal death)**. This is the death of a fetus before delivery when the gestation has reached at least 20 weeks or the weight is over 400 g. This Australian definition differs from the World Health Organization definition, which requires the stillborn infant to weigh at least 1000 g or to have reached at least 28 weeks gestation. Therefore, caution is required in comparing international rates. The stillbirth rate is 7.4 per 1000 births in Australia. Low birthweight occurred in 79% of stillborn babies, with 28% of these unexplained. The mean gestational age of stillborn babies was 27.4 weeks in 2007 compared with 38.9 weeks for live-born babies. Preterm birth occurred in 80.8% of stillborn babies, compared with 7.6% of live-born babies.

- **Neonatal death**. This is the death of a live-born baby of at least 20 weeks gestation or 400 g in weight within 28 days of delivery. In comparison, the WHO definition is the death of an infant of at least 1000 g or 28 weeks gestation that occurs within 7 days of birth. In 2007, the neonatal death rate (NDR) was 2.9 per 1000 live births. Congenital abnormality occurred in a higher proportion of neonatal deaths (31.3%) than fetal deaths (20.8%). Among neonatal deaths, congenital abnormalities accounted for 67.7% of babies born at 32–36 weeks and 37.3% of babies at 37 weeks or more. The second most common cause of fetal deaths was maternal conditions (18.1%) and the proportion was highest among babies of 20–27 weeks (22.4%). Spontaneous preterm birth was a common cause of neonatal death for babies born at 20–27 and 28–31 weeks.

- **Perinatal mortality rate (PMR)**. This is the total number of stillbirths and neonatal deaths per 1000 total births. In 2007, the PMR was 10.3 per 1000 births. Of these, 72% were fetal deaths. The PMR of babies born to Aboriginal or Torres Strait Islander mothers remains almost twice that of babies born to other mothers (20.1). PMR varied by sociodemographic, maternal and pregnancy risk factors. Young maternal age, maternal Indigenous status and multiple gestation were associated with higher rates of perinatal deaths. From data provided by four Australian states, the main cause of perinatal death was congenital abnormalities at 20–21 weeks gestation (38.5%). The leading cause of death at 22–27 weeks gestation was the category of maternal conditions (21.5%). Perinatal deaths of babies at 28–31 weeks, 32–36 weeks and 37–41 weeks were most commonly due to unexplained antepartum death. Maternal conditions accounted for 13.8% and spontaneous preterm birth for 10.8% of reported causes of perinatal death.

Stillbirth

- The investigation of a death should include a complete autopsy and detailed examination of the cord and placenta, and other investigations according to the clinical problem.
- Fetal death after the onset of labour has decreased by two-thirds. Antepartum deaths decreased to a lesser extent (46%) and currently make up approximately 65% of all fetal deaths. These patterns are similar in most developed countries and have resulted in a focus of attention towards reducing the antepartum stillbirth rate.
- In Australia over the past two decades, there has been no reduction in the rate of stillbirth. Stillbirths account for 70% of perinatal deaths, with approximately six babies each day stillborn. Stillbirth rates for Indigenous women are over twice that for non-Indigenous women.

Unexplained stillbirth
- The presence of fetal growth restriction in approximately 40%–50% of unexplained stillbirths is an important consideration for future prevention strategies.
- Some risk factors are modifiable. Risk factors include maternal overweight and obesity, age >35 years, smoking, primiparity, prolonged pregnancy and socioeconomic disadvantage.

Categories
The main categories of stillbirth, according to the Perinatal Society of Australia Perinatal Death Classification (PSANZ–PDC), system are:
- for singleton pregnancies (>70% of stillbirths):
  - unexplained antepartum death (28%)
  - congenital abnormality (20%)
  - maternal conditions (13%)
  - spontaneous preterm (10%)
- in multiple pregnancy:
  - twin–twin transfusion (35%)
  - spontaneous preterm (24%)
  - unexplained antepartum death (15%)
  - congenital abnormality (11%)

It is estimated that unexplained stillbirth is now 10 times that of sudden infant death syndrome (SIDS) (500 unexplained stillbirths each year compared with 50 SIDS deaths).

Birth asphyxia

There is no general agreement on the definition of birth asphyxia. The Australian and New Zealand Perinatal Society defines perinatal asphyxia as an event or condition during the perinatal period that is likely to severely reduce oxygen delivery and lead to acidosis, together with a failure of at least two organs consistent with the effects of asphyxia.

Asphyxia may be *long-term chronic partial* asphyxia due to poor placental function or *severe acute* asphyxia due to such conditions as placental abruption, cord prolapse or uterine rupture.

Indicators
- Obstetric indicators of asphyxia may include an abnormal cardiotocograph (CTG), fetal acidosis, and the presence of meconium liquor. The latter occurs in 0.5%–20% of all births and alone is an inadequate marker of perinatal asphyxia.
- CTG is a poor predictor of birth asphyxia. Although the false-negative CTG as a predictor of fetal acidosis is below 2%, the false-positive rate may be as high as 50%.
- Neonatal indicators are the Apgar score, delay in breathing, and hypoxic ischaemic encephalopathy. Apgar scores are poor predictors of birth asphyxia. Long-term studies on babies and children have shown that, although babies with very low Apgar scores (a score <3 at 5 minutes) have an increased risk of cerebral palsy, most infants with low Apgar scores do not develop cerebral palsy. Conversely, 75% of children with cerebral palsy have Apgar scores ≥7 at 5 minutes.

Cerebral palsy

Definition. Cerebral palsy covers a range of neurological impairments, characterised by abnormal control of movement or posture resulting from abnormalities in brain development or an acquired non-progressive cerebral lesion.

Incidence. In Australia, it is estimated that a child is born with cerebral palsy every 18 hours. Worldwide, the incidence is the same (1 in 400 births). There are 20,000 people with cerebral palsy in Australia. There is no prebirth test and no known cure. For most, the cause is unknown.

Aetiology
- Major associations of cerebral palsy are intrauterine growth restriction and extreme prematurity.
- Although the patterns of pathological response to brain injury are similar in all cases, it is usually impossible to determine the exact time of brain injury.
- Studies have claimed that at least 90%–94% of cerebral palsy cannot be related to intrapartum hypoxia.
- Other associated factors include fetal vascular events, intrauterine infective causes (rubella, cytomegalovirus, toxoplasmosis, listeriosis), genetic causes (chromosomal abnormalities, X-linked disorders), metabolic disorders (iodine deficiency), and lead and mercury toxicity. Postnatal cerebral palsy may be caused by meningitis, near-drowning episodes or complications of prematurity.
- In cases of cerebral palsy where intrapartum hypoxia was evident, many were found to have a preexisting neurological incident contributing to hypoxia.
- Less than 2% of cerebral palsy is caused by obstetric care alone.

Obstetric aspects of cerebral palsy
The Australian and New Zealand Perinatal Society suggests that to define the relationship of intrapartum events and cerebral palsy, the following are essential:
- evidence of metabolic acidosis in intrapartum fetal or umbilical arterial cord samples
- early onset of severe or moderate encephalopathy in infants of >34 weeks gestation
- cerebral palsy of the spastic quadriplegic or dystonic type, as well as:
  - a hypoxic event noted immediately before or during labour
  - a sudden rapid and sustained deterioration of the fetal heart rate pattern
  - Apgar scores of 0–6 for longer than 5 minutes
  - evidence of multisystem involvement
  - early imaging evidence of acute cerebral abnormality

Further reading and resources

Australian Institute of Health and Welfare (AIHW) National Perinatal Statistics Unit: www.npsu.unsw.edu.au/NPSUweb.nsf/page/ps22

Gibb D 2000 Birth asphyxia. Obstetrician and Gynaecologist 2:21–24

Goldenberg RL, Culhane JF 2007 Low birth weight in the United States. American Journal of Clinical Nutrition 85:S584–S590

Headley E, Gordon A, Jeffery H 2009 Reclassification of unexplained stillbirths using clinical practice guidelines. Australian and New Zealand Journal of Obstetrics and Gynaecology 49(3):285–289

Laws P, Sullivan EA 2009 Australia's mothers and babies 2007. Perinatal Statistics Series No. 23. Cat. No. PER 48 Sydney: AIHW National Perinatal Statistics Unit. Available at: www.aihw.gov.au/publications/per/per-48-10972/per-48-10972.pdf

MacLennan A 1999 A template for defining causal relationship between acute intrapartum events and cerebral palsy: international consensus statement. British Medical Journal 319:1054–1059

Perinatal Society of Australia and New Zealand 2009 Clinical practice guideline for perinatal mortality. Available at: www.psanz.com.au

Robson S, Leader L 2009 Unexplained stillbirth. O&G Magazine 11:1

Chapter 45

Hypertension in pregnancy

Nikki Whelan

Cardiovascular changes in pregnancy

There are significant physiological adaptations of the cardiovascular system to pregnancy. Blood volume rises from an average non-pregnant 2600 mL to 3800 mL at about 32 weeks gestation. The total red cell volume grows constantly until term from 1400 mL to 1700 mL, so there is a fall in haemoglobin concentration as gestation progresses. Cardiac output rises from 5 L/minute to 7.5 L/minute, mostly during the first trimester, and the heart rate rises by 10% with an average resting rate of 88 beats/minute. The peripheral resistance is lowered by a combination of increased vasodilatory substances during pregnancy and decreased sensitivity to vasopressor substances.

Blood pressure falls in the first trimester and is at its lowest in the second trimester. The reduction in diastolic blood pressure is about 10 mmHg by mid-pregnancy. Blood pressure rises to non-pregnant levels towards the end of the third trimester.

Uterine blood flow increases steeply from 24 weeks gestation.

Other factors affecting blood pressure in pregnancy include posture (via the supine hypotension syndrome) and uterine contractions, which raise blood pressure.

Definitions. *Hypertension* in pregnancy is defined as:
- systolic blood pressure ≥140 mmHg, and/or
- diastolic blood pressure ≥90 mmHg (Korotkoff 5)

These measurements should be confirmed by repeated readings over several hours. Elevations of both systolic and diastolic blood pressure have both been associated with adverse fetal outcome and therefore both are important.

Severe hypertension in pregnancy is defined as:
- a systolic blood pressure ≥170 mmHg, and/or
- diastolic blood pressure ≥110 mmHg

This represents a level of blood pressure above which cerebral autoregulation is overcome in normotensive individuals. It is generally acknowledged that severe hypertension should be lowered promptly, albeit carefully, to avoid cerebral haemorrhage and hypertensive encephalopathy.

Classification

Classifications of hypertensive disorders in pregnancy are:
- pre-eclampsia/eclampsia
- gestational hypertension

- chronic hypertension
  - essential
  - secondary
  - white coat
- pre-eclampsia superimposed on chronic hypertension

Pre-eclampsia

Incidence. While 20% of women are hypertensive at some stage of their pregnancy (blood pressure ≥140/90 mmHg), about 5%–10% of primigravid women and 2% of multiparous women fulfil a diagnosis of pre-eclampsia.

Definition. Pre-eclampsia is a multisystem disorder unique to human pregnancy, characterised by hypertension and involvement of one or more other organ systems and/or the fetus. Proteinuria is the most commonly recognised additional feature after hypertension, but should not be considered mandatory to make the diagnosis.

A diagnosis of pre-eclampsia can be made when hypertension arises after 20 weeks gestation and is accompanied by one or more of the following:
- renal involvement
  - significant proteinuria: dipstick proteinuria, subsequently confirmed by spot urine protein/creatinine ratio ≥30 mg/mmol
  - serum or plasma creatinine >90 μmol/L
  - oliguria
- haematological involvement
  - thrombocytopaenia
  - haemolysis
  - disseminated intravascular coagulation
- liver involvement
  - raised serum transaminases
  - severe epigastric or right upper quadrant pain
- neurological involvement
  - convulsions (eclampsia)
  - hyperreflexia with sustained clonus
  - severe headache
  - persistent visual disturbances (photopsia, scotomata, cortical blindness, retinal vasospasm)
  - stroke
- pulmonary oedema
- intrauterine growth restriction
- placental abruption

Pathophysiology

Two placental conditions predispose to the development of pre-eclampsia. Ischaemia results from the failure of the normal development of the uteroplacental circulation with the presence of small defective spiral arteries, which then may become blocked by acute atherosis or thrombosis. Excessive placental size also predisposes to pre-eclampsia, as seen in multiple pregnancy, hydatidiform mole, fetal triploidy and placental hydrops.

Maternal contribution to pre-eclampsia occurs when endothelial activation results in acceleration of the normal systemic inflammatory response, which is present in all pregnancies. Activation of leucocytes and the coagulation process, and subsequent metabolic changes, result in the clinical features which are typically seen in pre-eclampsia: hypertension, oedema, proteinuria, platelet dysfunction, clotting derangements and possibly eclampsia.

The specific placental factor or factors that generate the systemic inflammatory response of pre-eclampsia remain unknown, but recent research has highlighted the contribution of three circulating placental products: soluble fms-like tyrosine kinase 1 (sFlt-1), endoglin and placental growth factor.

Placentation also depends on the invasion of the placental bed by cytotrophoblasts. Immune tolerance must occur in this setting to allow a continued relationship between the mother and the fetus.

Hence, at least four factors are likely to contribute to the development of pre-eclampsia: placental, endothelial, inflammatory and immunological.

Risk factors associated with pre-eclampsia

Risk factors are listed in Table 45.1. Other factors associated with pre-eclampsia include chronic hypertension, preexisting renal disease, autoimmune disease, more than 10 years since a previous pregnancy, a short sexual relationship prior to conception, and other thrombophilias (e.g. Factor V Leiden and possibly periodontal disease).

Recurrence risk

Studies of the risk of recurrent pre-eclampsia in women with a history of a hypertensive disorder in a prior pregnancy show variable results. Recurrence rates vary from 6%–55%, with the greatest risk in women with early-onset pre-eclampsia and chronic hypertension. An Australian study suggests a 14% risk of developing pre-eclampsia, and also a 14% risk of developing gestational hypertension in their next pregnancy.

Clinical spectrum

Pre-eclampsia is a multisystem disorder with both maternal and fetal consequences.

Hypertension

Hypertension may be labile, often with flattened or the reverse of normal diurnal rhythm. This is thought to be due to decreased responsiveness to angiotensin II. Many of the complications of pre-eclampsia are due to arterial damage and loss of vascular autoregulation.

Table 45.1 Pre-eclampsia risk factors	
Risk factor	**Relative risk**
Previous history of pre-eclampsia	7.19
Antiphospholipid antibodies	9.72
Preexisting diabetes	3.56
Multiple pregnancy	2.91
Nulliparity	2.90
Family history of pre-eclampsia	2.90
Elevated body mass index (BMI) >25	2.47
Maternal age >40	1.96
Diastolic blood pressure >80 mmHg at first antenatal visit	1.38

Renal system

Glomerular swelling of endothelial cells and intracapillary cells known as endotheliosis is the main response to pre-eclampsia. This causes a reduced glomerular filtration rate, which slows urate clearance and raises serum creatinine levels. In uncomplicated pregnancy, glomerular filtration normally increases. A serum creatinine level of 0.09 μmol/L in pregnancy may predict renal involvement.

Proteinuria is often a late sign of pre-eclampsia and indicates poorer prognosis for the mother and fetus.

The commonest cause of nephrotic syndrome in pregnancy is pre-eclampsia. There is a reduced maternal plasma volume due to increased leakiness of capillaries, and hypoalbuminaemia predisposing to reduction in colloid oncotic pressure and raised fluid in interstitial spaces. The complications of fluid changes include pulmonary and laryngeal oedema, and acute renal failure.

Platelets

The reduction of platelets in pre-eclampsia is due to increased consumption and lowered platelet lifespan. However, this is an inconsistent feature of pre-eclampsia.

Coagulation

There is increased factor VIII consumption in early pre-eclampsia, and anti-thrombin III is lowered. Disseminated intravascular coagulation is a late and inconsistent feature of pre-eclampsia. The complications of coagulation/clotting changes include disseminated intravascular coagulation with widespread fibrin deposition, haemorrhage and necrosis.

Hepatic changes

- Liver dysfunction with elevated hepatic enzymes is often evident. Raised alkaline phosphatase is normal, due to the placental production, although raised transaminase levels reflect hepatic ischaemia of pre-eclampsia.
- Epigastric pain from the rare complication of subcapsular haematoma has associated mortality.
- The syndrome of haemolysis, elevated liver enzymes and low platelets is associated with microangiopathic haemolysis and is a variant of severe pre-eclampsia.

Central nervous system involvement

- Eclampsia has an incidence of <0.1%, with 50% occurring before labour. Most postpartum fits occur within 24 hours of delivery. Proteinuria increases the risk by seven to eight times.
- Hypertensive encephalopathy may be acute or subacute, with diffuse cerebral dysfunction, which improves with the lowering of blood pressure. The clinical presentation includes headache, nausea, vomiting and convulsions.
- Stroke in pre-eclampsia and or eclampsia is usually preceded by severe hypertension. In women who had experienced a stroke, 96% had a systolic blood pressure >160 mmHg, 21% had a diastolic blood pressure >105 mmHg and 13% had a diastolic blood pressure >110 mmHg; mean arterial pressure was >125 mmHg in 46% and >130 mmHg in 21% of women who had experienced a stroke.
- Only 11% women who experienced a stroke had a complete recovery without significant morbidity.
- Visual disturbance with cortical blindness occurs in 1%–3% of eclamptics and recovers with reduction in blood pressure.
- The cerebral pathology of eclampsia resembles hypertensive encephalopathy, with evidence of thrombosis, fibrinoid necrosis and microinfarction.

- Cerebral autoregulation is altered in hypertensive pregnant women, making them more sensitive to severe changes in blood pressure. Acute arterial hypertension can lead to damage to the blood–brain barrier with extravasation of fluid into the parenchyma resulting in cerebral haemorrhage and infarction. A mean arterial pressure of 140 mmHg (blood pressure 180/120) is an obstetric emergency and requires immediate treatment.

Placental and fetal involvement

Abnormal placentation reduces uteroplacental blood flow by changing the uteroplacental circulation from a low-resistance system to one of high resistance and underperfusion. The complications of this to fetuses are intrauterine growth restriction, death and complications of prematurity, when delivery is indicated.

Management of pre-eclampsia

Pre-eclampsia is a progressive disease that will inevitably worsen if pregnancy continues. Current therapy does not ameliorate the placental pathology, nor alter the pathophsiology or natural history of pre-eclampsia. Delivery is the definitive management and is followed by resolution, generally over a few days but sometimes over a much longer course. At a mature gestational age, delivery should not be delayed.

Prevention

- Prophylactic therapy with aspirin is associated with a reduction in the recurrence rate of pre-eclampsia, delivery prior to 34 weeks gestation, preterm birth and perinatal death. Risk reduction is greatest if therapy is commenced prior to 20 weeks gestation and if doses >75 mg are taken.
- The use of calcium supplementation has been demonstrated to reduce the risk of pre-eclampsia, especially in women with a low calcium intake. Calcium supplementation (1.5 g/day) should be offered to women at increased risk of pre-eclampsia, particularly those with a low dietary calcium intake.
- Randomised trials of antioxidants vitamins C and E have failed to show any significant benefit, and there was an increased risk of stillbirth and birthweight <2.5 kg in the treatment arm of the study. Hence, prophylactic treatment with vitamins C and E is not recommended.
- Heparin with and without aspirin has not been assessed using large randomised trials. At present, therefore, there is no evidence for this treatment in the absence of a thrombophilia or antiphosphlipid antibody syndrome.
- Observational studies have suggested that multivitamin supplementation containing folic acid may reduce the risk of pre-eclampsia, perhaps by improving placental and systemic endothelial function or by lowering blood homocysteine levels.
- Preconception counselling should be offered to all women at increased risk of pre-eclampsia, and particularly to women with preexisting disorders that may need to be stabilised prior to pregnancy.

Investigations

- initial assessment may be in a day assessment unit, unless severe hypertension, headache, epigastric pain or nausea and vomiting are present, which necessitate urgent admission
- urine dipstick testing for proteinuria, with spot protein/creatinine ratio if >1+ (30 mg/dL)
- full blood count
- urea, creatinine, electrolytes
- liver function tests

- ultrasound assessment of fetal growth, amniotic fluid volume and umbilical blood flow

Additional investigations that may be useful in certain women include urine microscopy on a mid-stream specimen, coagulation studies, blood film, lactate dehydrogenase, fibrinogen, investigations for underlying systemic lupus erythematosus, renal disease, antiphospholipid syndrome, thrombophilias, fasting plasma free metanephrines/normetanephrines and 24-hour urinary catecholamines.

Indications for delivery in pre-eclampsia or gestational hypertension
For indications for delivery in pre-eclampsia or gestational hypertension, see Table 45.2.

Antihypertensive therapy
Severe hypertension
Antihypertensive treatment (see Table 45.3) should be started in all women with a systolic blood pressure >170 mmHg or a diastolic blood pressure >110 mmHg because of the risk of intracerebral haemorrhage and eclampsia. A Cochrane review has concluded that there is no good evidence to support the use of any short-acting agent over any other and practice should therefore be guided by local experience and familiarity.

Mild to moderate hypertension
There is controversy regarding the treatment of mild to moderate hypertension in women with pre-eclampsia. No controlled trial to date exists. However, a small placebo-controlled study looked at treating women with mild hypertension. Placebo-treated women were delivered significantly earlier, mainly as a result of severe hypertension or premonitory signs of eclampsia, and there was more neonatal morbidity secondary to prematurity.

In the absence of compelling evidence, treatment of mild to moderate hypertension in the range 140–160/90–100 mmHg should be considered an option and will reflect local practice (see Table 45.4). Above these levels, treatment should be considered mandatory.

- First-line drugs include methyldopa, labetalol and oxprenolol.
- Second-line drugs are hydralazine, nifedipine and prazosin.

Table 45.2 Indications for delivery in pre-eclampsia or gestational hypertension

Maternal	Fetal
Gestational age >37 weeks	Severe intrauterine growth restriction
Inability to control hypertension	Non-reassuring fetal status
Deteriorating platelet count	
Deteriorating liver function tests	
Deteriorating renal function tests	
Placental abruption	
Persistent neurological symptoms	
Eclampsia	
Persistent epigastric pain, nausea or vomiting with abnormal liver function tests	
Acute pulmonary oedema	

- Angiotensin-converting enzyme (ACE) and angiotensin receptor blockers are contraindicated.
- All first-line and second-line drugs, plus enalapril, captopril and quinapril, are compatible with breastfeeding.

Intravenous fluids
Although maternal plasma volume is often reduced in women with pre-eclampsia, there is no maternal or fetal benefit to maintenance fluid therapy. As vascular permeability is increased in women with pre-eclampsia, administration of large volumes of intravenous fluids may cause pulmonary oedema and worsen peripheral oedema.

Management of eclampsia
The drug of choice for the prevention of eclampsia is magnesium sulfate. However, the case for its routine use in women with pre-eclampsia in countries with low maternal and perinatal mortality rates is controversial and is perhaps best determined by individual units monitoring their outcomes. In some units, the presence of severe headache, hyperreflexia with clonus, epigastric pain or severe hypertension are considered indications for prophylaxis.

Trial data suggest the use of magnesium does not appear to affect rates of caesarian section, infectious morbidity, haemorrhage or neonatal depression, nor the duration of labour (although necessitated higher doses of oxytocin).

Resuscitation
- **Usually self-limiting**. Intravenous diazepam (2 mg/minute to maximum of 10 mg) or clonazepam (1–2 mg over 2–5 minutes) can be used while MgSO4 is being prepared.
- **Magnesium sulfate**. The possible mechanisms of action include cerebral vasodilatation, thereby decreasing cerebral ischaemia or perhaps blocking neuronal damage associated with ischaemia. It prevents but does not terminate seizures. The dose includes an intravenous loading dose of 4 g over 10–15 minutes followed by an infusion of 1–2 g/hour for 24 hours. Side effects are hypocalcaemia, hyporeflexia and cardiac arrest. The Eclampsia Trial Collaborative Group found magnesium sulfate to be superior to phenytoin or diazepam in decreasing recurrent seizures, maternal mortality and intensive care admission.

Control hypertension
Stabilise blood pressure (see above).

Table 45.3 Antihypertensive agents for treatment of severe hypertension			
Drug	Dose	Route	Onset of action
Labetalol	20–50 mg	Intravenous (IV) bolus	5 minutes; repeat in 15–30 minutes over 2 minutes
Nifepidine	10–20 mg	Oral	30–45 minutes; repeat in 45 minutes
Hydralazine	5–10 mg	IV bolus	20 minutes; repeat in 30 minutes
Diazoxide	15–45 mg; maximum 300 mg	IV rapid bolus	3–5 minutes; repeat in 5 minutes

Table 45.4 Oral antihypertensives for moderate hypertension

Drug	Dose	Action	Contraindicatons	Practice points
Methyl dopa	250–750 mg three times a day	Central	Depression	Slow onset of action over 24 hours. Dry mouth, sedation, depression, blurred vision
Clonidine	75–300 µg three times a day	Central		Prompt onset of action; withdrawal effect; reduce over 7 days
Labetalol	100–400 mg three times a day	Beta-blockerMild alpha-vasodilator	Asthma, chronic airways limitation	Bradycardia, bronchospasm, headache, nausea, tingling scalp
Oxprenolol	20–160 mg three times a day	Beta-blocker with intrinsic sympatho-mimetic activity (ISA)	Heart block	
Nifedipine	20 mg twice a day–60 mg slow release twice a day	Calcium channel antagonist	Aortic stenosis	Severe headache, flushing, tachycardia, peripheral oedema, constipation
Prazosin	0.5 mg three times a day	Alpha-blocker		First dose effect orthostatic hypotension
Hydralazine	25–50 mg three times a day	Vasodilator		Flushing headache, nausea, lupus-like syndrome

Delivery

In the presence of eclampsia, there is no role for continuation of the pregnancy once the woman is stable.

When delivery is indicated, the mode of delivery depends on favourability of the cervix, the speed required for delivery and the fetal condition. In many cases, induction of labour and vaginal delivery is appropriate. In severe pre-eclampsia, prophylactic antihypertensive and anticonvulsant therapy are continued. Lumbar epidural is favoured for analgesia due to its ability to lower blood pressure and possibly increase uterine blood flow. Caution with epidural with strict investigation of platelet levels, coagulation profile and clotting times is important to avoid complications of bleeding and spinal haematoma. The use of general anaesthesia for caesarean section is associated with a marked hypertensive response to laryngoscopy and intubation.

Oxytocin in doses over 2 milliunit/minute intravenously acts as an antidiuretic and, although it is not contraindicated in severe pre-eclampsia, strict fluid balance must be adhered to.

Fetal wellbeing is monitored by continuous cardiotocography. The maternal pushing in the second stage should be shortened.

The use of ergometrine in the third stage is contraindicated, and the immediate postpartum period requires intensive monitoring of blood pressure, renal function and fluid balance.

Chronic hypertension in pregnancy

This is a major predisposing factor to pre-eclampsia, although alone it may not be associated with the maternal and fetal risks of pre-eclampsia. If superimposed on chronic hypertension, pre-eclampsia tends to recur in subsequent pregnancies, and it is therefore often difficult to differentiate between the two. A diagnostic guide includes decreasing platelet count, serum urate level (<0.30 mmol/L is unlikely to be pre-eclampsia), a 24-hour urinary protein concentration (except if hypertension is due to chronic renal failure) and liver biochemistry.

Management
- Cease therapy if hypertension is mild to moderate before pregnancy.
- Use a first-line drug where possible for controlling the hypertension.
- Watch closely for the development of pre-eclampsia, using the tests described above.
- Fetal monitoring should include an early dating ultrasound scan and 4-weekly growth scans in the third trimester, tracking growth, liquor volume and umbilical artery blood flow.
- Manage jointly with obstetric physicians.

Unusual causes of hypertension in pregnancy

Phaeochromocytoma
This is a tumour of the adrenal medulla associated with significant maternal and fetal mortality.
- Clinical presentation: sustained or paroxysmal hypertension; the patient complains of headache, palpitation, sweating, chest and abdominal pain, and visual symptoms.
- It may be familial or associated with other syndromes, such as multiple endocrine neoplasias, neurofibromatosis and thyrotoxicosis.
- Diagnosis: involves 24-hour urinary assessment for metanephrines, creatinine, vanillylmandelic acid and catecholamines. Diagnostic imaging using magnetic resonance and computed tomography are safe in pregnancy. Ultrasound is often inadequate to assess the adrenals. If phaeochromocytoma is diagnosed, examine for multiple endocrine neoplasia.
- Management: use alpha-blockers, and then beta-blockers. Surgery can remove the tumour, but there may be difficulties with the large uterus.

Coarctation of aorta
Cushing's syndrome
- rare in pregnancy
- clinical presentation: hypertension, pigmentation, striae, hyperglycaemia

- investigations: dexamethasone suppression test, computed tomography scan of the pituitary and adrenals

Conn's syndrome
- rare in pregnancy
- clinical presentation: hypokalaemia and hypertension (possibility of remission in pregnancy may be due to the antagonism of the action of aldosterone by progesterone)

Renal artery stenosis
Autoimmune connective tissue disorders
Women with systemic lupus erythematosus may present with hypertension, renal complications or superimposed pre-eclampsia.

Long-term consequences

Women who have been diagnosed with either pre-eclampsia or gestational hypertension are at an increased risk of subsequent cardiovascular morbidity, including hypertension and coronary heart disease. Recent studies suggest the relative risks for hypertension were 3.7 after 14 years follow-up, for ischaemic heart disease 2.16 after 12 years, for stroke 1.81 after 10 years, and for venous thromboembolism 1.87 after 5 years. Overall mortality after pre-eclampsia was increased 1.5-fold after 14 years.

It is recommended all women with hypertensive disease in pregnancy have an annual review for blood pressure and other cardiovascular risk factors.

Further reading

Askie LM, Duley L, Henderson-Smart DJ, Stewart LA 2007 PARIS Collaborative Group. Antiplatelet agents for the prevention of pre-eclampsia: a meta-analysis of individual patient data. Lancet 369 (9575):1791–1798

Australasian Society for the Study of Hypertension in Pregnancy 1993 Management of hypertension in pregnancy: executive summary. Medical Journal of Australia 158:700–702

Brown M 2003 Pre-eclampsia: a lifelong disorder. Medical Journal of Australia 179:182–184

CLASP Collaborative Group 1994 CLASP: a randomised trial of low dose aspirin for the prevention and treatment of pre-eclampsia among 9364 pregnant women. Lancet 343:619–629

Eclampsia Trial Collaborative Group 1995 Which anticonvulsant for women with eclampsia? Evidence from the Collaborative Eclampsia Trial. Lancet 345:1455–1463

Khong TY, Mott C 1993 Immunohistologic demonstration of endothelial disruption in acute atherosis in pre-eclampsia. European Journal of Obstetrics and Gynecology and Reproductive Biology 51:193–197

Levine RJ, Maynard SE, Qian C et al 2004 Circulating angiogenic factors and the risk of preeclampsia. New England Journal of Medicine 350:672–683

Magpie Collaborative Group 2002 Do women with pre-eclampsia and their babies benefit from magnesium sulphate? The Magpie Trial: a randomised placebo-controlled trial. Lancet 359: 1877–1890

Maynard SE, Min JY, Merchan J et al 2003 Excess placental soluble fms-like tyrosine kinase 1 (sFlt1) may contribute to endothelial dysfunction, hypertension, and proteinuria in preeclampsia. Journal of Clinical Investigation 111:649–658

Redman CWG 1991 The placenta and preeclampsia. Placenta 2:301–308

Redman CWG, Sacks GP, Sargent IL 1999 Preeclampsia: an excessive maternal inflammatory response to pregnancy. American Journal of Obstetrics and Gynecology 180:499–506

Roberts JM, Redman CWG 1993 Pre-eclampsia: more than pregnancy-induced hypertension. Lancet 341:1447–1451

Scott JS 1958 Pregnancy toxaemia associated with hydrops foetalis, hydatidiform mole and hydramnios. Journal of Obstetrics and Gynaecology of the British Empire 65:689–701

SOMANZ Society of Obstetric Medicine of Australia and New Zealand 2008 Guidelines for the management of hypertensive disorders of pregnancy. Available at: www.somanz.org

Therapeutic Guidelines 2008 Therapeutic guidelines: cardiovascular 2008, Version 5. Melbourne: Therapeutic Guidelines

Chapter 46

Diabetes in pregnancy

Nikki Whelan

Diabetes in pregnancy is either preexisting/pregestational diabetes or acquired gestational diabetes.

Physiology and pathophysiology

Maternal glucose homeostasis
- Normally, blood sugar levels are stable in all trimesters. This is achieved by doubling the insulin secretion from the end of the first trimester to the end of the third trimester.
- In early pregnancy, raised oestrogen and progesterone levels cause cell hyperplasia in the pancreas, which results in a rise in insulin secretion and an increase in fat stores.
- In the second and third trimesters, increases in the diabetogenic hormones human placental lactogen, prolactin and free cortisol cause insulin resistance and lipolysis. Therefore, the increased insulin concentration is counterbalanced by increasing insulin resistance, the mechanism of which is not clearly understood.
- Fasting blood glucose level (BGL) decreases, while postprandial BGL increases in pregnancy. The pregestational diabetic is at risk of hypoglycaemia in early pregnancy and ketoacidosis in later pregnancy, as the demand for insulin is increased.
- Fetal glucose homeostasis: maternal glucose crosses the placenta freely by facilitated diffusion. Therefore, the mother is responsible for regulating fetal blood sugar levels. Fetal insulin appears in the circulation at the end of the first trimester, but the exact role of fetal insulin is uncertain and it may act by promoting growth. It normally plays no role in blood glucose homeostasis. In response to fetal hyperglycaemia due to elevated maternal blood sugar, fetal pancreatic cells hypertrophy, leading to inappropriate release of insulin.

Pregestational diabetes

Effects on pregnancy
Maternal effects
Increased risks of:
- polyhydramnios
- pre-eclampsia
- placental abruption
- infection, including urinary tract and candidiasis

- diabetic ketoacidosis
- trauma during delivery
- caesarean section

Fetal effects

- Congenital malformation: pregestational diabetics (both type 1 and type 2) have an increased risk of fetal malformation with increasing levels of hyperglycaemia (see Table 46.1). Literature suggests only small increases in HbA1c are associated with increased risk.
- Type 1 diabetics with an HbA1c of 7.2% (normal range 6%) have double the risk of fetal malformation and type 2 diabetics may have twice the risk of fetal malformation of the non-pregnant population with a normal HbA1c. If their HbA1c rises to 7.3%, their risk of fetal malformation may be as high as 11%.
- Malformations include neural tube defects, cardiovascular and vertebral defects. The risk of malformation is proportional to imperfect metabolic control during organogenesis; improved blood sugar control decreases anomalies. Many malformations can be diagnosed by mid-trimester ultrasound.
- Abortion and perinatal mortality: diabetic women have higher abortion rates. An HbA1c of 6.5% increases the risk of spontaneous abortion by 3%. Perinatal mortality rates also rise in proportion to the rise in mean BGL. The exact mechanisms for the increased risk demise are uncertain.
- Abnormal fetal growth: there is an increase in the incidence of large-for-dates and small-for-dates fetuses, and consequently fetal morbidity. Macrosomia in all organs (except the brain) is due to an increase in cytoplasmic mass. Macrosomic babies are at risk of trauma during delivery, with definite risk of shoulder dystocia in the diabetic mother with a fetus >4000 g. Intrauterine growth restriction (IUGR) may be a complication of placental vasculopathy and may be related to underlying renal disease or the development of pre-eclampsia.
- Preterm delivery is common.

Neonatal effects

- Respiratory distress syndrome: carries six times the risk of non-diabetics. Fetal hyperinsulinaemia results in reduced pulmonary phospholipid production and a decrease in surfactant.
- Hypoglycaemia: 50% of babies of insulin-dependent diabetic mothers have blood sugar levels below 2 mmol/L due to fetal hyperinsulinaemia and discontinuation of the maternal glucose supply.
- Hypocalcaemia is present in 25%–50% of infants.
- Polycythaemia and jaundice: polycythaemia is due to an increase in erythropoietin caused by raised fetal insulin. Jaundice, which occurs in up to 50% of babies, is mainly due to elevated red cell destruction and immaturity of the liver.
- Macrosomia is common.

Table 46.1 Maternal diabetes and risk of congenital malformation	
Congenital malformation	Increased risk over non-diabetics
Cardiac	4 times
Neural tube defects	2–10 times
Gastrointestinal atresia	3–10 times
Caudal regression	200 times (though still rare)
Urinary tract	10 times

- Hypertrophic cardiomyopathy is usually reversible.
- Risk of diabetes: when one parent is diabetic, this is associated with a 3% risk of the offspring developing diabetes in 20 years. If both parents are diabetic, the risk is 20%.

Management
Prepregnancy counselling
General measures
- Stop smoking.
- Reduce alcohol intake.
- Review all medications, including complementary medications, for safety in pregnancy.
- Screen and vaccinate for infectious diseases, including rubella, varicella, bordetella pertussis and cervical human papillomavirus (HPV).
- Provide weight management, nutrition and exercise advice.
- Provide contraceptive advice until conception is desired.

Diabetes-specific measures
- The multidisciplinary team should include an obstetrician, physician, diabetes educator and dietician (wherever possible).
- Achieve optimal glycaemic control: HbA1c should be maintained in the normal range wherever possible. This should be possible in most women with type 2 diabetes, but may not be possible in all women with type 1 diabetes.
- The woman should take folic acid (5 mg daily).
- Medications include the use of the newer rapid-acting insulin analogues and insulin pump therapy. Oral agents should be ceased and switched over to insulin (e.g. basal bolus regimen). Although they are probably not teratogenic, the oral agents are not used routinely.
- Antihypertensive agents should be suitable for continued use in pregnancy.
- Statins should be ceased.
- Review diabetic complications, including retinopathy, nephropathy, macrovascular disease and autonomic neuropathy.
- Assess thyroid function and screen for other autoimmune diseases where appropriate.

Antenatal management
Management should be by a multidisciplinary team wherever possible.

Medical
- Assess BGL control with HbA1c and reinforce the necessity for regular self-monitoring of BGLs.
- Aims: fasting BGL of 4.0–5.5 mmol/L, 1 hour postprandial <8.0 mmol/L, and 2 hours postprandial <7.0 mmol/L.
- Monitor with HbA1c every 4–8 weeks.
- Advise that hypoglycaemia is common, especially overnight from 6–18 weeks, and that insulin requirements may increase substantially in late second trimester with increasing insulin resistance.
- Insulin requirements may reduce from 32 weeks gestation and should prompt assessment of fetal wellbeing if this is >5%–10%.
- Assess diabetic complications if no prepregnancy counselling has been performed, especially retinopathy (regular formal eye examinations) and nephropathy (24-hour urine analysis, spot albumin:creatinine ratio, dip stick urine analysis and serum electrolytes, creatinine and urea).

Obstetric management
- Offer nuchal translucency scan and serum screen at 12–13 weeks gestation for aneuploidy. If not performed, a dating scan should be performed.
- Perform a fetal morphology scan at 18–20 weeks and in selected cases repeat a morphology scan at 24 weeks, especially targeting the heart.
- Assess fetal growth and wellbeing at 28–30 weeks and at 34–36 weeks, or more frequently in the presence of medical or obstetric complications.
- Aim for delivery at term unless obstetric or medical complications arise (e.g. fetal macrosomia, polyhydramnios, poor metabolic control, pre-eclampsia or IUGR).
- Vaginal delivery is preferable, unless obstetric or medical contraindications exist (e.g. risk of shoulder dystocia increases with birthweight >4000 g).
- Anticipate the need for neonatal nursery admission if delivery is earlier than 36 weeks or poor metabolic control is present.

Labour
Monitor BGL 1–2 hourly, aiming for 4–7 mmol/L, which can be achieved with various regimens, including:
- insulin/dextrose infusion
- insulin/dextrose infusion if BGL is <4 mmol/L or >7mmol/L
- subcutaneous insulin injections
- insulin pump therapy

Postpartum
- Type 1 diabetes: insulin requirements fall rapidly postdelivery, and hence the primary goal is to avoid hypoglycaemia.
  - Close monitoring is needed.
  - Breastfeeding mothers need to be encouraged to test prefeeds and postfeeds to check for hypoglycaemia.
- Type 2 diabetes: many women can be managed with diet alone; some will need ongoing insulin therapy.

Contraception
There is no evidence that any present contraceptive methods are contraindicated in diabetes.

Gestational diabetes

Definition. This is the development of abnormal glucose tolerance during pregnancy in a woman who did not have diabetes before pregnancy.

Incidence. International criteria differ as to diagnosis, and so incidence ranges from 1%–10% at 26 weeks gestation. Most Australian centres report a 5%–9% incidence. These may include previously undiagnosed non-insulin-dependent diabetics. The Hyperglycaemia Adverse Pregnancy Outcome (HAPO) Study suggests there is a continuous, linear association between BGLs and major adverse pregnancy outcomes.

Diagnosis
The International Association of Diabetes in Pregnancy Group (IADPG) is developing a position statement on screening and diagnosis of hyperglycaemic disorders in pregnancy, based largely on the HAPO data. It is hoped this will standardise criteria for these definitions worldwide.

Gestational diabetes has increased perinatal morbidity, with characteristics for babies similar to preexisting diabetes. These include fetal macrosomia, neonatal hypoglycaemia, hyperbilirubinaemia and respiratory distress syndrome, with a probable long-term risk of obesity and diabetes.

Between 4% and 9% of women have plasma glucose >8 mmol/L at 2 hours after a non-fasting 75 g oral glucose load. The 95th percentile for true fasting BGL in pregnancy is >5.5 mmol/L.

WHO criteria
- impaired glucose tolerance: a fasting serum glucose of <7.8 mmol/L and/or a 2-hour blood sugar level >7.8 and <11.1 mmol/L after a fasting 75 g oral glucose load
- diabetes: a fasting BGL of ≥7.8 mmol/L and a 2-hour BGL of ≥11.1 mmol/L after a 75 g glucose load

Australasian Diabetes in Pregnancy Society criteria
- gestational diabetes: a fasting BGL of >5.5 mmol/L and a 2-hour BGL of >8.0 mmol/L after a 75 g glucose load (Australia) and >9.0 mmol/L (New Zealand)

Screening
Risk factors
- family history of type 2 diabetes, personal or family history of gestational diabetes or glucose intolerance
- past history of macrosomic baby >4000 g
- poor obstetric history (e.g. intrauterine fetal death)
- belonging to a high-risk ethnic group, such as Polynesian, Southern Asian (Indian), Middle Eastern or other Asian origin
- Australian Aboriginal or Torres Strait Islander background
- being overweight (body mass index >25) or obese (body mass index >30)
- maternal age >30 years
- previous abnormal glucose tolerance test (recurrence in 60%)
- multiple pregnancy
- glycosuria

Screening methods
- Risk factors only: with this method 30% of the population will have a glucose tolerance test and the false-negative rate is 40%.
- Random BGL sampling has poor sensitivity.
- Non-fasting glucose challenge: the screening test is performed at 24–28 weeks gestation with a non-fasting sugar load of 75 g. If >8.0 mmol/L is used as the cutoff level, 16% of the population will screen positive and 16% of these will have gestational diabetes. The false-positive rate is 10%.
- It is likely the IADPG will recommend abandoning the challenge test and move to a 75g oral glucose tolerance test (OGTT) with a fasting and a 1-hour level for diagnosis of gestational diabetes.
- International studies show the incidence of gestational diabetes is increasing over time, reflecting the increase in incidence of being overweight and obese in the world.
- Between 2000–01 and 2005–06, the incidence of confinements with gestational diabetes in Australia increased by 22%.

Management
Medical management
- a team approach with an obstetrician, endocrinologist, diabetic nurse educator and dietitian
- patient education mandatory

- modifying dietary habits and increasing physical activity levels (including resistance work)
- limit weight gain, especially in obese women (body mass index >30) to 5 kg
- monitoring by self-testing with:
  - fasting BGL of <5.5 mmol/L
  - 1-hour postprandial BGL of <8 mmol/L
  - 2-hour postprandial BGL of <7 mmol/L
- insulin treatment: shown to reduce the rate of large-for-gestational-age infants in pregnancies with levels consistently higher than above treated only by diet
- metformin: being used with caution in New Zealand and Australia following the MiG Study (a randomised control trial of metformin versus insulin for women who met the usual criteria for commencing insulin with no differences in major outcomes in the two arms); may be suitable for 50% of women with gestational diabetes who are currently being treated with insulin
- HbA1c levels (may be used as ancillary testing)
- in labour: regular BGL tests, especially in women treated with insulin and or oral agents (insulin or dextrose infusion are rarely necessary)
- immediately postpartum, cease insulin and monitor BGL
- postpartum glucose tolerance test: performed at 6 weeks
- 1–2 yearly fasting or OGTT for early detection of type 2 diabetes

Obstetric management
- Fetal growth and surveillance of fetal wellbeing: at 28–30 and 34–36 weeks gestation to monitor growth; more frequently if complications develop.
- Timing of delivery: if uncomplicated, await spontaneous labour, but avoid postdates.

Postpartum follow-up
- At discharge, counsel regarding contraception and recurrence risk. The woman with gestational diabetes has a long-term risk of developing non-insulin-dependent diabetes of up to 50%, compared with 7% of controls. Risk of progression to type 2 diabetes can be reduced by diet and exercise (up to 50%), metformin (up to 30%) and acrabose (up to 25%).

Further reading

Australasian Diabetes in Pregnancy Society 2005 Consensus guidelines for management of patients with type 1 and type 2 diabetes in relation to pregnancy. Medical Journal of Australia 183 (7): 373–377

Australian Institute of Health and Welfare (AIHW): Templeton M, Pieris-Caldwell I 2008 Gestational diabetes mellitus in Australia, 2005–06. Diabetes Series No. 10. Cat. No. CVD44. Canberra: AIHW

HAPO Study Cooperative Research Group 2008 Hyperglycemia and adverse pregnancy outcomes. New England Journal of Medicine 358 (19):1991–2002

Rowan JA, Hague WM, Wanzhen G et al for the MiG Trial Investigators 2008 Metformin versus insulin for the treatment of gestational diabetes. New England Journal of Medicine 358 (19):2003–2015

Chapter 47

Thromboembolism in pregnancy

Amy Mellor

Incidence. The incidence of venous thromboembolism (VTE) is 1 in 500–2000 pregnancies.

Significance. Pregnancy is associated with a 10-fold increase in risk of VTE compared with the non-pregnant population. VTE remains a leading cause of maternal mortality in developed countries. It results in approximately 1 death per 100,000 pregnancies.

The prevalence of VTE is distributed equally between the three trimesters. Although two-thirds of events occur antenatally, the daily risk is greatest in the postnatal period. The risk of VTE after caesarean section is approximately twice that of vaginal delivery. Deep venous thrombosis (DVT) is more common in the left leg. Pelvic vein thrombosis is more common in pregnancy than in the non-pregnant population.

Predisposing factors

All three components of Virchow's triad (venous stasis, endothelial injury and a hypercoaguable state) may be present in pregnancy.

Hypercoaguability
Pregnancy is associated with alterations in both thrombotic and fibrinolytic mechanisms. In the first trimester there is an increase in fibrinogen, prothrombin, and factors VII, VIII, IX and X. There is increased platelet aggregation and resistance to activated protein C. There is a reduction in protein S, factor XI and factor XIII. A reduction in fibrinolytic activity occurs due to a decrease in antithrombin levels and an increase in function of fibrinolytic inhibitors PAI-1 and PAI-2. After delivery there is an elevation in factors V, VII and X, and antithrombin levels return to normal.

Venous stasis
Compression of large veins by the gravid uterus and pregnancy-associated changes in venous capacitance result in a reduction in venous return from the lower limbs.

Risk factors
- previous VTE
- age >35, parity >4, obesity
- thrombophilia

- inherited: antithrombin deficiency, prothrombin gene mutation, factor V Leiden mutation, protein C deficiency, protein S deficiency
  - acquired: antiphospholipid antibodies
- operative delivery, prolonged labour
- immobilisation, infection, surgery, smoking, dehydration
- nephrotic syndrome, pre-eclampsia, cardiac disease

Clinical assessment

The clinical diagnosis of VTE is insensitive and non-specific. Few women with clinically suspected VTE have the diagnosis confirmed when investigations are employed. However, when clinical suspicion exists, treatment should be instituted until the diagnosis can be excluded by objective testing.

Signs and symptoms of VTE include leg pain and swelling, lower abdominal pain, low-grade pyrexia, dyspnoea, chest pain, haemoptysis and collapse.

Diagnosis

Deep venous thrombosis (DVT)
- Doppler ultrasound is the primary study for the diagnosis of DVT.
- Lack of compressibility is 95% sensitive and >95% specific for a proximal leg vein thrombosis. It is less sensitive for calf and pelvic vein thromboses.
- Venography is considered the gold standard investigation for suspected DVT. It is rarely used due to its invasiveness and attendant ionising radiation, and because Doppler ultrasound is almost as reliable.
- Magnetic resonance imaging (MRI) may be a useful modality in the diagnosis of pelvic vein DVT, with a sensitivity approaching 100% in the non-pregnant population. No adverse effects have been documented, though the safety of MRI in pregnancy remains unproven.
- The negative predictive value of a normal D-dimer falls progressively throughout pregnancy, making it less useful at later gestations.

Pulmonary embolism
- Arterial blood gas analysis is neither sensitive nor specific for the diagnosis of pulmonary embolism (PE). A normal result is common in the presence of a PE, while respiratory alkalosis is a common feature of pregnancy.
- A chest X-ray (CXR) should be performed when PE is suspected clinically. This may identify other pulmonary pathology (e.g. pneumonia), or may reveal features associated with PE (focal opacities, atelectasis, pulmonary oedema). However, in >50% of cases of PE, the CXR will be normal.
- When the CXR is normal, Doppler ultrasound of the lower limbs should be performed. If a DVT is found, no further investigation may be required, as the treatment of the two conditions is the same. However, fewer than 30% of patients with PE have evidence of DVT at presentation.
- If both the CXR and Doppler ultrasound are normal, a computed tomography pulmonary angiogram (CTPA) or ventilation-perfusion (V/Q) scan should be performed.
- CTPA is the investigation of choice due to its higher sensitivity and specificity and lower radiation dose to the fetus compared with V/Q scanning. Due to the high dose of radiation to maternal breasts, however, CTPA does carry an increase in lifetime risk of breast cancer.

Management
- Before anticoagulant therapy is commenced, blood should be drawn for a full blood count, coagulation screen, urea and electrolytes, and liver function tests. A thrombophilia screen may be performed, but the effects of pregnancy and thrombus on the results need to be considered.
- In clinically suspected VTE, treatment with low-molecular-weight heparin (LMWH) should be given until the diagnosis is excluded by objective testing.
- In the initial management of DVT, the affected leg should be elevated and a compression stocking worn. Mobilisation should be encouraged. A temporary inferior vena caval filter may be considered in cases of iliac vein thrombosis.
- In massive PE associated with cardiovascular compromise, immediate administration of intravenous unfractionated heparin (UH) is required. A loading dose of 80 units/kg should be followed by an infusion of 18 units/kg/hour. Thrombolytic therapy or urgent thoracotomy may be considered in certain cases.

Treatment
- LMWH is the treatment of choice for confirmed VTE. Administration is via subcutaneous injection twice daily, at a dose calculated from booking weight (e.g. enoxaparin 1 mg/kg twice daily). Anti-Xa monitoring is not warranted in routine cases. Treatment with therapeutic doses should continue for the remainder of the pregnancy and for 6 weeks postpartum, due to the risk of recurrence in this period.

Labour and delivery
- Women should be advised to cease anticoagulant therapy once labour has commenced. Therapeutic LMWH should be ceased 24 hours before planned delivery. A prophylactic dose can be given the night before a planned induction of labour or caesarean section. Regional anaesthesia should not be used until 24 hours after a therapeutic dose.
- For women at high risk of recurrence of VTE around the time of delivery, intravenous UH should replace LMWH 24 hours before intervention, and cease once labour is established or 6 hours prior to caesarean section. Protamine sulfate can be given to reverse the effect of heparin if the activated partial thromboplastin time (APTT) remains elevated at the time of delivery or abnormal bleeding occurs.
- The risk of haematoma at caesarean section in anticoagulated women is increased by about 2%. For this reason, wound drains, staples or interrupted sutures should be considered.

Postpartum
- The third stage of labour should be actively managed. Prophylactic doses of anticoagulant can be given 2–6 hours after vaginal and caesarean deliveries. A dose should not be given for 4 hours after removal of an epidural catheter, and removal should be delayed until 12 hours after the last dose. Therapeutic doses of anticoagulant can be administered 24 hours after vaginal delivery and 36–48 hours after caesarean section. Warfarin can be commenced after 48 hours. Heparin should be continued until the international normalised ratio (INR) is between 2 and 3 on two consecutive days.
- A thrombophilia screen should be performed once anticoagulation therapy has been ceased and follow-up arranged.

Prophylaxis
All women should be assessed for their risk of VTE early in pregnancy or preconceptually. Anticoagulant regimens are recommended based on the degree of risk for the individual.

- Women with a *history of VTE associated with a temporary risk factor and no thrombophilia* should receive prophylaxis for 6 weeks postnatally. If there has been more than one episode of VTE, a single unprovoked episode, an episode of VTE in an unusual site or a family history of VTE in a first-degree relative, antenatal prophylaxis should also be recommended.
- Women with a *history of VTE and a thrombophilia* should receive prophylaxis antenatally and for 6 weeks postpartum. Women with antiphospholipid antibodies and a history of VTE have a 70% chance of recurrence in pregnancy.
- Women with *no history of VTE and a thrombophilia* are treated according to the level of risk associated with their thrombophilia. Prophylaxis throughout pregnancy and for 6 weeks postpartum is recommended in antithrombin deficiency and for homozygosity or compound heterozygosity for factor V Leiden and prothrombin gene mutations. Women with a lower risk thrombophilia may require prophylaxis in the postpartum period only.
- Women with *no history of VTE or thrombophilia, but with three or more risk factors* for VTE (e.g. age >35, obesity, prolonged immobility) should be considered for prophylaxis during the antenatal period and for 3–5 days postpartum.

Anticoagulant agents
Low-molecular-weight heparin (LMWH)
- LMWH is the agent of choice for prophylaxis and treatment of VTE in pregnancy.
- It is at least as effective as, and safer than, UH, with improved bioavailability and a longer half-life, and less risk of haemorrhage, heparin-induced thrombocytopenia and osteoporosis.
- Monitor by anti-factor Xa assay if required (e.g. extremes of body mass index, renal disease).
- It does not cross the placenta, and is not contraindicated in breastfeeding.

Unfractionated heparin (UH)
- UH combines with antithrombin to accelerate the inactivation of thrombin, factor Xa and other factors.
- It is the agent of choice in massive PE associated with cardiovascular collapse.
- It may be used subcutaneously for prophylaxis or treatment of VTE where LMWH is contraindicated (e.g. allergy, renal failure).
- Dosage is titrated to achieve an APTT 1.5–2.5 times the normal value, which is monitored regularly for the duration of treatment.
- Platelet count and bone mineral density should be monitored with long-term use.
- It does not cross the placenta, and is not contraindicated in breastfeeding.

Warfarin
- Warfarin interferes with the action of vitamin K on coagulation factors II, VII, IX and X, protein C and protein S, rendering them inactive.
- Warfarin crosses the placenta and has a 5% chance of teratogenesis and increased risk of miscarriage if used in the first trimester. It is associated with fetal and neonatal haemorrhage (especially intracranial), intrauterine fetal death, and maternal haemorrhage when used later in pregnancy.
- It is safe to use postpartum from 2–3 days after delivery with close INR monitoring. It is not contraindicated in breastfeeding.

Further reading

Royal College of Obstetricians and Gynaecologists 2004 Thromboprophylaxis during pregnancy, labour and after vaginal delivery. Guideline No. 37, January

Royal College of Obstetricians and Gynaecologists 2007 Thromboembolic disease in pregnancy and the puerperium: acute management. Guideline No. 28, February

Schwartz DR, Malhotra A, Weinberger S 2008 Deep vein thrombosis and pulmonary embolism in pregnancy: epidemiology, pathogenesis and diagnosis. Up To Date, August

Schwartz DR, Malhotra A, Weinberger S 2008 Deep vein thrombosis and pulmonary embolism in pregnancy: prevention. Up To Date, October

Working Group on Behalf of the Obstetric Medicine Group of Australasia 2001 Position statement: anticoagulation in pregnancy and the puerperium. Medical Journal of Australia 175:258–263

Chapter 48

Cardiac disease in pregnancy

Michael Flynn

Incidence. Fewer than 1% of all pregnancies are affected by maternal cardiac disease.

Pathophysiology of cardiovascular changes in pregnancy

Intravascular volume
This is increased by 50% by early mid-trimester and peaks at 32–34 weeks gestation. In a woman with limited cardiac output secondary to cardiovascular disease, volume overload is poorly tolerated and congestive cardiac failure a risk.

Decreased peripheral resistance in pregnancy
This is important in the woman with potential right-to-left shunts, as the shunts tend to increase with lowered vascular resistance.

Cardiac output
- Cardiac output rises early in pregnancy, and is unrelated to rise in plasma volume.
- In labour, the cardiac output rises progressively from the first stage to an additional 50% in the late second stage, with an increase of over 7 L/minute. This great change, plus the dramatic shifts of fluid that occur at delivery, is poorly tolerated in women whose cardiac output depends on adequate preload (pulmonary hypertension) or those with fixed cardiac output (mitral stenosis).
- Epidural anaesthesia and general anaesthesia produce dramatic changes in cardiac output.

Maternal mortality risks in cardiovascular disease

Mortality is most likely in conditions where pulmonary blood flow cannot be raised secondary to obstruction. Maternal mortality risk may be classified into the following three groups.

Low risk (mortality <1 %)
- uncomplicated atrial septal defect, ventricular septal defect or patent ductus arteriosus
- mitral stenosis
- tricuspid incompetence

- corrected tetralogy of Fallot
- bioprosthetic valve

Medium risk (mortality <15%)
- mitral stenosis with atrial fibrillation
- artificial valve
- previous myocardial infarction
- aortic stenosis
- uncorrected tetralogy
- uncomplicated coarctation of aorta or Marfan's syndrome

High risk (mortality <50%)
- pulmonary hypertension
- Eisenmenger's syndrome
- complicated coarctation
- Marfan's syndrome with aortic dilatation
- peripartum cardiomyopathy

Fetal risks in maternal cardiovascular disease

Family history
- The presence of a congenital cardiac anomaly in either parent or sibling increases the risk of cardiac anomaly in the offspring to about 2%–4%, or twice that of the normal population. The risk rises to 10%–12% in mothers with defects, including atrial septal defect, ventricular septal defect, patent ductus arteriosus and tetralogy of Fallot. These have multivariant inheritance.
- Idiopathic hypertrophic subaortic stenosis is an autosomal dominant condition.
- Environmental risk factors include rubella virus and alcohol.

In women with cyanotic heart disease
The maternal haematocrit appears to correlate with perinatal outcome; a haematocrit of >65% is associated with poor outcome.

Management of cardiovascular disease in pregnancy

History
- The commonest symptom of heart disease is breathlessness on exertion, although this is unreliable in pregnancy.
- Syncope can occur with normal pregnancy, aortic stenosis, hypertrophic obstructive cardiomyopathy, tetralogy of Fallot and dysrhythmias.
- A history of rheumatic fever or previous investigation for a murmur are important.

Physical examination
- In normal pregnancy it is common for premature atrial and ventricular ectopics, oedema, loud first heart sound and third heart sounds to be present.
- An ejection systolic murmur may be present in up to 90% of women.

Investigations
- Chest X-ray in normal pregnancy shows slight cardiomegaly and increased pulmonary vascular markings.

- Electrocardiograph in normal pregnancy shows inversion in T waves, Q wave in lead III.
- Echocardiography is required to identify structural abnormalities.

Counselling

- Ideally, cardiovascular disease is identified and investigated before pregnancy, with the maternal risks evaluated and appropriate contraception advised.
- If termination of pregnancy is indicated, prostaglandin termination should be used with caution. Possible indications for termination include Eisenmenger's syndrome, primary pulmonary hypertension and pulmonary veno-occlusive disease.
- Risk factors for congestive cardiac failure need to be monitored and managed appropriately. Risks include infections, hypertension, obesity, multiple pregnancy, anaemia, arrhythmia and hyperthyroidism.

Endocarditis and pregnancy

- The efficacy of antibiotic prophylaxis against infective endocarditis in pregnancy has not been proven, although it is accepted that benefits override the possible risks.
- Women at risk include those with prosthetic heart valves, most congenital malformations, rheumatic mitral stenosis, hypertrophic cardiomyopathy, mitral valve prolapse with regurgitation, or past history of subacute bacterial endocarditis.
- A regimen may include intravenous (amoxy)ampicillin 1–2 g every 8 hours, together with gentamicin 1.5 mg/kg when labour commences and continuing for 24 hours.

Antenatal management

- Attend a combined obstetric and cardiac clinic.
- Ensure adequate rest.
- Watch for risks of congestive cardiac failure.
- Initiate anticoagulation therapy for patients with pulmonary hypertension, artificial valves or atrial fibrillation.

Labour

- Aim for spontaneous vaginal delivery at term, as induction of labour is associated with an increased risk of sepsis and caesarean section.
- Maintain a strict fluid balance.
- Adequate analgesia is essential, although epidural should be used with caution, especially in hypertrophic obstructive cardiomyopathy, aortic stenosis and Eisenmenger's syndrome.
- Avoid aortocaval compression.
- Shorten the second stage.
- If possible, avoid delivery in the lithotomy position.
- Avoid ergometrine.
- If possible, avoid caesarean section in the presence of cardiac failure.
- Oxygen supplementation is recommended.
- Avoid sympathomimetic drugs.
- Prevent endocarditis with intravenous antibiotics.
- Discuss with the woman the use of intensive monitoring and intensive care in labour.

Postpartum

- Maintain a strict fluid balance to predict cardiac failure associated with the major fluid shifts after delivery of the placenta.
- Continued oxygen postpartum is advised.

Congenital heart disease

Atrial septal defect
This is the commonest congenital anomaly, usually asymptomatic but occasionally associated with atrial fibrillation. Hypervolaemia in pregnancy can cause worsening in left-to-right shunting. This increases the burden on the right ventricle, which in turn may result in cardiac failure. Most patients tolerate pregnancy, labour and delivery well. In labour, general management includes the use of prophylactic antibiotics and avoidance of fluid overload, and the use of lumbar epidural is usually well-tolerated.

Ventricular septal defect
There is a risk of cardiac failure, arrhythmias and aortic regurgitation with large defects. If uncomplicated, the pregnancy, labour and delivery are tolerated well. The management is as for atrial septal defect.

Patent ductus arteriosus
While usually asymptomatic and well-tolerated in pregnancy, labour and delivery, the possibility of high-pressure, high-flow left-to-right shunting with large lesions may worsen prognosis.

Eisenmenger's syndrome
This is a syndrome arising from conditions of congenital left-to-right shunt, in which progressive pulmonary hypertension leads to shunt reversal or bidirectional shunting. In the antepartum period, reduced vascular resistance causes an increase in right-to-left shunting. This leads to a reduction in pulmonary perfusion, with hypoxia and deterioration of the fetal/maternal condition.

Hypotension in the woman with Eisenmenger's syndrome reduces right ventricular filling pressure and lowers perfusion in pulmonary beds. Therefore, reduction in blood pressure with haemorrhage or anaesthesia can lead to sudden death.

Management
- If corrected in childhood with no residual damage, there are usually no complications. If not, then pulmonary hypertension could decompensate during pregnancy.
- Advise the patient about the risks of continuing pregnancy.
- Avoid caesarean section and epidural anaesthesia.
- Initiate anticoagulation therapy.
- Avoid ergometrine and procedures that produce a sudden rise in venous return.

Coarctation of the aorta
The commonest site is at the origin of the left subclavian artery and can be associated with abnormal aorta, ventricular septal defect, patent ductus arteriosus and intracranial aneurysm in the circle of Willis.

Maternal mortality risk is dependent on whether there are associated vascular or cardiac lesions and on the increased risk of pre-eclampsia. There is a risk of dissection of aorta with hyperdynamic pregnancy state, and management involves treating hypertension aggressively.

Tetralogy of Fallot
This cyanotic heart condition consists of ventricular septal defect, overriding aorta, right ventricular hypertrophy and pulmonary stenosis. If uncorrected, the maternal mortality rises to 4%–15%.

Pulmonary hypertension

There is high maternal mortality during pregnancy or immediately postpartum. Avoid fluid overload, pulmonary congestion, heart failure and hypotension. It can lead to hypoxia and sudden cardiac death.

Acquired cardiac lesions

Rheumatic heart disease

This is the commonest heart disease in pregnancy.

Risks
- reduced ability to increase cardiac output in those with significant mitral stenosis
- endocarditis with mitral regurgitation
- sudden death with aortic stenosis
- pulmonary oedema with severe aortic regurgitation

Acute rheumatic fever
- is very uncommon in pregnancy
- presents with non-specific malaise, joint pains, anaemia, rash
- diagnosis includes raised antistreptolysin-O titre, electrocardiograph with prolonged PR and QT intervals, erythrocyte sedimentation rate >80 mm/hour (normal pregnancy <60 mm/hour)

Mitral stenosis
- This is the commonest rheumatic valvular lesion in pregnancy. The main problem is that ventricular diastolic filling against a valvular obstruction can cause a relatively fixed cardiac output and therefore risks acute cardiac failure and pulmonary oedema, and occasionally atrial fibrillation.
- Clinical symptoms include increasing shortness of breath and fatigue.
- On examination, there are signs of cardiac failure, atrial fibrillation, and the early diastolic rumbling murmur is heard.
- Atrial fibrillation is associated with a risk of thromboembolism, and requires anticoagulation therapy.

Management
- Cardiac output in mitral stenosis depends on adequate diastolic filling time and left ventricular preload. Therefore, tachycardia (from infections or blood loss) and fluid overload must be carefully avoided.
- Labour is a vulnerable time. Intrapartum fluctuations of cardiac output can be minimised with the use of epidural anaesthesia and a careful watch postpartum for fluid shifts.
- Antibiotic prophylaxis is indicated to avoid endocarditis.
- Immediately after delivery of the baby, there is a sharp rise in left atrial pressure, which may precipitate cardiac failure.

Mitral insufficiency

This may be secondary to rheumatic fever. However, the more common lesion is mitral valve prolapse. It is usually well tolerated in pregnancy, except for the risks of atrial fibrillation and endocarditis (therefore, require antibiotic prophylaxis in labour).

Aortic stenosis
- There is a higher maternal mortality in rheumatic compared with congenital aortic stenosis.

- It is not considered haemodynamically significant until the orifice is less than a third of normal size.
- In severe aortic stenosis, there is relatively fixed cardiac output, resulting in inadequate coronary artery and cerebral perfusion causing angina, syncope and sudden death. The times of greatest risk are delivery and pregnancy termination.
- It is very important to maintain adequate cardiac output. If hypotension occurs with blood loss, epidural or inferior vena caval occlusion, sudden death can occur.
- Surgical correction of the disease before conception greatly improves prognosis.

Aortic insufficiency
This is usually well tolerated in pregnancy, as tachycardia results in less time for regurgitation. Endocarditis prophylaxis is indicated in labour.

Cardiomyopathy
Hypertrophic obstructive cardiomyopathy
- This is a subaortic stenosis, with pathological appearances of hypertrophy and disorganisation of cardiac muscle.
- The woman presents with chest pain, syncope and arrhythmia.
- Diagnosis is made on echocardiography.
- The pregnancy is often well tolerated, and outcome is dependent on the severity of left ventricular outflow tract obstruction.
- Management includes beta-blocker if indicated, avoiding hypotension because of the risk of obstruction of left ventricular outflow tract, which occurs in aortocaval compression, and antepartum/postpartum haemorrhage.

Peripartum cardiomyopathy
- This rare cardiomyopathy may develop in the last month of pregnancy or the first 6 months postpartum, with a peak incidence in the second postpartum month.
- It is more common in older multiparous patients who breastfeed and have a history of hypertension, pre-eclampsia or multiple pregnancy with poor nutrition.
- Investigations include chest X-ray with non-specific cardiomegaly, electro-cardiography, showing non-specific changes or widespread abnormalities or arrhythmias, and echocardiography with a grossly dilated heart.
- Management includes anticardiac failure therapy, anticoagulation, and aiming for a vaginal delivery. Treat with diuretics and beta-blockers, decrease sodium intake, and use angiotensin-converting enzyme (ACE) inhibitors when delivered.
- The major cause of mortality is thromboembolism.
- Counsel the patient regarding the recurrence rate in future pregnancies. If the heart returns to a normal size within 12 months, there is less than a 15% mortality in the next pregnancy. If cardiomegaly persists until the next pregnancy, there is a 40%–80% associated mortality.

Marfan's syndrome
This is an autosomal dominant disorder characterised by a generalised weakness of connective tissue. It is associated with mitral or aortic regurgitation and dangerous weaknesses in the aortic root and aortic wall.

Maternal risks
- These include vascular aneurysms, especially rupture or dissection of the aorta or splenic artery, and abnormal aortic valve or aortic dilatation.
- Initial echocardiography evaluation includes the diameter of the aortic root. If the aortic root is <40 mm, the maternal mortality is <5%, but if the dilatation is >40 mm, the mortality reaches 50%.

Management
- Treat hypertension aggressively.
- Use beta-blocker medication if aortic dilatations are present, even without hypertension, as this reduces the pulsatile pressure and decreases the force of contraction of the heart, thereby reducing the rate of progress of aortic dilatation.
- Perform a caesarean section if there is evidence of aortic disease.

Myocardial infarction

The overall mortality in pregnancy is 35%, but mortality increases as pregnancy progresses. In young women, myocardial infarction in the puerperium is often associated with pre-eclampsia, possibly from dissection of coronary arteries.

Management
- Management is similar to that for non-pregnant patients.
- Delivery within 2 weeks of the infarction raises mortality.
- Labour must be intensively monitored.
- Continuous oxygen and epidural anaesthesia is indicated.
- Management includes elective shortening of the second stage with instrumental delivery.
- Ergometrine is contraindicated, as it may cause coronary artery spasm.

Chapter 49

Connective tissue disease in pregnancy

Amy Mellor

Systemic lupus erythematosus (SLE)

SLE is a multisystem autoimmune disease, involving direct attack by autoantibodies and deposition of immune complexes. It mainly affects women in the reproductive age group, making it a frequently encountered condition in obstetric practice. SLE has a prevalence of 1 in 5000–10,000 women, with a female to male ratio of 9:1. SLE is thought not to impair fertility. Pregnancy outcome for mother and offspring is best when the disease has been quiescent for at least 6 months prior to conception, and renal function is stable.

Pregnancy probably does not increase the rate of SLE exacerbation compared with the non-pregnant population. Flares occur equally across the trimesters, and are common in the immediate postpartum period. They present most commonly as fever, lymphadenopathy, skin and joint involvement, and renal impairment. Neurological, cardiovascular and respiratory manifestations may also occur. Exacerbation is more common when disease is active at the time of conception. Flare is associated with hypocomplementaemia and an increase in anti-double stranded DNA titres. One-third to one-half of SLE patients have antiphospholipid antibodies (aPL), and one-third have anti-Ro/SSA or anti-La/SSB antibodies.

Maternal effects
- pre-eclampsia: occurs in around 13% of patients with SLE, is much more frequent in women with preexisting renal disease and aPL, and can be difficult to distinguish from lupus nephritis
- lupus nephritis: associated with an increased risk of fetal loss and worsening of renal and extra-renal manifestations
- venous thromboembolism
- postpartum haemorrhage

Fetal effects
- intrauterine growth restriction (IUGR)
- intrauterine fetal death: risk is higher in women with active disease at conception, hypertension, renal disease, aPL, hypocomplementaemia, elevated anti-DNA antibodies and thrombocytopenia
- preterm birth: three times more common than in women without SLE

Neonatal lupus
- results from passive transfer of anti-Ro/SSA or anti-La/SSB antibodies
- causes complete heart block in the fetus/neonate in 2% of cases

- other features include rash, thrombocytopenia, hepatitis and haemolytic anaemia
- no congenital anomalies associated with SLE

Management
Pregnancy in women with SLE should be managed in a high-risk setting by an obstetrician and physician. Ideally, medication should be reviewed and disease management optimised preconceptually.

Initial investigations
- full blood count, renal function tests (including urinalysis, protein/creatinine ratio)
- aPL assays
- anti-Ro/SSA and anti-La/SSB antibodies
- C3 and C4 titres
- anti-double stranded DNA antibody titres

Ongoing management
- frequent auscultation of fetal heart with or without echocardiogram if heart block suspected
- monthly platelet count
- repeat aPL, complement, anti-double stranded DNA antibodies and renal function tests each trimester
- surveillance for exacerbation of disease, pre-eclampsia and IUGR
- regular surveillance of fetal wellbeing if complications arise
- delivery timed according to complications/fetal condition

Drug therapy
- The potential for medication to cross the placenta and cause fetal harm must be weighed against the risks of active disease to the mother and fetus.
- Low-dose aspirin with or without heparin should be considered in women with aPL.
- Non-steroidal anti-inflammatory drugs (NSAIDs) and azathrioprine should be used with caution.
- Glucocorticoids at the lowest possible dose to control disease activity are recommended for management of disease exacerbation. These increase the risk of gestational diabetes and adrenal suppression, necessitating hydrocortisone in labour.
- The safety of antimalarial drugs is uncertain.
- Cytotoxic agents are contraindicated in pregnancy.

Antiphospholipid syndrome (APS)

APS is characterised by arterial or venous thrombosis and specific pregnancy complications, in association with laboratory evidence of aPL.

Antiphospholipid antibodies (aPL)
The diagnosis of APS requires the presence of anticardiolipin antibody (aCL), lupus anticoagulant (LA) or antibody to B2-glycoprotein 1 on two occasions at least 12 weeks apart. Antibodies are present in 2% of the pregnant population.

Pregnancy complications
- complications are thought to arise primarily due to antibody-induced thrombosis in the uteroplacental circulation; antibodies also have a direct effect on placental trophoblast, resulting in reduced trophoblast invasion and human chorionic gonadotrophin (hCG) production

- intrauterine fetal death
- recurrent miscarriage after 10 weeks gestation (correlates with level of aCL immunoglobulin G (IgG))
- IUGR occurs in 30% of women with APS
- early, severe pre-eclampsia (stronger association with aCL than LA)
- maternal thromboembolic disease: 5% risk in women with APS

Management
- There is a paucity of data from large, well-designed trials into the management of pregnant women with APS.
- Women with known APS should be managed in a high-risk setting by an obstetrician and physician. Additional surveillance includes baseline renal and liver function tests, and serial growth and wellbeing ultrasounds.
- Low-dose aspirin has been associated with an increase in successful pregnancy outcome in some studies. It should be commenced as soon as possible from conception, and ceased at 36 weeks gestation.
- Heparin enhances the effects of antithrombin and other antithrombotic factors, and may also bind aPL to render them inactive. Meta-analysis shows the combination of heparin and aspirin significantly reduces the incidence of pregnancy loss compared with aspirin alone.
- Women with a history of thrombosis and aPL should receive thromboprophylaxis antenatally and in the postpartum period. These women are at high risk for recurrence and are generally on lifelong anticoagulation.
- Women with a history of early, severe pre-eclampsia or IUGR in a previous pregnancy can be recommended low-dose aspirin in the second and third trimesters.

Rheumatoid arthritis

Rheumatoid arthritis occurs predominantly in females, many of whom are in the reproductive age group.

Pregnancy
- About 75% of women experience improvement in rheumatoid arthritis symptoms. This is likely due to the immunological changes of pregnancy, resulting in a less inflammatory state.
- About 90% of women experience exacerbation of disease within the first 3 months after delivery.
- Reintroduction of medication in the immediate postpartum period is recommended.
- Pregnancy is generally uneventful, with no evidence of increased adverse outcome.
- Medication may need to be continued, or reintroduced if flare occurs.
- NSAIDs should be avoided in the third trimester to avoid premature closure of the ductus arteriosus.
- Prednisone at the lowest possible dose to control disease is the safest option.
- Sulfasalazine, azathioprine and hydroxychloroquine may be used in refractory cases.
- Elective caesarean section may occasionally be necessary where joint disease precludes vaginal delivery.

Further reading

Bermas BL 2007 Rheumatoid arthritis and pregnancy. Up To Date. September
Lockshin MD, Salmon JE, Erkan D 2009 Pregnancy and rheumatic diseases. In: Creasy RJ, Resnik R (eds) Maternal–fetal medicine: principles and practice, 6th edn. Philadelphia: Saunders Elsevier, pp. 1079–1087

Lockwood CJ, Schur PH 2008 Management of pregnant women with antiphospholipid antibodies or the antiphospholipid syndrome. Up To Date, November

Lockwood CJ, Schur PH 2008 Obstetrical manifestations of the antiphospholipid syndrome. Up To Date, October

Schur PH, Bermas BL 2008 Pregnancy in women with systemic lupus erythematosus. Up To Date, October

Chapter 50

Haematology and pregnancy

Amy Mellor

Haematologic changes in pregnancy

Plasma volume increases during pregnancy by up to 50%, and is maximal at around 34 weeks gestation. Red blood cell mass increases by only 17%, resulting in a relative haemodilution. This leads to a reduction in haemaglobin, haematocrit and red blood cell count, without changing the mean corpuscular volume or mean corpuscular haemaglobin concentration.

Iron requirements increase throughout pregnancy, with 60 mg/day of elemental iron needed during the second and third trimesters. Folate requirements increase from 50μg/day in the non-pregnant woman to around 400 μg/day. Pregnancy has minimal impact on vitamin B_{12} levels, as most adults have a 2–3-year store available.

Platelet count remains in the normal range for most pregnant women, though the average is slightly lower than in the non-pregnant population. The lower limit of normal is between 106 and 120 x10^9/L. Pregnancy is associated with a leucocytosis due to an increase in circulating neutrophils. The average white blood cell count in the second and third trimesters is between 9 and 15 x10^9/L.

Anaemia in pregnancy

Anaemia is a reduction in red cell mass relative to plasma volume, measured as the amount of haemaglobin (Hb) per litre of blood volume. Anaemia in pregnancy is defined as an Hb <110 g/L in the first and third trimesters, and <105 g/L in the second trimester. Around 20% of women are anaemic in the third trimester of pregnancy. Anaemia should be investigated and treated, as severe anaemia has been associated with miscarriage, preterm birth, intrauterine growth restriction (IUGR) and fetal death.

Causes of anaemia
- microcytic: iron deficiency, haemoglobinopathies, chronic disease
- normocytic: haemolysis, haemorrhage
- macrocytic: vitamin B_{12} or folate deficiency

Iron deficiency
- Iron requirements average around 1000 mg over the course of a normal pregnancy; 300 mg is required for the fetus and placenta, 500 mg for the expansion of maternal Hb, and 200 mg is lost through the gut, urine and skin.

- Iron deficiency is responsible for 75% of cases of anaemia in pregnancy.
- Prevalence may approach 50% of pregnancies.
- It results in a microcytic, hypochromic anaemia with low plasma iron, high iron-binding capacity and low serum ferritin.
- Treatment is with oral iron (e.g. 325 mg of ferrous sulfate) once to three times daily.
- Absorption is enhanced by administration of 500 mg of vitamin C.
- Side effects of iron include nausea, vomiting, abdominal pain, constipation and diarrhoea.
- Parenteral administration via intravenous or intramuscular routes is rarely required (malabsorption syndromes, severe anaemia with intolerance to oral preparations). Anaphylaxis occurs in 1%.

Folic acid deficiency
- This is much more common than vitamin B_{12} deficiency as a cause of megaloblastic anaemia. It occurs due to poor nutrition or decreased absorption.
- Findings include macrocytic (or normocytic), normochromic anaemia with hypersegmentation of leucocytes. Reticulocyte count is normal or low. White blood cell and platelet counts are often reduced.
- It is defined as red blood cell folate level <165 ng/mL or serum folate <2 µg/L. Vitamin B_{12} is within the normal range.
- Treatment is with oral folic acid, 1–5 mg/day.

Vitamin B_{12} deficiency
- Deficiency is rare except in strict vegans and women with intrinsic factor deficiency.
- It may manifest as neurological defects. It is critical that women with vitamin B_{12} deficiency not be treated with folic acid alone, as neuropathy may worsen.
- Treatment is with 1 mg of intramuscular vitamin B_{12} daily for 1 week, then weekly for 4 weeks.

Thalassaemia

Thalassaemia is an inherited defect in Hb, resulting from decreased globin chain production. Both alpha-thalassaemias and beta-thalassaemias result in defective synthesis of HbA. Alpha-chain synthesis is controlled by two pairs of genes on chromosome 16, and alpha-thalassaemia results from one or more gene deletions. Beta-chain synthesis is controlled by one pair of genes on chromosome 11, and beta-thalassaemia results mostly commonly from a point mutation.

Alpha-thalassaemia
- Alpha-thalassaemia is most common in South-East Asian populations.
- A single gene deletion is known as the 'silent carrier' state and is clinically undetectable.
- Two genes are deleted in alpha-thalassaemia minor, resulting in a mild hypochromic, microcytic anaemia.
- A deletion of three alpha genes results in HbH disease, the most severe form compatible with life. Abnormally high levels of HbH (β4) and Hb Barts (γ4) accumulate, resulting in severe haemolytic anaemia.
- In the homozygous state, all four genes are deleted. The fetus is unable to synthesize HbF or any adult Hb, resulting in high output cardiac failure, hydrops and fetal death. This is associated with significant maternal morbidity and mortality if pregnancy continues.

Beta-thalassaemia
- Beta-thalassaemia is autosomal-recessive and occurs most commonly in Mediterranean populations.
- Beta-thalassaemia minor or trait results in a variable clinical picture, depending on beta-chain production. If both parents are carriers, there is a 25% chance of a child affected with beta-thalassaemia major.
- In homozygous beta-thalassaemia or beta-thalassaemia major, unimpeded beta-chain production results in severe haemolytic anaemia. The fetus is protected by the production of HbF. This protection disappears after birth, with the infant becoming anaemic by 3–6 months of age.

Screening and treatment
- All pregnant women should have a full blood count with red cell indices as screening for thalassaemia. A mean corpuscular volume (MCV) <80 fL in the absence of iron deficiency necessitates further testing, as does a significant family history or high-risk ethnicity.
- Hb electrophoreisis identifies the presence of excessive or deficient amounts of globin chains. More than 3.5% of HbA_2 ($\alpha_2\delta_2$) suggests beta-thalassaemia, while a normal amount of HbA_2 with an MCV <80 fL suggests alpha-thalassaemia.
- The definitive diagnosis of alpha-thalassaemia requires DNA analysis.
- When an abnormality is identified, the father should be tested to determine the risk of disease to the fetus. Diagnosis can be made by analysis of fetal DNA obtained through chorionic villus sampling, amniocentesis or fetal blood sampling. Genetic counselling to discuss treatment options should follow. Preimplantation genetic diagnosis can also be used by at-risk couples.
- Pregnant women with thalassaemia require adequate iron and folate intake. Severe disease may necessitate regular blood transfusion.

Thrombocytopenia in pregnancy

Gestational thrombocytopenia
- Gestational thrombocytopenia occurs in 5% of women and accounts for more than 70% of cases of maternal thrombocytopenia.
- The platelet count rarely falls below 80 $\times 10^9$/L, and lies between 130 and 150 $\times 10^9$/L in the majority of cases.
- It is defined by the following criteria:
  - mild, asymptomatic thrombocytopenia
  - no history of thrombocytopenia outside of pregnancy
  - occurs in the latter stages of pregnancy
  - no association with fetal thrombocytopenia
  - spontaneous resolution after delivery
- It may be a mild and transient manifestation of idiopathic thrombocytopenic purpura (ITP) (see below).
- There is no associated increased risk to the mother or fetus/neonate, so routine obstetric management should be employed.
- The maternal platelet count should be checked postnatally to ensure resolution.

Idiopathic thrombocytopenic purpura (ITP)
ITP is a syndrome in which antibody-bound platelets are destroyed by the reticuloendothelial system, predominantly in the spleen. The rate of destruction exceeds that of production in the bone marrow, resulting in thrombocytopenia. The

diagnosis is one of exclusion, being no definitive clinical or laboratory parameters. The condition may be difficult to distinguish from gestational thrombocytopenia when first encountered in pregnancy.

ITP and pregnancy
- Prevalence of ITP is 1–5 per 10,000 pregnancies.
- The platelet count nadir occurs most commonly in the third trimester.
- The course of ITP is not changed by pregnancy. ITP impacts upon pregnancy by increasing the risk of maternal haemorrhage. Immunoglobulin G (IgG) antibodies can cross the placenta and cause thrombocytopenia in the fetus/neonate.

Treatment
- Treatment of the mother does not affect the fetal platelet count, so should be based on maternal need only.
- Asymptomatic women with platelets >30 x10^9/L do not require treatment until delivery is imminent.
- First-line treatment is with corticosteroids (prednisone 1 mg/kg/day). Once platelets are normal, the dose can be tapered until the lowest possible dose to maintain platelets >50 x10^9/L is reached.
- Intravenous immunoglobulin (IVIg) can be used in cases refractory to steroids, or in emergency situations.
- Splenectomy is the most effective treatment for severe symptomatic ITP, but should be avoided in pregnancy if possible. Indications may include ongoing bleeding or a platelet count <10 x10^9/L despite treatment with steroids or IVIg. When necessary, splenectomy is ideally performed in the second trimester.

Delivery
- Platelet counts of >50 and >80 x10^9/L are considered safe for vaginal delivery and caesarean section respectively.
- Local protocols vary, but a platelet count >80 x10^9/L is generally considered safe for regional anaesthesia.
- Labour and delivery is managed normally, with caesarean section reserved for routine obstetric indications. Fetal scalp electrodes, fetal blood sampling and vacuum extraction should be avoided in case of fetal thrombocytopenia.

Neonatal issues
- Around 10% of neonates born to mothers with ITP are thrombocytopenic at birth. The risk of neonatal intracranial haemorrhage during delivery is <1%.
- Cord blood should be tested for platelet count at delivery. If <20 x10^9/L or abnormal bleeding occurs, treatment is with IVIg.
- Neonatal platelet count reaches a nadir 2–5 days after delivery due to an increase in splenic activity. Levels should be rechecked at this time if abnormal at delivery or if clinical signs of thrombocytopenia are present.

Thrombotic thrombocytopenic purpura

- characterised by thrombocytopenia, microangiopathic haemolytic anaemia, fever and neurological and renal dysfunction
- caused by profound intravascular platelet aggregation, resulting in multiorgan ischaemia
- associated with absence of plasma enzyme ADAMTS13
- incidence in pregnancy of 1 in 25,000

- can be difficult to distinguish from severe pre-eclampsia/HELLP syndrome (i.e. H—haemolysis, EL—elevated liver enzymes and LP—low platelets); diagnosis is clinical
- can present any time in pregnancy or postpartum
- 33% chance of perinatal mortality
- unlike pre-eclampsia, delivery does not result in resolution of disease
- treatment is with plasmapheresis, which has increased the maternal survival rate to around 80%

Further reading

Bowden DK 2001 Screening for thalassaemia. Australian Prescriber 24:120–123

British Committee for Standards in Haematology, General Haematology Task Force 2003 Guidelines for the investigation and management of idiopathic thrombocytopenic purpura in adults, children and in pregnancy. British Journal of Haematology 120:574–596

George JN, Knudtson EJ 2009 Thrombocytopenia in pregnancy. Up To Date, January

Kilpatrick SJ 2009 Anemia and pregnancy. In: Creasy R, Resnik R (eds) Maternal–fetal medicine: principles and practice, 6th edn. Philadelphia: Saunders Elsevier, pp. 869–884

Lockwood CJ, Silver RM 2009 Coagulation disorders in pregnancy. In: Creasy R, Resnik R (eds) Maternal–fetal medicine: principles and practice, 6th edn. Philadelphia: Saunders Elsevier, pp. 825–854

Mueller BU 2007 Prenatal testing for the hemoglobinopathies and thalassemias. Up To Date, January

Paidas MJ 2009 Hematologic changes in pregnancy. Up To Date, January

Chapter 51

Gastrointestinal disorders in pregnancy

Michael Flynn

Abdominal pain in pregnancy

Pain arises either from inside an organ or the covering visceral peritoneum or, later, involvement of parietal peritoneum. Visceral pain is poorly localised, as it is mediated by the autonomic nervous system. With parietal peritoneum, localisation is more specific.

Pain pathways of pelvic organs
- Sensory afferent pathways from the body of the uterus travel via sympathetic nerves to T10–L1.
- The cervix is supplied by sympathetic nerves to T10–L1 and parasympathetic nerves to S2–S4.
- Pain pathways from the ovary travel via sympathetic nerves to T10.

Causes of abdominal pain in early pregnancy
- abortion
- impacted retroverted uterus at 10–14 weeks gestation, with the pain caused by urinary retention (management is by draining the urine and laying the woman prone or lateral)
- fibroids (torsion tends to occur in the puerperium; red degeneration is most common at 12–18 weeks gestation; presenting complaint is of tenderness over a mass, with mild fever and nausea/vomiting; management is with rest and analgesia)
- fallopian tube: ectopic pregnancy, torsion, salpingitis
- ovary: ovarian tumour/mass; complications: rupture, haemorrhage or torsion
- pelvic soft tissue (round ligament pain may commence from early second trimester; management is with rest, analgesia and warm packs)
- others: gastrointestinal (e.g. appendicitis) and urinary tract (e.g. infection, stone)

Causes of abdominal pain in late pregnancy
- uterine: contractions, placental abruption
- gastrointestinal tract: heartburn (occurs in 70%–80% of pregnant women), constipation, peptic ulcer disease, cholelithiasis (occurs in 3%–5% of pregnant women, but is mostly asymptomatic), pancreatitis, acute appendicitis (incidence of about 1 in 2500 pregnancies; has a significant association with premature labour), acute obstruction (from bands/adhesions, volvulus, hernia), inflammatory bowel disease
- other causes: renal (pyelonephritis, calculus), malignancy

Gastro-oesophageal disorders

Gastro-oesophageal reflux
- This is due to a combination of changes in lower oesophageal pressure, raised intragastric pressure and failure of acid clearance. The incidence is up to 80% in the third trimester.
- Initial management of reflux is with dietary change, upright posture and antacids.
- In established gastro-oesophageal reflux, the use of proton pump inhibitors (esomeprozole) is indicated.

Nausea and vomiting
- This is present in up to 85% of early normal pregnancies. Women with hyperemesis often have higher levels of serum human chorionic gonadotrophin (hCG).
- The nausea and vomiting commonly occurs at 6–16 weeks gestation, but 20% persist beyond this time.
- Hyperemesis does not affect birthweight. The incidence of abortion, stillbirths and premature delivery is lower in these women.

Management of hyperemesis gravidarum
- between 7 and 11 weeks; rarely severe
- fluid resuscitation and electrolyte restoration
- avoidance of trigger events
- ginger and vitamin B_6 have some effect
- antiemetics, including metoclopramide and prochlorpromazine, and anti-histamines, have been used as first-line management safely
- ondansetron: used successfully as second-line management
- glucocorticoids: used in severe hyperemesis, especially after the fetal palate has been formed
- investigations: mid-stream urine for urinary infection; pelvic ultrasound scan to exclude gestational trophoblastic disease and multiple pregnancy; full blood examination and electrolytes; liver function tests and thyroid function tests looking for hypochloraemic alkalosis
- differential diagnosis of persistent hyperemesis: includes hepatitis, pancreatitis, gastrointestinal obstruction, peptic ulcer disease, thyroid disease and adrenocortical insufficiency

Gastrointestinal disorders

Peptic ulcer disease
Incidence. Incidence is 1 in 4000.

Peptic ulcer disease rarely occurs for the first time in pregnancy. If it is present before pregnancy, there is often a reduction in symptoms. Peptic ulceration can increase in severity with pre-eclampsia and during the puerperium.

Management of peptic ulcer disease is similar to that in non-pregnant patients, with proton pump inhibitors forming the mainstay of treatment.

Coeliac disease
Gluten-sensitive enteropathy is often associated with subfertility in those with untreated coeliac disease. Untreated disease in pregnancy has an increased risk of recurrent abortion, intrauterine growth restriction (IUGR) and megaloblastic anaemia.

Management of coeliac disease in pregnancy includes a gluten-free diet, iron and folate supplementation, and fetal monitoring.

Inflammatory bowel disease
Fertility correlates with disease activity. Pregnancy itself does not increase the risk of relapse of inflammatory bowel disease.

Acute exacerbations are managed by admission to hospital, stool cultures, rest, withholding food and drink, corticosteroids and salazopyrine.

Hepatic disorders in pregnancy

Liver function tests in pregnancy
- There is no change in serum bilirubin and transaminase levels, although reduced total protein and albumin levels are normal.
- The increase in serum alkaline phosphatase is secondary to placental production.

Intrahepatic cholestasis of pregnancy
Incidence. Intrahepatic cholestasis affects up to 2% of pregnancies.

Presentation. Pruritus and mild jaundice present in the third trimester. Pruritus usually resolves within 48 hours of delivery. It starts at the soles and palms of the hands, and then spreads to the rest of the body.

Risk factors
- There is a family history in 45% of cases.
- It can recur with the use of the oral contraceptive pill and with future pregnancies.
- It is often worse with multiple pregnancies. Pre-eclampsia must be excluded.

Effect on pregnancy
- There is an increased risk of preterm delivery and perinatal mortality if not treated.
- In 10%–20% of cases, there is meconium liquor.

Investigations
- liver biochemistry (raised liver transaminase and bilirubin)
- raised fasting bile acids (this is the diagnostic feature of this disease)
- full blood count, urea/electrolytes and urate
- coagulation profile (raised prothrombin time may occur)
- hepatitis serology
- autoantibody screen
- antimitochondrial antibodies (primary biliary cirrhosis)
- ultrasound scan to exclude cholelithiasis

Pathophysiology
- altered bile acids and progesterone metabolism

Treatment
- coagulation monitoring
- vitamin K supplementation
- antihistamines
- ursodeoxycholic acid (UDCA) 10–16 mg/kg daily until delivery
- close monitoring (consider delivering early)

Acute fatty liver of pregnancy
Incidence. Incidence is 1 in 12,000 deliveries, with associated maternal and fetal mortality. It does not tend to recur.

Risk factors
- primiparity, obesity, pre-eclampsia and multiple pregnancy
- association with long-chain 3-hydroxyacyl CoA dehydrogenase (LCHAD)

Presentation
- abdominal pain, especially epigastric 50%
- nausea and vomiting in 75% of cases
- headache, pruritus
- jaundice in over 90% of cases
- hypertension in 50% of cases with oedema, proteinuria
- fever, ascites, pancreatitis
- progression to hepatic coma and renal failure possible

Investigation
- full blood examination (reveals a raised white cell count with neutrophilia, reduced platelets and haemolytic anaemia)
- coagulation profile (shows evidence of disseminated coagulopathy)
- electrolytes and renal function (elevated urea, creatinine and markedly raised urate)
- liver biochemistry (elevated bilirubin, but not markedly so; markedly elevated aspartate transaminase)
- hepatitis serology
- blood sugar levels (hypoglycaemia is common)
- ultrasound: microvascular fat deposits

Management
- Treat complications of hypoglycaemia and hypertension, and general supportive management.
- Exclude severe pre-eclampsia and prompt delivery required.
- 10% glucose and fresh frozen plasma/cryoprecipitate may be considered.
- Fetal morbidity is 90%, but with early recognition and treatment >70% survive.

Acute viral hepatitis
There does not appear to be an overall increase in congenital abnormalities if acute hepatitis occurs in pregnancy. Common causes are hepatitis A, B and C, herpes virus (simplex, varicella, cytomegalovirus) and Epstein-Barr virus.
Hepatitis A virus is usually self-limiting, with no increased fetal risks.

Chronic hepatitis
Chronic active hepatitis may be due to autoimmune diseases. In pregnancy, there is a risk of IUGR, fetal death, prematurity and pre-eclampsia. There does not appear to be an increased risk of fetal malformation.

Cirrhosis
- There may be a decrease in fertility secondary to oligomenorrhoea.
- Pregnancy is complicated by an increased incidence of abortion and intrauterine fetal death.
- Other complications of cirrhosis may also occur, such as bleeding oesophageal varices.
- Management: avoid increasing portal pressure, cease alcohol, increase carbohydrate consumption, lower protein and supplement with vitamins. In labour, shorten the second stage. Take precautions against the risk of postpartum haemorrhage. Avoid caesarean section because of large collateral circulation and adhesions.

- Primary biliary cirrhosis: antimitochondrial antibodies are present in over 95% of cases.
- There are no prospective studies to assess the effects of disease in pregnancy.

Causes of fulminant hepatic failure in pregnancy
- viral hepatitis
- acute fatty liver of pregnancy
- severe pre-eclampsia
- haemolytic uraemic syndrome
- paracetamol overdose

Gallbladder and biliary tract

Dilatation of the gallbladder is found in pregnancy. However, anecdotal evidence of an increased risk of developing cholesterol stones in pregnancy has not been substantiated.

Acute cholelithiasis and cholecystitis in pregnancy requiring cholecystectomy occurs in about 1 in 1000 deliveries. The prevalence of asymptomatic gallstones in pregnancy is 2%–10%, which is similar to the rate in non-pregnant women.

Further reading

Calhoun BC 1992 Gastrointestinal disorders in pregnancy. Obstetrics and Gynecology Clinics of North America 19:733–744

Chamberlain G 1991 Abdominal pain in pregnancy. British Medical Journal 302:1390–1394

Mullaly BA, Hansen WF 2001 Intraheptic cholestasis of pregnancy: review of the literature. Obstetrical and Gynecological Survey 57:47–52

Samuels P, Cohen A 1992 Pregnancies complicated by liver disease and liver dysfunction. Obstetrics and Gynecology Clinics of North America 19:745–763

Chapter 52

Neurological disease in pregnancy

Michael Flynn

Epilepsy and pregnancy

Incidence. Epilepsy occurs in 0.5%–1% of the population. Over 90% of women with epilepsy have a normal pregnancy.

Effects of epilepsy on pregnancy
- reports of fetal bradycardia after generalised seizure
- increased risk of childhood epilepsy of 3%–4% if one parent has epilepsy
- increased association with pre-eclampsia, preterm delivery, low birthweight, higher perinatal mortality and congenital malformations due to the epilepsy and the anticonvulsant drugs; fetal effects include cerebral palsy, seizures and mental retardation

Effects of pregnancy on epilepsy
- About 50% remain stable, with improvement in seizure frequency in 25% and deterioration in 25% of women.
- The deterioration is attributed to hormonal and metabolic changes and diminished compliance with drug therapy.
- In about 70% of patients, serum levels of anticonvulsants fall in early pregnancy and return to prepregnancy levels by 4 weeks postpartum; so if seizure activity increases, it is often in the first two trimesters.
- If epilepsy presents for the first time in pregnancy, rigorous investigation is required to exclude other neurological abnormalities.

Pharmacokinetics of anticonvulsants in pregnancy
- Drug absorption may be lowered with vomiting in early pregnancy.
- Volume of distribution is increased due to raised plasma volume and total body water, and results in a reduced steady state of plasma levels.
- Increased fat stores will lower lipid-soluble drug excretion.
- Phenytoin and valproate are highly protein-bound. With the reduction of albumin in pregnancy, there is a lower percentage of bound drug. Therefore, unbound levels in plasma remain constant, but total plasma levels are reduced.
- The glomerular filtration rate rises, raising the clearance of renally excreted drugs.
- Hepatic hydroxylation of phenytoin is increased, and this causes a reduction in free drug.
- Non-compliance due to maternal fears of teratogenicity often reduces plasma levels of drug.

Teratogenicity of anticonvulsants
- In a woman with epilepsy treated with a single anticonvulsant, the fetus has a risk of congenital malformation of 7%, compared with 3% in non-epileptics. There may be a higher incidence with polypharmacy.
- The defects include orofacial clefts, cardiovascular anomalies, neural tube defects (which are commonly primary myelomeningocele and anencephaly, and especially if valproate is taken in the first trimester), microcephaly and digital hypoplasia.
- Epilepsy pregnancy registries indicate valproate at doses >1100 mg/day confer significant risk compared to other doses and other drugs.

Other maternal effects of anticonvulsants
- reduced folate levels
- increased vitamin D metabolism with phenytoin and phenobarbitone, and risk of hypocalcaemia

Fetal/neonatal effects of anticonvulsants
- reduced fetal thyroxine as phenytoin competes for thyroxine-binding sites
- increased risk of haemorrhagic phenomenon of the newborn (mostly internal bleeding, secondary to decreased levels of vitamin K-dependent clotting factors as a result of drug-induced liver enzyme induction)
- increased drowsiness, jitteriness, irritability and poor suckling in the neonate

Anticonvulsants and breastfeeding
- Although all anticonvulsants except valproate cross the placental barrier, breastfeeding is not contraindicated.
- Neonatal serum levels are 40%–80% of maternal levels, and drowsiness may be a problem.

Anticonvulsants and contraception
- There is an increased risk of pregnancy and contraception failure secondary to hepatic enzymatic induction from anticonvulsants (carbamazepine, phenytoin, phenobarbitone, primidone, oxcarbazepine and topiramate >200 mg/day). There is no interference for gabapentin, lamotrogine, valproate and levetiracetam.
- The higher dose oestrogen (50 μg ethinyloestradiol) pill is required.

Management of epilepsy in pregnancy
Before conception
- If seizure-free for 2 years, consider withdrawing therapy. When possible, this should be 6 months prior to pregnancy.
- Aim for monotherapy or at least lowest possible dose.
- With the exception of valproate, there is no agreement as to which anticonvulsant drug should be used. It is appropriate to avoid valproate, especially at doses >1100 mg, if epilepsy is controlled by other medications.

Pregnancy
- Adopt a combined approach with the obstetrician and neurologist.
- Continue current anticonvulsant therapy and folate. Do not change therapy in established pregnancy solely to decrease teratogenicity.
- Plasma levels of free anticonvulsant drugs should be monitored where available.
- At 18 weeks gestation, a detailed fetal morphology ultrasound scan is required to assess for neural tube defects and orofacial clefts.

- Vitamin K 20 mg/day orally in the last 2–3 weeks of pregnancy may help reduce the risk of haemorrhagic disease of the newborn.
- Intramuscular vitamin K injection for the neonate is indicated.

Delivery
- Seizures during labour and delivery should be treated with intravenous benzodiazepines. Magnesium sulfate is not first-choice management, but may be used if eclampsia is suspected.

Postpartum
- Return to prepregnancy medication dose.
- Advise on the importance of sleep and rest.

Cerebral and spinal tumours

Prolactinoma
- Hyperprolactinaemia stimulates an increase in dopamine secretion, thereby inhibiting the release of gonadotrophin-releasing hormone (GnRH). Most women will be infertile unless treated.
- During normal pregnancy, the pituitary increases in size by 50%–70% secondary to lactotroph hyperplasia, and prolactin levels rise. Pituitary tumours are also likely to expand in pregnancy.

Management
- Institute combined obstetrician/neurologist management.
- Review regularly to assess growth of prolactinoma.
- Microadenoma causing hyperprolactinaemia: bromocriptine or cabergoline is withdrawn after pregnancy is confirmed and reinstated after delivery without significant risk of disease progression.
- Macroadenoma: the risk of expansion in pregnancy is <10%. It is recommended that pregnancy only be attempted when the tumour has shrunk to at least the confines of the sella turcica.
- Combined management during pregnancy with endocrinologists and neurosurgeons is indicated. The common complaints of tumour expansion are visual field defects and headaches. There is no evidence of teratogenesis with bromocriptine. Surgical management in pregnancy may be required.
- In symptomatic women, induction of labour at 38 weeks is indicated with elective use of forceps.

Neurofibroma
An acoustic neuroma can expand in pregnancy, as can cutaneous neurofibromatosis. This condition is associated with hypertension.

Neuropathies

Carpal tunnel syndrome
This is a common condition in pregnancy due to fluid retention, and resolves mostly in the postpartum period. It is often symptomatic at night, and management is initially with splints and physiotherapy. If these bring no improvement, then orthopaedic review and hydrocortisone injections or surgery may be indicated.

Bell's palsy
This is more common in pregnancy, especially in the last trimester with increasing oedema. Management is with corticosteroids, optimally within 1 day of onset. It is probably associated with increased risk of eclampsia.

Paraplegia

Antenatal care involves an increased incidence of urinary tract infections and constipation.

Management in labour
- Management is dependent on the level of spinal cord lesion.
- If the spinal cord is divided above T10, labour will be painless.
- If the division is above T5–T6, there is a risk of autonomic hyperreflexia. This is an autonomic and somatic hyperreflexia in response to intense sensory stimulation. In labour, uterine contractions can overstimulate the splanchnic sympathetic bed and release catecholamines, which results in hypertension, arrhythmia, headache, facial flushing and sweating. This response can be prevented by epidural and spinal anaesthesia to the level of the umbilicus (T10).

Multiple sclerosis in pregnancy

Effects of pregnancy on multiple sclerosis
- Pregnancy is generally considered to provide a stabilising effect on multiple sclerosis. This is thought to be due to the altered immune state in pregnancy.
- Relapses are common in the first 3–6 months postpartum.
- There is no significant effect on fertility or fetal wastage.
- When combining both the protective effect of pregnancy and postpartum risk period, there seems no change to multiple sclerosis relapse rate or long-term disability from pregnancy.

Management
- General measures include rest, counselling, preventing urinary tract infections and treating anaemia.
- Epidural anaesthesia has no effect on the disease.
- No contraindications exist to breastfeeding.
- Acute exacerbations of the disease are treated with glucorticoids.

Further reading

EURAP Study Group 2006 Seizure control and treatment in pregnancy: observations from the EURAP epilepsy pregnancy registry. Neurology 66:354–360
Vukusic S, Hutchinson M, Hours M et al 2004 Pregnancy and multiple sclerosis (the PRIMS study): clinical predictors of post-partum relapse. Brain 127:1353–1360

Chapter 53

Thyroid disease in pregnancy

Michael Flynn

Incidence. In developed countries, 2 in 1000 pregnancies are complicated by hyperthyroidism and 9 in 1000 pregnancies are complicated by hypothyroidism.

Thyroid physiology and pregnancy

- During normal pregnancy, the thyroid gland grows in size due to gland hyperplasia and increased vascularity.
- Circulating levels of iodine are reduced in pregnancy. This may be secondary to reduced renal tubular absorption, maternal–fetal transfer and fetal storage. There is a daily requirement of inorganic iodine 250 μg. This is increased from the non-pregnant state of 150 μg. Iodine is absorbed from foods such as salt, milk, dairy products, seafoods and eggs. Miscarriage rates are increased in iodine-deficient women. Iodine supplementation is recommended for all women except those with Graves' disease or a past history of hyperthyroidism.
- Thyroid-binding globulin production rises throughout pregnancy as a result of increased oestrogen and remains raised postpartum. Because of this, more T3 and T4 are protein-bound, thus raising total T3 and T4 levels.
- There may be a reduction in free T3 and T4 as pregnancy progresses. In late pregnancy, this may be in the non-pregnant hypothyroid range. Therefore, when low free T3/T4 levels are present in pregnancy, thyroid-stimulating hormone (TSH) is required for a diagnosis of hypothyroidism. Free thyroxine concentrations correlate to thyroid function.
- TSH levels fall in the first trimester. Free thyroid hormones are raised in about 70%–75% of women with hyperemesis, suggesting a relationship between high human chorionic gonadotrophin (hCG) levels and thyroid stimulation (hCG and TSH have the same alpha subunit with different beta subunits; hCG may be a TSH agonist).
- Fetal thyroid commences functioning at 10–12 weeks gestation; however, it is the maternal thyroxine mostly supplying fetal needs until the third trimester when the fetal thyroid is sufficiently mature to be independent. In this trimester, the placenta acts as a barrier to maternal TSH, T4 and T3, and the fetal axis acts independently of the mother. The placenta freely transports iodine and thyrotrophin-releasing hormone. Fetal blood sampling correlates to fetal status most reliably. After birth, fetal TSH levels

rise markedly due to a thyrotrophin-releasing hormone surge and decrease to normal over 3 days. The fetal dependence on maternal iodine continues during breastfeeding.

Maternal–fetal interactions

- Thyroid antibodies: microsomal and thyroglobulin antibodies cross the placenta, but are not cytotoxic to fetal thyroid cells.
- TSH receptor antibodies are immunoglobulin G-type antibodies and therefore cross the placenta with a risk of neonatal complications.
- Antithyroid antibodies, if present, can increase the risk of miscarriage.

Hypothyroidism

- Autoimmune thyroid disease is diagnosed by destructive antibodies (antithyroid perroxidase antibodies and antithyroglobulin antibodies). The underlying thyroiditis is known as Hashimoto's disease. Prevalence is unknown, although antibodies may be present in 5% of women of childbearing age.
- It is possible that women with normal thyroid function when not pregnant are at risk of developing hypothyroidism in early pregnancy when the thyroid gland cannot increase the required production for pregnancy.
- Always use TSH, free thyroxine (T4) for diagnosis and this should be monitored approximately every 6 weeks:
  - Raised TSH, decreased free T4 and positive thyroid autoantibodies are diagnostic of hypothyroidism.
  - Mild elevation TSH and normal free T4 are diagnostic of subclinical hypothyroidism likely to become hypothyroid as pregnancy progresses.
  - The presence of antithyroid antibodies and normal TSH and free T4 is controversial, but requires frequent monitoring in pregnancy.
- Treat with thyroxine to maintain TSH in the low–normal range. Most pregnant women will increase their thyroxine dose to approximately 50% of preconception dose. In the postpartum, thyroxine requirements decrease.

Congenital hypothyroidism
Incidence. It occurs in 1 in 4000 live births.
   It constitutes part of the neonatal screening test.

Hyperthyroidism

Incidence. It affects 2 in 1000 pregnancies.

Causes
- Graves' disease (the commonest cause in pregnancy)
- gestational trophoblastic disease
- toxic nodular goitre
- Hashimoto's disease
- subacute thyroiditis
- rare: hyperemesis gravidarum, hydatidiform mole, struma ovarii

Effects on pregnancy
There is an increase in low birthweight infants and a small rise in the neonatal mortality rate.

Graves' disease
This is caused by thyroid hyperactivity due to TSH receptor-stimulating antibody.

Maternal effects during pregnancy
- In 80% of cases, the woman remains euthyroid throughout pregnancy.
- Episodes of thyrotoxicosis can occur in the first trimester and postpartum, and treatment is required during these times.
- In 20% of cases, thyrotoxicosis remains stable during pregnancy and requires treatment throughout.

Fetal/neonatal effects
- Fetal thyrotoxicosis may occur, as the antibody readily crosses the placenta.
- Goitre may be seen on ultrasound. Fetal blood sampling can be performed.
- Even after treatment of the mother with thyroidectomy, there may be persisting antibodies.
- There is an increased risk of intrauterine growth restriction (IUGR) and premature labour.
- Fetuses at risk can be evaluated by assessment of maternal antibody concentrations and fetal heart rate. Fetal tachycardia begins from about 25 weeks gestation.
- Neonatal Graves' disease is seen in 10%–20% of neonates of mothers with Graves' disease. These babies suffer from tachycardia, poor weight gain and accelerated bone ossification.

Management of thyrotoxicosis in pregnancy
Failure to treat is associated with an increased risk of pre-eclampsia, premature labour, thyroid storm, congestive cardiac failure and perinatal mortality. The aim is to achieve the euthyroid state as early as possible (i.e. preconception) to minimise risks. The symptomatic woman requires treatment throughout pregnancy.

Investigations
Investigations include increased serum free T4 and decreased TSH.

Medical management
- Propranolol is used in acute events. The small risk of IUGR is outweighed by control of maternal tachycardia, tremor and anxiety.
- Both propylthiouracil (PTU) and carbimazole cross the placenta and there is no difference in placental transfer or teratogenicity of either. Both these drugs block thyroid hormone synthesis and produce immunosuppression. PTU is preferable in lactation, with less fetal transfer and is indicated in maternal doses of <150 mg a day. The fetal risks of both drugs are fetal goitre and transient hypothyroidism. Both drugs can cause maternal agranulocytosis.
- If treated with antithyroid drugs, monitor thyroid function tests for fetal status, but the risk is low.
- If treated with surgery or radioiodine therapy, measure TSH receptor antibodies early; if high, then repeat in the last trimester.
- If still under treatment with antithyroid drugs, then repeat TSH receptor antibodies in the last trimester.
- Radioactive iodine is contraindicated in pregnancy.
- Surgical management: if possible, delay this until the second trimester.
- Antenatal management: includes combined management with endocrinology clinic.
- Check thyroid function tests monthly and adjust medications to keep serum T4 at upper limit of normal.
- Fetal monitoring is indicated in the third trimester for assessment of fetal growth and fetal hyperthyroidism.

Labour and delivery
Notify the paediatrician, as the neonate requires monitoring for hyperthyroidism.

Postpartum thyroiditis

Incidence. About 10% of women develop subclinical postpartum thyroiditis.

Clinical presentation
- Symptoms typically develop 1–3 months postpartum.
- It often commences with symptoms of mild hyperthyroidism and then mild hypothyroidism at about 3–6 months postpartum, which then resolves.
- If symptoms persist, Hashimoto's thyroiditis is likely.

Aetiology
- Thyroiditis is associated with microsomal antibodies in 50%–80% of cases.
- It is considered an autoimmune disorder, with 20%–25% of women having a first-degree relative with autoimmune disease.
- Type 1 diabetics have a three-fold risk.

Recurrence
There is a 10% recurrence risk in future pregnancies.

Further reading

American Endocrine Society 2007 Clinical guidelines: management of thyroid dysfunction during pregnancy and the postpartum. Chevy Chase: American Endocrine Society

Hall R, Richards O, Lazarus JH 1993 The thyroid and pregnancy. British Journal of Obstetrics and Gynaecology 100:512–515

Lazarus JH, Kokandi A 2000 Thyroid disease in relation to pregnancy: a decade of change. Clinical Endocrinology 53:265–278

Chapter 54

Renal disease in pregnancy

Michael Flynn

Physiology

In pregnancy there is a rise in renal blood flow and a subsequent rise in glomerular filtration rate (GFR) by up to 50%, which is present from the first trimester. There is a slight fall in GFR in the last 3 weeks of pregnancy. This increase in GFR causes a fall in serum creatinine and urea levels to lower than non-pregnant levels.

Changes in renal tubular function result in a fall in serum urate levels in early and mid-pregnancy, with levels rising again in the third trimester. Similarly, up to 50% of normal women will have glycosuria at some point in pregnancy, as the rise in GFR exceeds the tubular capacity to reabsorb glucose.

Anatomically, in pregnancy the kidney enlarges and the renal pelves and ureters dilate. The right side enlarges more than the left due to the dextrorotation of the uterus.

Urinary tract infections
Acute pyelonephritis occurs in 1%–2% of all pregnancies (*see Ch 30*).

Chronic renal disease

Pregnancy outcome in chronic renal disease is dependent on renal function and blood pressure before pregnancy.

Mild renal disease is defined as serum creatinine <125 μmol/L preconception. There is usually a successful outcome. Pregnancy usually does not affect the long-term progress of the disease, although proteinuria is common. Hypertension is usually not a feature.

Moderate renal disease is preconception serum creatinine between 125 and 250 μmol/L. Most pregnancies are complicated by intrauterine growth restriction (IUGR) and hypertension. Close monitoring is required. A definite group will have irreversible decline in renal function. The risk is especially in uncontrolled hypertension. The major predictor of permanent decrease in renal function from pregnancy is hypertension and prepregnancy serum creatinine, rather than underlying aetiology. Fetal demise due to uncontrolled hypertension, and prematurity, is higher. Prematurity is secondary to severe pre-eclampsia and IUGR. Women with underlying renal disease have a risk of earlier and more severe pre-eclampsia.

Severe renal disease is serum creatinine >250 μmol/L. Although pregnancy is possible, many women are subfertile due to chronic disease and amenorrhoea. Pregnancy poses a significant risk to mother and baby, and general advice is to avoid pregnancy before renal transplant. There is a tendency to worsen more rapidly in the postpartum.

Management of chronic renal disease in pregnancy
There should be joint management with the renal physician.

Prepregnancy counselling
- Counselling includes general health advice.
- In mild impairment, pregnancy is unlikely to change the underlying disease (except scleroderma and polyarteritis nodosa).
- Control of hypertension is essential.
- Review medications and avoid those contraindicated in pregnancy (including angiotensin-converting enzyme inhibitors, angiotensin receptor blockers and some immunosuppressive drugs).
- Advise on possible pregnancy outcomes.
- Pregnancy is not common among long-term dialysis patients, and there is no advantage to any dialysis route.

Antenatal management
- baseline assessment of serum creatinine, urea, electrolytes, creatinine clearance and 24-hour urinary protein
- ultrasound scan: 18-week fetal morphology assessment
- mid-stream urine specimen to exclude infection
- serial assessment of renal function, and specifically hypertension and superimposed pre-eclampsia
- fetal surveillance in the third trimester
- admission for stabilisation if hypertension severe
- aim: delivery at 38–40 weeks (although preterm delivery is indicated for fetal reasons, substantial deterioration of renal function, uncontrollable hypertension or eclampsia)

Most of the risks of pregnancy are associated with hypertension and superimposed pre-eclampsia.

Nephrotic syndrome in pregnancy

The commonest cause of nephrotic syndrome in pregnancy is pre-eclampsia. Greater than 5 g/day proteinuria is associated with significantly higher perinatal mortality and morbidity. If the nephrotic syndrome is not due to pre-eclampsia, the pregnancy may continue to 38–39 weeks gestation if blood pressure and renal function are near normal before pregnancy and the fetus seems well.

Management includes a high-protein diet and fetal monitoring. Diuretics are contraindicated, as they exacerbate the decreased intravascular volume.

Pregnancy and renal transplant

Incidence. About 2% of women with a renal transplant become pregnant. The success rate of an ongoing pregnancy may be higher than 90%.

There is a 30% chance of developing hypertension, pre-eclampsia, or both. It is likely that pregnancy will not have any long-term effect on survival of allograft.

Prepregnancy advice

Advise to use contraception for 2 years after a transplant, after which immuno-suppressive therapy will be reduced to maintenance levels. Neither prednisone nor azathioprine is likely to affect pregnancy and pregnancy is then not contraindicated, provided there is stable renal function and normotension.

Pregnancy

- Immunosuppressive medication should be maintained.
- A glucose tolerance test is indicated.
- There are increased risks of IUGR (20%–40%) and preterm delivery (40%–60%).
- The transplanted pelvic kidney is not injured during vaginal delivery.

Further reading

de Sweit M 1995 Medical disorders in obstetric practice, 3rd edn. Oxford: Blackwell Science

McKay DB, Josephson MA, Armenti VT et al 2005 Reproduction and transplantation: report on the AST Consensus Conference on Reproductive Issues and Transplantation. American Journal of Transplantation 5:1592–1599

Chapter 55

The puerperium

Michael Flynn

Definition. The puerperium is the period from the completion of the third stage of labour to the return of the prepregnant physiological state. It is said to last 6 weeks.

Physiology. Involution of the uterus is due to catabolism of the uterine muscle bulk, with the fundal height decreasing from the level of the umbilicus on day 1 postpartum to not being palpable abdominally on days 10–14. It returns to a non-pregnant size within 4 weeks. The cervix involutes with the uterus and the os is closed by 2–3 weeks. The endometrium starts to regenerate 2–3 days postpartum.

The lochia or vaginal discharge is usually red (lochia rubra) for 2–14 days, then serous (lochia serosa) for up to 20 days, and gradually ceases by 4–8 weeks (lochia alba). Ovulation is often inhibited in breastfeeding before 10 weeks; if lactation is suppressed, it may occur at 7–10 weeks.

Afterbirth pains are tonic contractions of the uterus. They are increased in multiparas and with breastfeeding. Diuresis occurs 2 days after birth, and there is a return of plasma volume and other blood parameters to normal within 2 weeks.

Abnormal postpartum bleeding

Normal duration of blood loss is a mean of 24 days, with approximately 10% of women still bleeding at 8 weeks. Treatment is investigation with ultrasound to exclude retained pregnancy tissue prior to antibiotic treatment and, if required, surgical management with curettage.

Puerperal infections

Incidence. Puerperal infections occur in 2% of women after delivery.

Sites
- The genital tract is the commonest site of infection.
- Other sites include respiratory, wound and breast.
- Milk fever can occur with engorgement on days 3–4 but does not imply infection.
- A urinary tract infection is uncommon unless catheterisation has been performed.
- On days 2–5 postpartum, the infection is commonly genital or urinary tract (*Escherichia coli* or haemolytic *Streptococcus*).
- During week 2 postpartum, sites are more likely wound, breast or complicated pelvic infections.
- Deep venous thrombosis and pulmonary embolism are possible.

Postpartum endometritis
Risk factors
- prolonged rupture of membranes
- emergency caesarean section
- excessive blood loss
- prolonged surgery
- multiple vaginal examinations
- preterm delivery

Microbiological causes (mostly polymicrobial)
- 60% anaerobic endometritis: *Peptostreptococcus, Bacteroides, Clostridium*
- 40% aerobic causes: *Streptococcus, Enterococcus, E. coli, Staphylococcus aureus*
- *Bacteroides fragilis,* which may cause invasive anaerobic endometritis, often with adnexal involvement
- *Mycoplasmas* common although pathogenesis unsure

Management
- General examination should specifically assess the patient for infections of the breast, uterus, genital tract, chest, abdomen/wound and urinary tract. Deep venous thrombosis may present as a febrile illness.
- Microbiological assessment includes urine and blood for culture. Microbiological cultures of the genital tract are often not helpful, as the infective organisms are usually vaginal commensals.
- In the woman who is febrile with no other clinical symptoms and signs, empirical therapy of amoxycillin/potassium clavulanate 500/125 mg orally every 8 hours may be tried.
- If fever persists for more than 48 hours, add erythromycin 500 mg orally every 8 hours, as *Mycoplasma* may be involved.
- In the clinically unwell woman, intravenous therapy is indicated. A combination of (amoxy)ampicillin, gentamicin and metronidazole is used.

Breast infection
Incidence. Breast infection occurs in 1%–5% of postpartum infections.

Causes
- mostly *S. aureus*
- *Streptococcus*
- *E. coli*
- usually nosocomial, with transfer from infant to nipple (the causative organism can often be isolated from milk or pus)

Treatment
- The aim of early treatment with antibiotics is to avoid abscess formation.
- Breastfeeding should be continued or the breast manually emptied to avoid milk stasis and further abscess risks.
- Oral antibiotic treatment consists of flucloxacillin 500 mg to 1 g every 6 hours, dicloxacillin or cephalexin 500 mg to 1 g every 6 hours.
- Failure of antibiotic therapy may represent the presence of an abscess.

Breastfeeding

Physiology of lactation

During pregnancy, breast tissue is stimulated and hypertrophy of alveolar lobular structures occurs. Oestrogen, progesterone and prolactin are required for growth of the milk-collecting ducts. The milk production is inhibited in pregnancy by high levels of oestrogen and progesterone.

Milk production is regulated by prolactin, which causes glandular cells to secrete milk in response to a suckling reflex. Oxytocin is also released by suckling, although by different neuroendocrine pathways. Oxytocin acts on myoepithelial cells to induce milk ejection. The 600 mL breast milk made per day contains all vitamins except for vitamin K.

Establishing and maintaining lactation is complex, but several studies demonstrate beneficial effects of early contact of mother with baby. There appears to be no critical period for the first feed in the establishment of lactation. Colostrum, a yellow fluid, is made in the first 2 days. It differs from breast milk due to its increased fat globules and higher mineral and protein content. Immunoglobulin A can also be found.

Correct positioning of the baby on the breast is crucial to the avoidance of sore nipples and the successful establishment of feeding. In the correct position, the nipple forms the distal third of a teat and the baby's lower jaw and tongue are opposed to breast tissue, which makes the milk flow.

Frequency and duration of feeds
- Babies who are allowed to regulate their own feeds tend to gain weight more quickly and maintain breastfeeding longer than those on feeding schedules.
- There is no reason to restrict feeding duration, as small-volume high-caloric milk is present at the end of the feed.
- There is no evidence to support the use of routine supplemental formula or fluids.
- The combined oral contraceptive pill increases breastfeeding failure, and the progesterone-only pill is indicated in the postpartum period.

Common breastfeeding problems
- Nipple trauma: this is usually due to incorrect positioning, and education is required.
- Breast engorgement: this occurs when the volume of milk exceeds the capacity of alveoli to store it. Management involves correct positioning of the baby and the use of firm breast support.
- Insufficient milk: although a common reason for ceasing breastfeeding, objective evidence suggests that only 1%–5% of lactating mothers have inadequate milk supply. The treatment includes unrestricted feeding and dopamine antagonists (metoclopramide).

Lactational amenorrhoea
- This is due to a suckling-induced change in hypothalamic sensitivity to the negative feedback of ovarian steroids.
- Inhibition of lactation occurs with the combined oral contraceptive pill and smoking.
- Bromocriptine may suppress lactation if required.

Common postpartum problems

- Anaemia: postpartum anaemia occurs in 25%–30% of women, and sustained iron intake is recommended.

- Perineum: breakdown of sutures occurs in 2%–3% of cases, and primary resuturing with antibiotic cover may be appropriate. Dyspareunia is more common with episiotomy.
- Urinary problems include voiding difficulty and urinary tract infections.
- Constipation and haemorrhoids are also potential problems.

Postnatal mood disorders

During the lifetime of a woman, the postpartum period is the time of highest risk for psychiatric illness. Postpartum mood disorders are common and are usually divided into three diagnostic categories:
- the 'blues'
- postnatal depression
- postpartum psychosis

The 'blues'
- This is a common, minor and usually self-limiting condition, occurring in up to 80% of new mothers.
- The peak incidence is at days 3–5 postpartum.
- Symptoms include weepy, flat, emotional lability and feelings of inadequacy.
- Support is required.

Postnatal depression
- Clinical depression associated with pregnancy may occur both antenatally and postnatally. However, it most commonly follows birth.
- Incidence is 1%.
- Symptoms include: a mood that is not reactive to circumstances and is lowest in the morning; decreased appetite, energy, interest, concentration and confidence; sleep disturbance; alteration of the mother's feelings for the baby; panic attacks; feelings of inadequacy; bonding failure.
- The Edinburgh Postnatal Depression Scale can be used as a screening device for postnatal depression.
- Management includes recognition, appropriate referral for psychiatric assessment and management, and a social support structure.
- Management is advanced by antenatal identification of at-risk groups: those with a previous history of depression or severe premenstrual syndrome; recent significant life event (significant bereavement or relationship break-up); recent migrants; low or high maternal age; low socioeconomic status.
- As both psychological and biological aetiologies are present, a multifactorial treatment regimen, including psychotherapy, social service and pharmacological treatment, is required.

Postpartum psychosis
- Incidence is 0.2%.
- Postpartum psychosis is mostly affective, and rarely does schizophrenia present for the first time in this situation.
- Recurrence rate: if significant psychosis in the previous pregnancy is not resolved before the subsequent pregnancy, recurrence is highly likely. If the psychosis has resolved, the risk for the next pregnancy is 50%.
- Symptoms include delusions, hallucinations and extremes of behaviour.
- Management includes psychiatric admission to a specialised mother-and-baby unit. Treatment with neuroleptics, antidepressants, lithium or electroconvulsive

therapy may be required. Breastfeeding is avoided if lithium or polypharmacy is used. Social support for the family and partner is required.
- Early psychiatric referral is advisable in the next pregnancy.

Further reading

Glazener C, MacArthur C 2001 Postnatal morbidity. Obstetrician and Gynaecologist 3:179–183

Appendix

Objective Structured Clinical Examinations (OSCEs) in obstetrics

Miriam Lee
Amy Mellor

Case 1

Information for candidate

Dear Doctor,

Thank you for seeing Daisy, aged 33. She is currently at 12 weeks gestation in her fourth pregnancy. Her antenatal blood results suggest she is Rhesus immunised. She had a normal delivery at term 2 years ago, and has had two previous miscarriages.

Yours sincerely,
Dr Edwards
(General Practitioner)

Antenatal screen

Blood group	O Rh-negative
Antibody screen	Anti-D titre 1 in 8
FBC	Hb 138, platelets 284
Hep B S Ag	negative
Hep C Ab	negative
HIV	negative
Rubella IgG	non-immune (0 IU/mL)
Syphilis	negative
MSU	no growth

Encounter 1
'You are meeting Daisy in your consulting rooms. You have read the referral letter. I will play the role of the patient and you the obstetrician. Please proceed.'

Encounter 2
'You are reviewing Daisy in clinic. She is now at 22 weeks gestation. A blood test done 2 days ago shows an anti-D titre of 1 in 128. Please proceed.'

Gestation	8/40	12/40	16/40	20/40	22/40
Titre	1 in 8	1 in 8	1 in 16	1 in 16	1 in 128
Anti-D (IU/mL)	2	2	3	3	15

Encounter 3
Part A
At 28 weeks, Daisy has had an uncomplicated intrauterine blood transfusion, with a postprocedural fetal Hb of 127 g/L. Six hours later while on the antenatal ward she has become distressed. You are the consultant on call. The registrar on call has just reviewed the patient and is calling you for advice.

'I'm sorry to bother you Doctor, but it's late and I can't get hold of the maternal–fetal medicine specialist. Daisy has increasing abdominal pain and can't feel any fetal movements. On examination, her uterus is tense with palpable uterine activity. What should I do?'

Part B
You are now in the delivery suite. The cardiotocography (CTG) shows a sinusoidal pattern. Daisy asks:

'What do we do now Doctor?'

Encounter 4
You are reviewing Daisy 3 days later on the postnatal ward. She has delivered via caesarean section a 1200 g female who is doing well in the nursery after an exchange transfusion. Daisy says:

'Doctor, this pregnancy has been very stressful. I'd like my tubes tied as soon as possible.'

Information for examiner
Case summary
A 33-year-old, G4P1 is referred by her general practitioner at 12 weeks gestation with an anti-D titre of 1 in 8. At 22 weeks, the titre rises to 1 in 128. At 28 weeks, the patient is found to have an abnormal CTG after an intrauterine fetal blood transfusion.

Competencies tested
- management of a Rhesus isoimmunised pregnancy
- reassurance and explanation to an anxious patient
- management of a rising titre, outlining a plan of surveillance, including possible fetal blood sampling and in utero transfusion
- management of a possible fetomaternal haemorrhage after in utero transfusion and consideration of delivery
  If requested:
- husband's blood group: A Rh-positive (Rh CCDdEe)

Encounter 1
History
- currently 12 weeks gestation; planned pregnancy
- two miscarriages before first child; early first trimester—complete
- spontaneous vaginal delivery (SVD) at term two years ago, 3000 g female; anti-D not given after delivery as 'antibodies already present' (titre 1 in 8)
- no history of blood transfusion
- nil significant medical, surgical, gynaecological or psychiatric history
- sister had a pulmonary embolus after SVD
- normal Pap smear 1 year ago
- taking folate
- nil allergies, non-smoker, non-drinker
- happily married, is a librarian

Examination
- healthy-looking Caucasian female of stated age
- body mass index: 21
- observations normal, urinalysis no abnormalities detected
- examination unremarkable

Expectations of candidate
- outline management of Rhesus disease
- maternal–fetal medical (MFM) referral if titre >1 in 32
- monitor titres 4 weekly, then fortnightly
- check partner's blood group
- discuss possibility of fetal blood sampling, middle cerebral artery (MCA) surveillance, intrauterine transfusion, early delivery, neonatology involvement
- consider thrombophilia screen, given family history of venous thromboembolism
- offer screening for aneuploidy
- recommend rubella vaccine postpartum

Encounter 2
Expectations of candidate
- identify need for referral to MFM subspecialist
- organise ultrasound to check for evidence of hydrops/MCA Dopplers
- outline likely management
- reassure outcome likely to be good

Encounter 3
Part A: Expectations of candidate
- state: 'I will come in and review'
- request a CTG be commenced

Part B: Expectations of candidate
- identify possible fetomaternal haemorrhage or abruption
- recognise sinusoidal pattern on CTG
- organise urgent caesarean section
- notify neonatal team

Encounter 4
Expectations of candidate
- targeted postnatal history and examination (breasts, lochia, calves)
- discuss natural history of disease; husband's genotype is CCDdEe, so 50% chance in future pregnancy, but likely to be more severe
- discuss alternative contraception options
- do not arrange permanent contraception at this stage; arrange follow-up in 6 weeks to further discuss

Scoring for case 1	
Encounter	**Mark**
Encounters 1 and 2	
• Explain Rh disease	____ out of 1
• Request husband's genotype	____ out of 1
• MFM referral	____ out of 1

(Continued)

Scoring for case 1—Cont'd	
Encounter	Mark
• Monitoring (titres, MCA Dopplers)	____ out of 1
• Discuss possible management options (fetal transfusion, early delivery)	____ out of 1
• Discuss prognosis (risk of anaemia, fetal death in utero)	____ out of 1
• Complications of intrauterine transfusion (emergency caesarian section, 1% mortality)	____ out of 2
• Rubella vaccine	____ out of 1
• Thrombophilia screen	____ out of 1
Encounter 3	
• Identify complication of transfusion	____ out of 1
• Organise urgent caesarian section	____ out of 2
Encounter 4	
• Discuss natural history of Rh disease	____ out of 1
• Delay before arranging tubal litigation	____ out of 1
Global competence	____ out of 5
TOTAL SCORE	**____ out of 20**

Case 2

Information for candidate

You are a consultant obstetrician in a city hospital. You have been contacted on the telephone by a GP obstetrician from a small country hospital approximately 150 km away. The GP has informed you that a 19-year-old Aboriginal primigravid woman has just presented to his hospital in active labour. He had just examined the woman 30 minutes ago. He found that she was coping well with the pain of the contractions. Abdominal examination revealed fundal height of about 38 weeks with cephalic presentation. On vaginal examination, she was 8 cm dilated, the head at right occipito anterior (ROA) position and the level of the head at spines. There were no forewaters palpable. The CTG has been reassuring and her labour seems to be progressing well.

Part 1

The examiner will play the role of the GP.

Examiner: *'The reason I called was that this lady has had only one antenatal visit during her pregnancy. At that stage, she was about 22 weeks and antenatal bloods and ultrasound results were performed. She has prior to this pregnancy presented at the hospital with pneumonia and it was noted from her records that she has rheumatic heart disease with mitral regurgitation. Can you tell me what precautions should be undertaken for this patient?'*

Part 2

You have now been contacted again by the midwife at the hospital who has been asked by the GP obstetrician to call you. He successfully delivered the baby 5 minutes ago.

The examiner will play the role of the midwife.

Examiner: *'Hello Doctor, when Dr Jones attempted to deliver the placenta, a large lump started to protrude from the vagina. The patient also complains of severe abdominal pain and is bleeding quite heavily. The placenta has not been delivered.'*

Scoring for case 2	
	Mark
Part 1: Intrapartum management	_____ out of 6
• If analgesia required, epidural recommended; is effective; decreases cardiac output	
• Prophylactic antibiotics: ampicillin and gentamicin	
• Shorten second stage to decrease maternal effort	
• Syntocinon: less venous constriction	
Part 2: Uterine inversion	_____ out of 9
• Symptoms: patient complains of severe abdominal pain during management of third stage of labour	
• Mass protruding from cervix and fundus of uterus indented; large blood loss	

(Continued)

Scoring for case 2—Cont'd		
	Mark	
• Management: — call for help: diagnose uterine inversion — stop cord traction; leave placenta in place — cease any syntocinon infusion — resuscitate with intravenous fluid — attempt replacement with hand — if not successful, use hydrostatic method described by O'Sullivan: infuse warm saline into vagina with fluid running 1 m above patient; block off vaginal orifice to prevent fluid leak — once uterus is replaced, remove placenta manually in operating theatre — when stage 3 complete, use syntocinin		
Global competence	_____ out of 5	
TOTAL SCORE	**_____ out of 20**	

Case 3

Information for candidate
Part 1
Mrs KD presents at her second antenatal visit. This is her ultrasound result:

Anomoly scan
Transabdominal; good view
Fetal measurements
BPD	45.9 mm
OFD	56.6 mm
HC	165.7 mm
AC	135.4 mm
FL	29.3 mm

Gestational age: 19 weeks and 6 days
Heart motion seen.
Fetal movements visible.
Presentation is cephalic and amniotic fluid is normal. The cord has 3 vessels.
Placenta is anterior, not low and the structure is normal.

Fetal anatomy
The following were visualised and appear normal: head, brain, face, spine, neck and skin, skeleton, chest, four-chambered heart and great vessels. There is an omphalocoele. There are features suggestive of possible horseshoe kidneys.

The examiner will play the role of the patient.
Mrs KD: *'Hello Doctor. How were my test results? Can you tell me what that means?'*
The candidate gives the results to the patient.
Mrs KD: *'Are there any more tests I can do to know if there is anything wrong with my baby? I don't know how my husband and I can handle not knowing if there is something wrong with our baby.'*

Part 2
Mrs KD, who is now 22 weeks, presents 1 week after the amniocentesis with a history of per vaginal fluid loss for 1 week. The preliminary fluorescence in situ hybridisation (FISH) aneuploidy screen panel reviewed a male fetus with no abnormality detected. The patient was informed of the results when they were first available. The examiner will play the role of the patient.
Examiner: *'Doctor I have had small amount of fluid leak down below for 1 week. It started about 3 days after the amniocentesis. Initially, there was very slight loss and then I started to notice it more, and even though the amount is small it has been constant up till yesterday. I am very worried. What do you think is happening?'*

Ultrasound
Transabdominal; good view
Fetal measurements
BPD	50.9 mm
HC	168.9 mm
AC	140.24 mm
FL	30.1 mm

Gestational age: 21 weeks and 1 day
No heart motion seen.
No fetal movements visible; consistent with intrauterine fetal death.

Presentation is cephalic and amniotic fluid index is <1 cm. The cord has 3 vessels. Placenta is anterior, not low and the structure is normal.

Part 3

You are now reviewing Mrs KD in the labour ward. She has had 1600 mg of misoprostol over 24 hours followed by 10 hours of intravenous syntocinin, and the cervix on vaginal examination is found to be tightly closed, posterior and firm. The examiner will play the role of the patient.

Examiner: *'Doctor, how much longer will this be? I feel very uncomfortable with crampy pains down low.'*

Scoring for case 3	
	Mark
Part 1: Explanation	_____ out of 3
• Adequate explanation of the nature of the abnormalities found on the ultrasound scan	
• Advise amniocentesis and explanation of the procedure and risks involved	
Part 2: Recognise the possibility of PPROM	_____ out of 8
• Examination of the patient: speculum and ultrasound	
• On examination temperature is 36.6°C, pulse is 80 beats per minute	
• Speculum reveals small pool of fluid in posterior fornix	
• Perform transabdominal ultrasound	
• Explanation of clinical findings and results to patient	
• Advise treatment plan in form of induction of labour for intrauterine fetal death	
• Intravenous syntocinon or misoprostol	
Part 3: Recognise that induction of labour has failed	_____ out of 4
• Advise hysterotomy	
• Explanation of procedure to patient	
• Further implications for patient	
Global competence	_____ out of 5
TOTAL SCORE	_____ **out of 20**

Index

Page numbers followed by 'f' denote figures; those followed by 't' denote tables